Nurse-Midwifery
Health Care for Women and Newborns

Nurse-Midwifery

Health Care for Women and Newborns

Edited by

Constance J. Adams, R.N., C.N.M., Dr.P.H.

Professor
Rush University College of Nursing
Chairperson
Department of Obstetric and Gynecological Nursing
Rush-Presbyterian-St. Luke's Medical Center
Chicago, Illinois

Grune & Stratton
A Subsidiary of Harcourt Brace Jovanovich, Publishers
New York   London
Paris   San Diego   San Francisco   São Paulo
Sydney   Tokyo   Toronto

Library of Congress Cataloging in Publication Data
Main entry under title:
Nurse-midwifery: health care for women and newborns.
  Includes bibliographies and index.
    1. Obstetrical nursing. 2. Obstetrics. 3. Midwives.
I. Adams, Constance J. [DNLM: 1. Nurse midwives.
WY 157 N9735]
RG951.N865   1983   618.2   83-5666
ISBN 0-8089-1570-3

Grune & Stratton, Inc.
111 Fifth Avenue
New York, New York 10003

Distributed in the United Kingdom by
Grune & Stratton, Inc. (London) Ltd.
24/28 Oval Road, London NW 1

Library of Congress Catalog Number 83-5666
International Standard Book Number ISBN 0-8089-1570-3

Printed in the United States of America

To my parents, Betty and Edward Adams, who continue to hold family health and togetherness above all else.

Contents

Acknowledgments

The editor extends sincere appreciation to Joyce Roberts, R.N., C.N.M., Ph.D., for demonstrating her commitment to nurse-midwifery through the many hours and thoughts she devoted to the development of a proposal for this text.

Preface

Nurse-midwifery is not only a very special way to practice nursing, it is also an opportunity for women to receive primary health care from well-prepared professional nurses. This book has been designed to identify major issues that influence the practice of nurse-midwifery in the United States and document the present state of knowledge about various aspects of these issues.

The first section of this book attempts to put nurse-midwifery in its proper perspective within our health care system. Women in their reproductive years are characterized according to several social and health parameters, their major health problems are identified, and their needs for health care services are outlined. Providers of women's health care services are discussed in terms of preparation and credentials, quality assurance, and need versus availability. The growth and development of nurse-midwifery in the United States are addressed in the context of developments in the total health care system.

Major issues confronted by nurse-midwives when making management decisions are addressed in the second section. Issues confronted in all aspects of nurse-midwifery clinical management are considered.

The text focuses on reproduction as a normal process, maintenance of optimal health, early identification of potential problems, and family-centered care. Providing women and their families with the information needed in all phases of the reproductive process is a major focus in each chapter.

The terms *nurse-midwife* and *certified nurse-midwife* are used interchangeably throughout this book. Nurse-midwives, as referred to within the text, are nurses who have been certified by the American College of Nurse-Midwives (ACNM) or nurses who have successfully completed an educational program in nurse-midwifery and will soon be certified by the ACNM. Although information in the text has been directed to these individuals, students in nurse-midwifery educational programs should find the content to be particularly helpful. It is hoped that other professionals with a commitment to high-quality women's health care will also find the information useful.

Constance J. Adams, R.N., C.N.M., Dr.P.H.

Contributors

Constance J. Adams, R.N., C.N.M., Dr.P.H.
Professor, Rush University College of Nursing
Chairperson, Department of Obstetric and Gynecological Nursing
Rush-Presbyterian-St. Luke's Medical Center
Chicago, Illinois

Diane B. Boyer, R.N., C.N.M., Ph.D.
Associate Professor and Head, Department of Nursing
Luther College
Decorah, Iowa

Julia Harrison-Coughlin, R.N., C.N.M., M.S.N.
Nurse-Midwifery Service
Illinois Masonic Medical Center
Chicago, Illinois

Ann M. Koontz, R.N., C.N.M., M.S., Dr.P.H.
Maternal Health Care Consultant
Division of Maternal and Child Health
Bureau of Health Care Delivery and Assistance
Health Resources and Services Administration
U.S. Department of Health and Human Services
Rockville, Maryland

Teresa Marchese, R.N., C.N.M., M.S.N.
Instructor, Growing Family/Nurse-Midwifery
School of Nursing, Graduate Program
Georgetown University
Washington, D.C.

Virginia Michels, R.N., C.N.M., M.S.N.
Assistant Professor, Graduate Nurse-Midwifery Program
College of Nursing, University of Illinois
Chicago, Illinois

Sarah J. Naber, R.N., C.N.M., M.S.N.
Instructor, Graduate Nurse-Midwifery Program
College of Nursing, University of Illinois
Doctoral Student, Department of Nursing Sciences
Graduate College, University of Illinois
Chicago, Illinois

Nurse-Midwifery
Health Care for Women and Newborns

Demographic and Professional Factors

Nurse-midwives have demonstrated their ability to provide optimal health care for women who are at low risk of experiencing medical or obstetrical complications. It is important that the services of nurse-midwives are understood and evaluated in terms of the health care needs of all women of reproductive age and in terms of the providers available to meet these needs. This section characterizes women of reproductive age according to several social and health parameters and discusses major health problems and health care needs. Health care providers are discussed in terms of preparation, credentialing, quality assurance, and need versus availability.

Constance J. Adams

1

Women in their Reproductive Years

Early in 1981 it was estimated that about 228 million people were residents of the United States.[99] Almost 52 million of these individuals were women between the ages of 15 and 44 years, traditionally referred to as the childbearing years. More than 3.6 million babies were born alive to these women and about 45,000 of them died before one year of age. Approximately 36,000 additional pregnancies of at least 20 weeks gestation resulted in the death of each fetus before birth.[136]

REPRODUCTIVE PROFILE

Data on births and deaths in the United States are collected, tabulated, and published annually at the National Center for Health Statistics in volumes entitled *Vital Statistics of the United States*. It usually takes 4−6 years before publication of a volume pertaining to any specific year because of the extensive amount of detailed information contained in each volume. Published data are estimates based on 100 percent reporting of births and deaths in selected states and differing percentages of reporting in the other states. Provisional estimates of the numbers of births, marriages, divorces, and deaths in the United States are published for each month in the *Monthly Vital Statistics Report* with only a 3−4 month delay. The following description of the reproductive profile for women in the United States is based on information obtained from the volume entitled *Vital Statistics of the United States,*

1977[135,136,137] and the *Monthly Vital Statistics Report* for February of 1981,[99] unless otherwise indicated (through p 10).

Births

During 1977 an estimated 3,326,000 babies were born alive to women in the United States—2,691,000 to white women and 544,000 to black women. The remaining babies were born to women of all other races. Completeness of this reporting was estimated to be 99.3 percent.

The overall live-birth rate in 1977 was 15.4/1000 total pop. This rate was lower than that of 16.0/1000 pop. estimated for the 12-month period ending with February of 1981. Birth rates for white women have been consistently lower than those for women of other races. In 1977 the live-birth rates were 14.4/1000 pop. for white women, 21.7/1000 pop. for black women, and 21.9/1000 pop. for women of all other races. The highest birth rate for white women was among those 25−29 years old—113.8/1000 pop.—while the highest rates for black women and women of all other races were among those 20−24 years old—147.7 and 145.7, respectively. Lowest birth rates were experienced by women 45−49 years old from all racial groups and were 0.2/1000 pop. for white women and 0.5 for all other women. Adolescent women 10−14 years old experienced an overall live-birth rate of 1.2/1000 pop. The rate for white females in this age group was 0.6/1000 pop., while rates for black females and females from all other races were 4.7 and 4.3, respectively.

Black women tend to bear more children than other women. In 1977 the birth rate among women who had a fourth or greater live birth was 13.3/1000 pop. for black women, 7.2/1000 pop. for white women, and 6.2/1000 pop. for all other women.

Mean intervals, in months, between termination of the last pregnancy and delivery of the enumerated live birth increase steadily as maternal age increases. In 1977 this mean interval was estimated to be 22.3 months for women less than 20 years old and 88.9 months for women 40 or more years old.

About 74 percent of all live births in 1977 were to women who had completed at least 12 years of schooling. Approximately 45 percent of all live births to white women and 40 percent of all live births to black women were to women who had completed exactly 12 years of schooling. In addition, about 32 percent of the births to white women and 20 percent of the births to black women were to women who had completed more than 12 years of schooling. As many as 14 percent of all live births to white women and 5 percent of those to black women were to women who had completed 16 or more years of schooling.

An estimated 515,700 live-born infants were born illegitimately in 1977. About 220,100 of these births were to white women and about 281,600 were to black women. White women contributed about 80 percent of the total live births in 1977 and almost 43 percent of the illegitimate live births, while black women contributed about 18 percent of the total live births and 55 percent of the illegitimate live births. Mothers 15−19 years old contributed about 46 percent of the illegitimate live births, and mothers less than 15 years old produced approximately 10,100 additional illegitimate live births. The total contribution to illegitimate live births by mothers less than 20 years old was about 48 percent.

Rates of illegitimate live birth are strikingly different for white women than they are for women from other races. In 1977 the rate of illegitimate live births for white women was 13.7/1000 unmarried white women, while it was 84.5 for all other unmarried women. The highest rates of illegitimacy in all racial groups were for women 18−19 years old with a rate of 18.8/1000 unmarried white women 18−19 years old and 117.0/1000 unmarried women from all other races who were 18−19 years old. The illegitimate live birth rate for black women 18−19 years old was 125.9/1000 unmarried black women in this age group. In all racial groups rates of illegitimate live birth declined as maternal age increased after 19 years of age.

Pregnancy data for 1977 submitted to the National Center for Health Statistics indicated that about 1.4 percent of all women who delivered live babies during that year were known to have had no prenatal care. Information about prenatal care was not recorded for an additional 109,779 women, or 3.7 percent of the women who delivered live babies during 1977. Of the women who did have at least one prenatal visit, about 71 percent began prenatal care by the end of the third month of pregnancy and an additional 20 percent began prenatal care by the end of the sixth month of pregnancy. Estimates indicate that about 95 percent of white mothers and 90 percent of black mothers had at least one prenatal visit. White women of all ages and women of all races who were 25−34 years old tended to begin prenatal care earlier than all other women.

About 234,884 babies, or seven percent of the babies born alive in 1977, had a birth weight of 2500 g or less (low birth weight). Only about 6 percent of the babies born to white mothers had a birth weight of 2500 g or less, while almost 13 percent of the babies born to black mothers had a birth weight of 2500 g or less. Mothers reported to have had no prenatal care delivered babies with birth weights of 2500 g or less twice as frequently as mothers known to have had at least one prenatal visit.

Infant Deaths

Approximately 46,975 babies died before one year of age in 1977, resulting in an infant mortality rate of 14.1/1000 live births. It was estimated that 33,199, or almost 71 percent of all of the infant deaths, were among babies born to white women and that 12,863, or about 27 percent of all of the infant deaths, were among babies born to black women. About one in five of these babies was reported to have had at least one congenital anomaly and about three out of four of them died before 28 days of age. The neonatal mortality rate in 1977 for infants less than 28 days old was 9.9/1000 total live births.

Small infants—designated by a birth weight of 2500 g or less, or of less than 37 weeks gestational age at birth—have been found most vulnerable to death within the first 28 days of live.[21,78,146] A birth weight of 2500 grams or less, in particular, has been reported as the single most important factor associated with infant loss at an early age.[20,23,70] Rates of neonatal and infant death have been shown to be greater among babies born to mothers from low socioeconomic status population groups than mothers from middle or high socioeconomic status groups;[21,70,81] to mothers from racial groups other than white;[21,22,70,82] to mothers less than 20 years old or more than 34 years old than mothers between 20 and 34 years old;[21,22,134] to mothers with total birth orders of greater than three than from one to three;[4,21,22,134] to mothers with a positive history of reproductive loss than a negative history;[22,82,96,117] or to mothers who had experienced intervals of less than one year between pregnancies as opposed to longer periods of time.[31,70] Infants of plural births have been designated to be at a particularly high risk of neonatal death because of the considerably greater incidence of low birth weight in this group of babies compared with single live-born infants.[4,20,23]

Interrelationships between these factors and neonatal or infant death have been shown to be most complex. For example, babies born to mothers who are less than 20 years old have a greater than average risk of early death, but there is also a higher than average risk of prematurity among this group of babies than among those born to mothers who are 20 or more years old; the reported incidence of neonatal or infant death is greatest among prematurely born babies.[21,23,146] Teenage motherhood occurs most frequently among females from low socioeconomic groups and races other than white, two population categories in which high rates of premature birth and early infant loss are experienced.[21,70,81,134]

Fetal Deaths

Many of the same sociodemographic and reproductive history factors that have been associated with neonatal and infant deaths have also been associated with fetal deaths that occur at 20 or more weeks of gestation.[31,95,96,97,117] An estimated 33,053 fetuses of at least 20 weeks gestational age died before birth in 1977. About 71 percent of these deaths occurred to fetuses of white mothers and the remainder occurred to fetuses of mothers from all other races. The fetal death ratio among fetuses of at least 20 weeks gestational age was 8.3/1000 live births for white women and 14.8/1000 live births for women from all other races. Numbers of fetal deaths of at least 20 weeks gestational age in each racial group were almost as high as the numbers of neonatal deaths within the same racial groups.[136,137]

Due to underreporting of early pregnancy losses, it is difficult to estimate the number of women who become pregnant each year but do not carry their pregnancies to 20 weeks of gestation. Some authorities have suggested that spontaneous abortions occur at a rate of one in five pregnancies.[41,122] In addition, it has been estimated that as many as 1.3 million legal abortions were performed in the United States during 1978.[91] About one-third of the women who have induced abortions each year are less than 20 years old and another one-third are 20−24 years old. Pregnant adolescents less than 15 years old and pregnant women more than 40 years old tend to have induced abortions more frequently than they have live births.[36] Abortion ratios are highest for unmarried women and for women who are either nulliparous or of grand multiparity. The number of illegal abortions performed in the United States each year remains unknown, however, it is believed to have declined dramatically since liberalization of abortion laws.[91]

Maternal Deaths

Maternal deaths are deaths assigned to the category "Complications of pregnancy, childbirth, and the puerperium" in the *Manual of the International Statistical Classification of Diseases, Injuries, and Causes of Death, 1975*.[83] Although the numbers of women in the United States who die from conditions directly related to pregnancy have declined considerably since the early 1900s, women do still die from pregnancy-related conditions. In 1977 pregnancy-related complications were reported as the major cause of death for about 373/total pop. women and the maternal mortality rate was 11.2/100,000 live births.[137]

Recent evidence suggests that many more women die from pregnancy-related complications than reported on death certificates.[113] Information on all live births to Georgia residents was compared with information on all deaths of Georgia women between the ages of 10 and 44 years at the time of their death in 1975, 1976, or the first two months of 1977. The birth certificates of babies delivered by these women were matched to the maternal death certificates and then additional information about each mother was obtained from medical examiners' reports, physician and hospital records, police reports, and family members of each deceased mother. After all pertinent clinical information had been compiled, the investigators decided, by consensus, which of the deaths could be reasonably attributed to pregnancy or delivery. The maternal mortality rate based on the additional information was 50 percent higher than the rate based only on death certificate information.

Based on data pertaining to first-trimester abortions performed in the United States from 1972 through 1974, it was estimated that the first-trimester abortion death rate was 1.2/100,000 for women 15−24 years old, 1.4/100,000 for women 25−34 years old, and 1.8/100,000 for women 35−44 years old.[129] Risk of death from second-trimester abortions is higher than it is for first-trimester abortions,[18,19] however, approximately 84 percent of all legal abortions are performed prior to the 13th week of pregnancy.[36] Data from the Center for Disease Control indicate that 27 women died from all abortions in the United States during 1976 and 16 of these deaths resulted from illegal abortions.[1]

MAJOR CAUSES OF DEATH

In 1978 the life expectancy for individuals born in the United States was 77.2 years for women and 69.5 years for men.[91] Although women have a greater life expectancy and lower mortality rates in each age group than men, women eventually die from the same major causes of death as men. The four leading causes of death for women in the United States are diseases of the heart, cancer, cerebrovascular diseases, and accidents.[137]

Diseases of the Heart

Approximately 322,368 females died from diseases of the heart during 1977, and 4,018 (about 1.2%) of these deaths were among women between the ages of 15 and 44 years.[137] Ischemic heart disease accounted for about 52 percent of the deaths among women 15−44 years old and acute myocardial infarction accounted for an additional 30 percent of the deaths among these women.

When rates of mortality due to diseases of the heart in women were adjusted for age, a 44.9 percent decline was noted for women from races other than white between 1950−1977 and a 38.8 percent decline was noted for white women during the same period of time.[57] Recent declines in heart disease mortality rates among women have been attributed to improved medical management of hypertensive disorders, decreased consumption of fats, increased physical activity, better medical emergency services, and more efficient use of coronary care units.[56,68,143]

Data from the Framingham study, a classic study of 5209 men and women over a period of 25 years, indicate that women have about one-half the risk that men of the same age have of developing a "major cardiovascular event" between the ages of 15 and 44 years.[68] Several authors have interpreted this to mean that women have some biologic protection,[68,91] however, environment must also have a strong effect since the wives of men who developed coronary heart disease had double the risk of developing heart disease themselves than the wives of men who did not develop coronary heart disease. Women who developed diabetes during the 25 year period were found to have at least a doubled risk of cardiovascular mortality than the women who did not develop diabetes.

About one-half to two percent of all pregnant women are affected by heart disease.[66,100] Maternal mortality has been reported to be as high as 3 percent among mothers with severe heart disease and perinatal mortality as high as 50 percent in instances of persistent cardiac decompensation.[66] The risk of stillbirth among women with heart disease is much greater than the risk of neonatal death.[100]

Cancer

Cancer is the second highest cause of death for all women in the United States, but is the leading cause of death among women 30-54 years old.[137] In 1977 about 176,227 females died from malignant neoplasms and 10,090 (about 5.7%), of these deaths were among women between the ages of 15 and 44 years. Malignant neoplasms of the breast accounted for almost 27 percent of the cancer deaths among women 15-44 years old; malignant neoplasms of the genital organs accounted for about 15 percent; malignant neoplasms of the digestive organs accounted for 12 percent; and malignant neoplasms of the respiratory system accounted for just over 10 percent of these deaths.

Age-adjusted mortality rates among all women who died from malignant neoplasms were about 18 percent lower for white women in 1977 than in 1950 and about seven percent lower for women from all other races.[57] Mortality rates among all females are increasing sharply from cancer of the lung—the major site for malignant neoplasms of the respiratory system—and are increasing slightly from cancer of the breast, ovary, pancreas, and large intestine, as well as from leukemia.[91] Mortality rates for females seem to be decreasing from cancer of the stomach and uterus, inculding cancer of the cervix.

Breast cancer is the leading cause of cancer death among women of childbearing ages and it has been estimated that one in 13 American women will develop breast cancer at some point in life.[91] About 107,000 new cases of breast cancer were diagnosed in 1979. Women who have already had breast cancer are at greatest risk of developing it again and women whose mothers or sisters had breast cancer are at greater risk of developing it than all other women who have never had breast cancer.[76] There is also some evidence that women who have never given birth and women whose diets are high in animal fats also have a higher risk of developing breast cancer than women in general. Advances in early detection and treatment of breast cancer have reduced mortality rates for females less than 50 years old, but mortality rates for women 50 or more years old have increased.

Estimates from the American Cancer Society indicate that about 50 percent of all deaths from uterine cancer are specifically from cancer of the cervix.[77,112] These estimates also indicate that in 1978 about 20,000 new cases of cancer of the cervix were diagnosed, with about 7400 deaths from cancer of the cervix in that year. The American Cancer Society projects that about two percent of all women will develop cervical cancer by the time they are 80 years old.[77]

About 16/100,000 total pop. females in the United States died from cancer of the respiratory system in 1977 and the majority of these deaths were specifically due to lung cancer.[57] Age-adjusted mortality rates for malignant neoplasms of the respiratory system indicate that there was a 220 percent increase in mortality rates for white women between 1950 and 1977 and a 300 percent increase for women from all other races during the same period.[57]

Cerebrovascular Diseases

An estimated 104,583 females died from cerebrovascular diseases in 1977 and 1943 (1.9%) of these deaths were to women between the ages of 15 and 44 years.[137] Deaths from cerebral hemorrhage accounted for about 28.7 percent of these deaths among women 15−44 years old and deaths from cerebral thrombosis accounted for an additional 5.2 percent. During the 10 year period between 1968 and 1977, mortality rates for women from cerebrovascular diseases declined from about 65/100,000 total pop. to about 44/100,000 total pop.

Accidents

Accidents are the leading cause of death among persons from 1−34 years of age.[137] Many mothers and children die as the result of accidents. During 1977 an estimated 31,267 females died as the result of accidents and 10,430 (33.4%) of these deaths were among women between 15 and 44 years old. About 7289 (70%) of these deaths among women 15−44 years old were due to motor vehicle accidents. Mortality rates due to accidents among females declined from about 29/100,000 total pop. in 1968 to about 23/100,000 total in 1977. Women between the ages of 15 and 19 years old had the highest mortality rates due to accidents, particularly motor vehicle accidents, and these mortality rates declined as the ages of women increased.

MAJOR HEALTH PROBLEMS

Major health problems encountered by women in the United States include misuse of alcohol, misuse of drugs, obesity, smoking, and stress. These problems are complex and, although they will be discussed separately for the most part, are frequently interrelated.

Misuse of Alcohol

Data pertaining to alcoholism, or the consumption of excessive quantities of alcohol, are difficult to interpret. Definitions for the term ''alcoholism'' vary, data have been obtained from a variety of sample population groups—which makes it difficult to compare findings—many study groups have been small in number, and methodologies for obtaining and interpreting data have been inconsistent. Most studies designed to obtain information about alcohol consumption have focused on men and, as a result, most treatment programs have been designed to meet the needs of men.[91,102,114,116]

In general, the term "alcoholism" refers to the chronic or repetitive consumption of alcoholic beverages to the extent that it interfers with one's economic, social, phycial, or mental functioning.[114] It has been estimated that about 61 percent of all adult females in the United States consume alcoholic beverages compared to 76 percent of all adult males.[114] It is thought that the incidence of heavy or problem drinking among women is considerably lower than the incidence of heavy or problem drinking among men.[114] Conservative estimates of the number of women who have alcohol-related problems range from 1.5−2.25 million.[91,114] Several authors, however, consider these numbers to be severe underestimates[6,102,114] and it has been suggested by the President's Commission on Mental Health that as many as 40 percent of the women in this country may abuse alcohol.[110] Underestimates of the magnitude of alcohol-related problems among women are thought to be due to the greater social stigma associated with alcoholic women than with alcoholic men,[114] as well as the wide-spread use of male-oriented criteria for diagnosis and treatment.[102,114,116] There seems to be a trend toward increasing misuse of alcohol among women,[6] particularly among women less than 30 years old and 50 or more years old.[91,102] An estimated 50,000 women die each year from alcohol-related conditions such as homicide, suicide, cirrhosis of the liver, and alcoholic psychosis.[91]

Women seem to be more likely than men to begin drinking excessive amounts of alcohol with the onset of depression, in the face of sex-role conflicts, and following immediate and lasting crises such as divorce, death of a family member, a child leaving home, reproductive loss, limited economic resources, or sole responsibility for child rearing.[6,10,11,29,102,114,115,118] Alcoholism secondary to depression seems to occur in about 27 percent of all alcoholic women.[6,139] Self-esteem among alcoholic women has been found to be lower than self-esteem among nonalcoholic women and lower than self-esteem among alcoholic men[8,10,88] Alcoholic women tend to withdraw from meeting their responsibilities and from participation in social activities.[60,74] They also tend to have weaker defense mechanisms against stress than nonalcoholic women. Many alcoholic women exhibit antisocial behaviors such as breaking established rules, teasing or mistreating other individuals, or engaging in petty thievery.[60]

Major physical problems encountered by female alcoholics include hypertension, obesity, liver disease, anemia, ulcers, and gastrointestinal hemorrhage.[5] Alcoholic beverages contain many calories and alcoholism often results in poor nutritional status since all of the nutrients necessary for the maintenance of health are frequently not consumed each day.[38] Alcohol is also an irritant to the lining of the gastrointestinal system. There is some evidence indicating that alcoholic women may experience more reproductive-related problems, such as infertility and reproductive loss, than nonalcoholic women. In three different studies 61−78 percent of the alcoholic women reported having had obstetric or gynecologic problems and 34−53 percent of the nonalcoholic women reported having had such problems.[6,7,141] Some women have reported that consumption of alcohol increases their sexual desires and enjoyment.[8,9,141] It is not known whether these feelings are the result of the effects of alcohol psychologically and physiologically or whether the reporting of these feelings may be a way of rationalizing drinking behaviors.

It has been estimated that as many as 50 percent of all alcoholic women also use other drugs in addition to alcohol.[43] These drugs are usually stimulants, opiates, hypnotics, or antianxiety drugs, and are usually obtained from physicians by prescription.[13,119] During interviews of women in an alcoholic treatment center, the women who were known to abuse drugs in conjunction with abuse of alcohol reported more suicide attempts, antisocial behaviors, and psychiatric care than alcoholic women who were not drug abusers.[119]

During pregnancy the alcohol blood level in the fetus is as high as it is in the mother.[66] The most commonly recognized problem in the offspring of alcoholic women is mental retardation.[38] In addition, the risks of stillbirth, low birth weight, and defects affecting the brain and central nervous system have been found to be higher among newborns of mothers who consume alcoholic beverages during pregnancy than among mothers who do not consume any alcoholic beverages during pregnancy.[91,124] Mothers who consume large amounts of alcohol consistently during pregnancy have also been found to have a higher risk of delivering babies with heart valve defects, brain cell abnormalities, and various facial abnormalities than mothers who do not consume large quantities of alcohol during pregnancy. Data are not yet available on the long-term prognosis for infants of alcoholic mothers but it seems likely that it is less than desirable when an infant with growth failure and mental retardation is cared for by a mother who is depressed and tends to neglect her responsibilities.

Misuse of Drugs

Estimates of the number of women in the United States who misuse drugs have been more difficult to obtain and interpret than estimates of the number of alcoholic women. Definitions for the terms "misuse" or "abuse" vary and the meanings of the terms "addiction," "addicting drugs," and "dangerous drugs," are often ambiguous. Individuals representative of the general population have been asked questions about patterns of drug use. However, drug addicts are often not accessible in such interviews because many of them are transients, in a hospital, or in jail.[24] In addition, heroin use is illegal and socially unacceptable, which may pressure individuals being interviewed into concealing any addiction to it.

Data from the Drug Abuse Warning Network, an organization sponsored jointly by the Drug Enforcement Administration and the National Institute on Drug Abuse, indicate that, at some time in their lives, about 32 million women will use tranquilizers, about 16 million women will use sedatives, and about 12 million women will use stimulants.[91] It is estimated that only about one-half as many men as women will use these drugs at some time in their lives.[91] An estimated 62,500 women are thought to be addicted to heroin and they represent about 25 percent of all heroin addicts.[91] About 67 percent of all prescriptions for psychotropic drugs such as Valium and Librium are written for women.[109,110] Females accounted for about 43 percent of all identified drug-related deaths in 1977[137] and at least 60 percent of all emergency room visits for drug-related problems are made by females.[59] Over 1000 females were interviewed in a recent household survey conducted in Baltimore, Maryland, and one in five reported having used some form of over-the-counter medication other than vitamins in the two days preceding the interview.[17] Over-the-counter medications used by these females were found to be primarily pain relievers.

Although the number of female drug addicts in the United States has been estimated to be quite low, it has been suggested that drug abuse among women in this country is increasing rapidly.[33,109,126] Increases in illicit use of drugs have been noted particularly among young women and women with liberal values and life-styles. Many women have reported that initiation into illicit drug use and continued reliance upon drugs have been the result of encouragement by men.[109]

It has been suggested that women use prescription and nonprescription drugs more frequently than men either because they experience more morbidity and discomfort or because they have a keener perception of their own symptoms and are more willing to take medications for relief than men.[91] Women do make more visits to physicians than men, which is most likely the reason that women receive more prescriptions than men. Physicians do tend, however, to prescribe more psychotropic drugs for women than they do for men.[33,126] There is some evidence suggesting that women report symptoms of anxiety and stress, as well as other diffuse symptoms, more frequently than men and that there is a greater likelihood that a physician will determine such symptoms to be psychosomatic when reported by a woman.[91]

Symptoms of drug abuse include drowsiness, irritability, mental confusion, and impairment of coordination.[72] Drug abuse not only increases the individual's risk of accidents, suicide, and homicide, but contributes to family disruption and poor school or work performance.[58] It also has potential for development of chronic disease. Pregnant addicts tend not to obtain prenatal care until late in pregnancy, if at all, and are at much greater risk of abortions, stillbirths, premature births, and delivery of babies who experience neonatal complications than pregnant women who are not addicted to drugs.[91]

Obesity

Although there are established measurements of obesity, differences of opinion exist about what constitutes an ideal weight and what percentage of weight above the ideal weight is detrimental to a woman's health. A weight in excess of 20 percent over an ideal weight has most frequently been considered to be the point at which obesity is identified.[54,73] Recent evidence, however, suggests that the medical risks of developing chronic disease and the risk of accidents among women may not increase appreciably until the ideal weight is exceeded by 30 percent.[80]

It has been estimated that about one in four women in the United States between 15 and 44 years of age is overweight. This estimate is based on a weight in excess of 20 percent over an ideal weight subscribed to by several insurance companies,[54,73] as well as measures of skinfold thickness.[91] Obesity is more prevalent among black women than among white women[39] and is about six times more prevalent among women from low socioeconomic status population groups than among women from high socioeconomic status groups.[45,104]

Fatness and leanness appear to run in families. About 42 percent of all adult obese women were obese as children[131] and husbands and wives frequently are both either fat or lean.[45] Family tendencies to be either fat or lean may be partly due to attitudes and habits regarding food and exercise.

Obesity is the major nutritional problem among women in the United States.[39] Excessive calorie intake does not assure that all of the required nutrients are consumed each day and healthy body functioning is dependent upon them. Women whose weight is in excess of 30 percent above their weights are at a much higher risk of developing hypertension, coronary heart disease, cancer, or diabetes mellitus and of encountering accidents than women without this degree of excess weight.[49,80,86,105] Many overweight women also experience menstrual irregularities and hirsutism.[86] Psychotherapeutic data suggest that obese women frequently suffer from a distorted body image, alienation, and feelings of despondency, dependency, and manipulation.[14] Resulting reactions to such feelings are often exhibited through hostile behaviors.

Women who are obese when they become pregnant face increased risks of hypertensive disorders and diabetes mellitus and these disorders are known to have adverse effects on pregnancy outcome.[27,105,130] Restricted intake of certain dietary nutrients during pregnancy has potential for limiting a mother's capacity to make the physiological adjustments required during pregnancy and fetal development may be compromised.[107] Obese women tend to have longer gestations and heavier babies than women who are not obese.[51,101] Increased risk of prolonged labor among obese women has been reported in the literature[69] but not consistently.[51,106] Some researchers have noted increased rates of cesarean section among obese women[44] while others have found no differences in cesarean section rates among obese and nonobese mothers[34,106]

The risks of developing medical and psychological problems associated with obesity in women can be dramatically reduced with weight loss.[39,49] About 60−75 percent of those individuals who try to lose weight have some degree of success but only about five percent of them are able to maintain a weight loss over time.[125] Rates of success with weight loss are highest when the obesity is of adult onset, when weight reduction is approached in gradual steps using a diet that is nutritionally adequate and sufficiently filling, and when some form of psychologic support is consistently available.[39]

Smoking

Since 1955 there has been an enormous increase in the incidence of cigarette smoking among women and in the number of women who die each year from lung cancer. In 1979 women accounted for about 25 percent of all lung cancer deaths and the risk of death from lung cancer among women who smoke has been estimated to be as high as five times greater than the risk of death from lung cancer among women who do not smoke.[91] The greatest increases in the incidence of smoking among women during the past 25 years have been noted in the relatively young age groups. Among women born during the decade from 1951–1960, the average age of onset of smoking was 16 years and the number of women between 17 and 24 years of age who smoke is currently greater than the number of men between the ages of 17 and 24 years who smoke.[91] Although the overall percentage of individuals in the total population of the United States who smoke is decreasing, this percentage is decreasing at a slower rate for females than it is for males.[37] Between 1964 and 1977 smoking rates for girls between the ages of 13 and 19 years doubled while smoking rates for boys in this same age group remained stable.[87]

A strong dose-related association has been noted between smoking and the risk of developing lung cancer[42] or other undesirable respiratory symptoms.[142] Although some variation in individual susceptibility to the harmful effects of smoke on the respiratory system has been acknowledged,[142] there appears to be increased risk of developing respiratory problems with increased daily duration of the smoking habit, number of cigarettes smoked daily, and the amount of smoke inhaled.[42] Lung cancer is of major concern since the malignant lesion grows rapidly and afflicted women often experience rapidly fatal disease courses after symptoms become apparent. An estimated one-third of all such lesions have been found to be incurable before they are even evident radiologically.[37]

Respiratory problems are not the only adverse effects in women that have been associated with cigarette smoking. The incidence of cerebrovascular disease has been reported to be from 38–114 percent higher in women who smoke than in women who do not smoke,[37] and cigarette smoking has been found to be a major independent factor in risk of fatal and nonfatal heart attacks, as well as sudden death in women.[91] It has been noted that cessation of smoking will greatly reduce a woman's risk of mortality or morbidity from coronary heart disease, chronic bronchopulmonary disease, and lung cancer.[37]

Growth retardation has been associated with maternal smoking during pregnancy[94] and frequently results not only in spontaneous abortion, fetal death, or neonatal death, but in conditions, such as hypoglycemia, with potential for causing permanent morbidity in afflicted children.[2] The mean birth weight of babies born to mothers who smoked during pregnancy has been reported to be from 150−250 g less than the mean birth weight of babies born to mothers who did not smoke during pregnancy, and mothers who smoke while pregnant have been found to deliver babies with a birth weight of less than 2500 g almost twice as frequently as mothers who do not smoke while pregnant.[2,26,38,55,93,94,128] Mothers who smoke during pregnancy have also been found to experience placental abruption, placenta previa, bleeding during pregnancy, and premature or prolonged rupture of the fetal membranes significantly more often than mothers who do not smoke during pregnancy.[2,38] All of these conditions are associated with high risks of perinatal loss. Many children born to mothers who smoked while pregnant have been found to exhibit measurable deficiencies in physical growth, as well as in intellectual and emotional development.[103] These deficiencies were not found to be attributable to any risk factors other than smoking during pregnancy. There is some preliminary evidence which indicates that individuals born to mothers who smoked during pregnancy may be at greater risk of developing cancer at some time in their lives than those born to mothers who did not smoke during pregnancy.[63]

In spite of the known risks associated with smoking during pregnancy, it has been estimated that as many as one-half of all pregnant women smoke.[75] It appears that the risks of undesirable pregnancy outcome become even higher among women who smoke during pregnancy when they are also of low socioeconomic status, are poorly nourished, or have poor obstetric histories.[26,90]

Among women who smoke, cessation of smoking during pregnancy appears to reduce the risks of undersirable pregnancy outcome. Data from an extensive investigation of 8193 pregnancies indicated that the babies born to mothers who stopped smoking during pregnancy had no signs of growth retardation even though smoking is known to cause permanent damage to uterine arteries.[94]

Stress

All women are exposed to stress in one form or another periodically throughout life. Difficulty in coping with stress is frequently an underlying factor in the development of alcoholism, drug abuse, obesity, and dependence on cigarettes. It is not clear from the literature whether women actually experience more stress than men or whether the higher incidence of mental disorders among women is due to sex-linked differences in reporting and interpreting symptoms of stress. Inequality of women within the United States has been suggested as one major factor responsible for increasing the vulnerability of women to stress and, therefore, the potential for development of mental disorders.[33] Many women continue to feel that they experience discrimination in business, politics, the law, and the home despite the 1974 amendment to the Civil Rights Act of 1964 which prohibits discrimination on the basis of sex.[33,89,110,126]

More than 50 percent of all women in the United States are employed outside of their homes[110] and it has been estimated that as many as 60 percent will be paid for work outside of their homes by 1990.[35] Most employed women are in the lowest paying occupations and many are at the bottom of achievement ranking systems. Almost 90 percent of all employed women in this country earned less than $9000 during 1977, while only 49 percent of all employed men earned less than $9000 during the year.[133] An estimated one in four women, compared with one in 18 men, lived on an annual income of less than $4000 in 1977.[110] About 32 percent of all households headed by women in 1977 and 51 percent of those headed by black women had incomes lower than the federally designated poverty level.[91]

Housework, child care, and care of the elderly remain primarily the woman's responsibility whether or not she is employed outside of her home.[110] Although many women have accepted the challenges of new roles and responsibilities, the activities required for maintaining a home have not been shared equally by men. Many women are forced into responsibility for two full workdays in every 24 hour period.[67,110] Role strain has been found to be particularly high among women with strong commitments to both their career and domestic responsibilities.[67]

Only a few women in the United States are in positions with substantial political influence. As a result, political capacity to improve the status of women in society is severely limited. Females comprise about 3.5 percent of the United States House of Representatives membership and about two percent of the United States Senate membership.[110] Fewer than 10 percent of all state legislators are female.

The legal system in the United States provides little support for divorced women in need of money to pay for living expenses and the divorce rate is higher than that of any other country.[91] In the 12-month period ending with February of 1981, an estimated 1,182,000 divorces took place in this country.[99] In 1975 only 14 percent of all divorced women received alimony.[120] As many as 44 percent of all single mothers received money for child support at least one time during 1975, however, only about 21 percent of these mothers received money for child support on a regular basis.[110,120]

Within the home, women not only continue to have major responsibility for all domestic activities, but many women are subjected to physical abuse by their husbands. The Federal Bureau of Investigation has indicated that about 1.5 million cases of wife abuse are brought to the attention of the Bureau each year.[110] It has been suggested that as many as one-half of all marriages in the United States involve some form of physical abuse of the wife.[127]

More women than men in the general population of the United States report that they experience symptoms of depression and almost twice as many women as men are admitted to hospitals for treatment of depression.[110] About 120 females per 100,000 are treated for depression each year in outpatient settings, which is more than twice the number of males treated for depression each year in such settings. There is some evidence suggesting that physicians tend to label questionable symptoms reported by women to be psychogenic instead of organic, particularly when anxiety is an accompanying symptom,[3,89] and it is known that twice as many women are given prescriptions for tranquilizing drugs than men.[110]

The profile of a woman at greatest risk of developing mental disorders due to stress might read: divorced, black, completed nine years of education, raising four young children, works full-time as a nursing assistant, has a total annual income of $6000.[33,52,133] Unmarried women have been found to have a lower incidence of mental illness than unmarried men, however, married women have a higher incidence of mental illness than married men.[91] Symptoms of depression among married women are most common among women whose children are living with them[110] and the child rearing period of a woman's life has been equated with less life-satisfaction, more stress, and more overt mental illness than other periods of life.[120] It has been suggested that women are more likely than men to have emotional problems because the traditional role of wife and mother is often confining, demanding, and boring.[50,140,144] Divorced mothers have been found to be significantly less satisfied with the state of their lives than their divorced husbands.[120] Loneliness and isolation, particularly in conjunction with economic deprivation, have potential for development of serious mental health problems among single mothers.[33]

Although better employment opportunities have reduced the stress experienced by some women due to boredom and isolation in traditional female roles, new role expectations impose new kinds of stress. No matter how desirable the changes presently occurring in role expectations for women may be, rapid changes disturb one's psychologic equilibrium and may result in symptoms of stress.[92,108,138]

Emotional stress during pregnancy may be associated with increased risk of fetal malformations. Data pertaining to 1263 study births of women who had been refused permission for abortion were compared with data from each birth subsequent to a study birth in the same setting.[12] The incidence of fetal malformations was found to be 1.8 percent in the study group and only 1.1 percent in the control group. It was not known whether this difference might have been due to direct physiological responses to stress or to indirect physiological responses resulting from attempts to provoke abortion, improper nutrition, excessive smoking, or abuse of alcohol or drugs on the part of some mothers.

OTHER CONCERNING HEALTH PROBLEMS

Other health problems of particular concern to women include exposure to violence through rape and battering, as well as the problems resulting from sexually transmitted diseases.

Exposure to Violence

Rape has recently been acknowledged as the most rapidly increasing violent crime in the United States[30] and reported increases in the incidence of forcible rape of females between 1960 and 1976 ranged from 60–121 percent.[53] According to the Federal Bureau of Investigation, more than 67,000 forcible rapes occurred in 1978.[91] It is speculated that incidents of rape are severely underreported because of the additional stresses placed on female victims who do report having been raped.[53,72,91] These stresses include the ordeal of a pelvic examination, police questioning, and the possibility of having to appear in court for questioning if the rapist is found and indicted.[84,91] Rape victims are also frequently exposed to lack of support from the police, hospital personnel, and family members.[84]

Victims of rape have been found to be responsible for fewer precipitation behaviors, such as manner of dressing or interacting, than victims of other kinds of violent crimes.[72] Precipitation behaviors are thought to be involved in only about four percent of all rapes compared with 22 percent of all homicides, 14 percent of all assaults, and almost 11 percent of all armed robberies. About 33 percent of all rapes are planned single rapes; 13 percent are planned pair rapes; 24 percent are planned group rapes; and 30 percent are spontaneous rapes.[72] About 58 percent of all rapists are the victim's relative or close friend, or an individual recognized by the victim. More than one-half of all rapes occur in the victim's or rapist's home. About three-fourths of all rapes occur in urban areas. More than 50 percent of all rapists have had no prior criminal record and approximately 4.5 percent are rape repeaters.

Almost 60 percent of the forcible rapes of females are of those between 11 and 24 years old.[72] The incidence of forcible rape decreases as age increases after 24 years. Violence, such as beating, stabbing, and choking, is thought to take place in at least one out of five incidents. Women are often physically injured during rape and sometimes the injuries are severe. Life-threatening injuries such as subdural hematomas or ruptured internal organs are sometimes encountered and occasionally life is lost.[53]

The physical injuries from rape can be serious, and most women find the emotional repercussions to be very traumatic. Burgess, in 1974,[16] delineated symptoms for acute and long-term phases of the "rape trauma syndrome". During the acute phase of the syndrome many women experience insomnia or disorganized sleep patterns with nightmares, decreases in appetite, nausea when thinking about the incident, somatic complaints related to the area of the body that was the major focus of attack, overwhelming fears of physicial injury, mutilation, or death, and feelings of degradation, shame, guilt, or humiliation. Even in the long-term reorganization phase of the syndrome there continues to be disruption in one's patterns of daily living. Many women who have experienced rape have been found to have significantly less satisfaction with sexual relationships after the rape than women who have never been victims of rape.[15,32,71] Victims who are given opportunities to articulate their feelings about the experience of rape seem to be able to cope with their fears and return to their normal routines faster than victims who are not given such opportunities.[61,65]

The most violent institution, group, or setting that a typical woman is likely to encounter is her own family.[123] Physical assaults by husbands on their wives represent a serious problem of intrafamily violence (second only to child abuse) and may occur in as many as one-half of all marriages in the United States.[123,127] Data from a nationally representative sample of 2143 couples indicated that the number of physical assaults on wives by their husbands increased within a period of one year as the number of stresses experienced by the husbands increased.[123] Level of education was not found to be a factor associated with wife battering; however, low income and employment in low status occupations were found to be highly associated with such abuse.

Men who batter their wives tend to have certain characteristics in common, including jealousy, inadequate impulse control, and inability to tolerate frustration.[46] Early exposure to violence and inadequate parent−child relationships appear to be important in influencing the social development of such men.[46,47,48,62] Many women feel that they must tolerate battering because reporting such incidents to the police would only result in further violence.[46] High levels of anxiety resulting from the ever-present threat of violence frequently result in symptoms of depression. Battered women commonly have vague somatic complaints and may express feelings of incompetence, powerlessness, or even numbness.[53] Many battered women react to being battered by physically abusing their children and some battered women are suicidal because they feel it is their only option for having control over their destinies.[53,79]

Sexually Transmitted Diseases

As many as one in ten females in the United States may be afflicted with venereal disease, or infectious disease transmitted sexually.[121] In one study of patients with venereal disease, it was found that more than 66 percent of the patients had contracted the disease after only one sexual contact.[25] Less than 50 percent of all sexually transmitted diseases occur in women but more than 90 percent of the resulting complications occur to them and their offspring.[91] Increasing numbers of sexually transmitted pathogenic organisms are being identified, and the incidence of infections caused by many of them has risen dramatically since the early 1950s.[64,91] More than one million new cases of gonorrhea, considered to be the most serious infectious disease in the United States, are diagnosed in females each year.[40,64] Genital herpes simplex virus infection, which is always present once it is contracted because there is no known effective treatment or cure, has emerged as the most prominent sexually transmitted disease of the early 1980s and it has been found to affect at least 20 percent of all sexually active individuals. Major reasons given for the dramatic increases noted in the incidence of venereal disease in the United States include the steady increases in the percentages of young adults who are sexually active coupled with an increase in the median age of first marriage.[147,148]

Sexually transmitted diseases sometimes have devastating effects on human fertility and reproduction, as well as on maternal and infant morbidity. It is thought that as many as 50,000 women in the United States become involuntarily sterile each year as a direct result of gonococcal pelvic inflammatory disease[91] and, during 1977, more than 20,000 ectopic pregnancies among women in this country were attributed to salpingitis.[132] Salpingitis is a frequent complication of sexually transmitted disease. Risk of involuntary infertility has been found to be almost 20 percent higher among women who have had one or more episodes of salpingitis than among women who have never had salpingitis, and risk of ectopic pregnancy has been found to be about 10 times higher in women who have had one or more episodes of salpingitis than in women who have not had any such episodes.[64]

Pelvic inflammatory disease is the major complication encountered by females who contract a sexually transmitted disease and about 270,000 new cases are diagnosed among females in the United States each year.[91] Pain is the universal symptom in pelvic inflammatory disease and infections may involve the fallopian tubes, ovaries, or pelvic peritoneum, veins, or connective tissue. Approximately 20 percent of all gynecologic problems have been found to be a result of pelvic inflammatory disease.[85] Genital herpes virus infection is thought to be responsible for about 90 percent of all vesiculoulcerative lesions of female genitalia[40] and has been found to be three times more prevalent in pregnant women than in women who are not pregnant.[28]

Insults to the health of children born to mothers who have a sexually transmitted disease are often much more severe than the symptoms of morbidity encountered by the mothers themselves. It has been estimated that more than 10,000 children born in the United States each year are left with major health problems such as deafness, blindness, cerebral palsy, epilepsy, or mental retardation as a result of maternal infection. Mothers with an active genital herpes virus infection during pregnancy have a three to five-fold increased risk of spontaneous abortion over that for mothers without an active infection, an increased risk of premature delivery if the infection is primary, and an increased risk of congenital malformations among offspring infected in utero.[98] These congenital malformations frequently include microencephaly, retinal dysplasia, patent ductus arteriosus, and intracranial calcification. Severe mental retardation is not uncommon among these children.

NEEDS FOR HEALTH CARE SERVICES

Statistics on the major causes of mortality among females in the United States and about selected health problems encountered by many of them during their lives are important as a basis for understanding the complexities underlying the needs of women for health care services during their reproductive years. Statistics, however, do not fully illustrate these complexities. All women should have access to professional health care services through which health status is monitored, minor health concerns are alleviated, potential health problems are prevented, and medical problems are treated. Although very few women in this country die from obstetric or gynecologic problems, many of them enter the health care system with reproductive-related concerns.[37] It is frequently the professional specializing in women's reproductive health care who has major impact on women's attitudes toward utilizing available health care services for a variety of personal needs.

Of concern is the fact that many women in the United States are not satisfied with the health care services they have received and their numbers seem to be increasing.[37,91] To these women, care providers often seem unresponsive, repressive, and even punitive. Recently, members of the New York County Medical Society became concerned about whether an anti-doctor feeling really exists among women and they decided to discuss the issue openly with representatives from the National Council of Women of the United States, the League of Women Voters, the National Organization for Women, the Young Women's Christian Association, the Legal Defense and Education Fund of the National Organization for Women, *Ms.* magazine, and the National Women's Health Network.[145] It was learned that many women feel that they receive insufficient information about what is happening to their bodies, therapeutic regimes recommended for them, or the alternative options for treatment available to them. Some of the women involved in these discussions also expressed concerns about the lack of sensitivity on the part of some physicians to the health care needs of women.

In order to resolve the concerns that many women have about the health care services available to them, it has been recommended that women be encouraged to become better health care consumers.[111] This can be accomplished by being well enough informed to ask questions, to request further explanation or a second opinion, to refuse proposed diagnostic or treatment measures, or to change physicians. Women seeking health care services and the providers of these services must communicate openly if optimal resolutions for the health care needs of individual women are to be a reality.

REFERENCES

1. Abortion Surveillance, Annual Summary 1977. Atlanta, Ga., USPHS Center for Disease Control, 1979
2. A Report of the Surgeon General. Washington, D.C., DHEW Publication No. (PHS) 79-50066, 1979
3. Armitage K, Schneiderman L, Bass R: Response of physicians to medical complaints in men and women. JAMA 241:2186-2187, 1979

4. Armstrong RJ: A Study of Infant Mortality from Linked Records: by Birth Weight, Period of Gestation, and Other Variables, United States, 1960 Live-Birth Cohort. Washington, D.C., Vital and Health Statistics, Series 20, No. 12, 1972

5. Ashley MJ, Olin JS, LeRiche WM: Morbidity in alcoholics: evidence for accelerated development of physical disease in women. Arch Intern Med 137:883−887, 1977

6. Beckman L: Women alcoholics: a review of social and psychological studies. J Stud Alcohol 36:797−819, 1975

7. Beckman LJ: Beliefs about the causes of alcohol-related problems among alcoholic and nonalcoholic women. J Clin Psychol 35:663−670, 1979

8. Beckman LJ: Perceived antecedents and effects of alcohol consumption in women. J Stud Alcohol 41:518−530, 1980

9. Beckman LJ: Reported effects of alcohol on the sexual feelings and behavior of women alcoholics and nonalcoholics. J Stud Alcohol 40:272−282, 1979

10. Beckman LJ: Self-esteem of women alcoholics. J Stud Alcohol 39:491−498, 1978

11. Beckman LJ: Sex-role conflict in alcoholic women: myth or reality. J Abnormal Psychol 87:408−417, 1978

12. Blomberg S: Influence of maternal distress during pregnancy on fetal malformations. Acta Psychiatr Scand 62:315−330, 1980

13. Borgman RD: Medication abuse by middle-aged women. Social Casework 54:526−532, 1973

14. Bruch H: The Golden Cage. Boston, Harvard Press, 1978

15. Burgess AW, Holmstrom LL: Rape: sexual disruption and recovery. Am J Orthopsychiatry 49:648−657, 1979

16. Burgess AW, Holmstrom LL: Rape: Victims of Crisis. Bowie, Md., Robert J. Brady, 1974

17. Bush PJ, Rabin DL: Who's using nonprescribed medicines? Med Care 14:1014−1023, 1976

18. Cates W, Grimes DA, Smith JC, et al: Legal abortion mortality in the United States. JAMA 237:452−455, 1977

19. Cates W, Smith JC, Rochat RW, et al: Assessment of surveillance and vital statistics data from monitoring abortion mortality, United States, 1972−1975. Am J Epidemiol 108:200−206, 1978

20. Chase HC: Infant mortality and weight at birth: 1960 United States birth cohort. Am J Public Health 59:1618−1628, 1969

21. Chase HC: A Study of Infant Mortality from Linked Records: Comparison of Neonatal Mortality from Two Cohort Studies, United States. Washington, D.C., Vital and Health Statistics, Series 20, No. 13, 1972

22. Chase HC: A study of risks, medical care, and infant mortality. Am J Public Health 63:1−56, 1973 Supplement

23. Chase HC, Byrnes ME: Trends in "Prematurity", United States: 1950−67. Washington, D.C., Vital and Health Statistics, Series 3, No. 15, 1972

24. Cohen S: Narcotism: dimensions of the problem. Ann NY Acad Sci 311:4−9, 1978

25. Darrow WW: Changes in sexual behavior and venereal diseases. Clin Obstet Gynecol 18:255−267, 1975

26. Deibel P: Effects of cigarette smoking on maternal nutrition and the fetus. JOGN Nurs 9:333–336, 1980

27. Edwards KE, Dickes WF, Alton IR, et al: Pregnancy in the massively obese: course, outcome, and obesity prognosis of the infant. Am J Obstet Gynecol 131:479–483, 1978

28. Edwards MS: Venereal herpes: a nursing overview. JOGN Nurs 7(5):7–15, 1978

29. Evinson RC, Altman H, Sletten TW, et al: Factors in the description and grouping of alcoholics. Am J Psychiatry 130:49–54, 1973

30. Federal Bureau of Investigation: Uniform Crime Reports. Washington, D.C., US Department of Justice, 1977

31. Fedrick J, Adelstein P: Influence of pregnancy spacing on outcome of pregnancy. Br Med J 4:753–756, 1973

32. Feldman-Summers S, Gordon PE, Meagher JR: The impact of rape on sexual satisfaction. J Abnorm Psychol 88:101–105, 1979

33. Fishel A: Mental health, in Fogel CI, Woods NF (eds): Health Care of Women. St. Louis, CV Mosby Co, 1981, pp 582–627

34. Fisher JJ, Frey I: Pregnancy and parturition in the obese patient. Obstet Gynecol 11:92–94, 1958

35. Flaim P, Fullerton HN: Labor force projections to 1990. Three possible paths. Monthly Labor Rev 101:25–35, December 1978

36. Fogel CI: Abortion, in Fogel CI, Woods NF (eds): Health Care of Women. St. Louis, CV Mosby Co, 1981, pp 524–538

37. Fogel CI: Assessment of health status, in Fogel CI, Woods NF (eds): Health Care of Women. St. Louis, CV Mosby Co, 1981, pp 118–136

38. Fogel CI: High-risk pregnancy, in Fogel CI, Woods NF (eds): Health Care of Women. St. Louis, CV Mosby Co, 1981, pp 171–191

39. Fogel CI: Nutrition, in Fogel CI, Woods NF (eds): Health Care of Women. St. Louis, CV Mosby Co, 1981, pp 450–483

40. Fogel CI: The gynecologic traid: discharge, pain, and bleeding, in Fogel CI, Woods NF (eds): Health Care of Women. St. Louis, CV Mosby Co, 1981, pp 220–256

41. Fogel CI: The unwanted pregnancy, in Fogel CI, Woods NF (eds): Health Care of Women. St. Louis, CV Mosby Co, 1981, pp 209–219

42. Frame PS, Carlson SJ: A critical review of periodic health screening using specific screening culture. J Fam Pract 2:29–36, 123–129, 189–194, 283–289, 1978

43. Freed EX: Drug use by alcoholics: a review. Int J Addict 8:451–473, 1973

44. Freedman MA, Wilds PL, George WM: Grotesque obesity: a serious complication of labor and delivery. South Med J 65:732–736, 1972

45. Gain S: Levels of education, level of income and level of fatness in adults. Am J Clin Nutr 30:721–725, 1977

46. Gayford J: Wife battering: a preliminary survey of 100 cases. Br Med J 1:194–197, 1975

47. Gayford J: Battered wives: Part I. Nurs Mirr Midw J 143:62–65, 1976

48. Geracimos A: How I stopped beating my wife. Ms 5:53, August 1976

49. Gordon T: Diabetes, blood lipids, and the role of obesity in coronary heart disease risk for women. Ann Intern Med 87:393–397, 1977

50. Gove WR: Sex, marital status and mortality. Am J Soc 79:45−67, 1973
51. Gross T, Sokol RJ, King KC: Obesity in pregnancy. Obstet Gynecol 56:446−450, 1980
52. Guttentag M, Salasin S, Legge WW: Women's utilization of mental health services studied. Evaluation 3:30−31, 1976
53. Harris C: Women and violence, in Fogel CI, Woods NF (eds): Health Care of Women. St. Louis, CV Mosby Co, 1981, pp 139−145
54. Hashim SA: Hunger and satiety in man, in Winick M (ed): Nutritional Disorders of American Women. New York, John Wiley & Sons, 1977, pp 107−118
55. Haworth JC, Ellestad-Sayed JJ, King J, et al: Relation of maternal cigarette smoking, obesity, and energy consumption to infant size. Am J Obstet Gynecol 138:1185−1189, 1980
56. Health, United States, 1978. Hyattsville, Md., DHEW (PHS) Publication No. 79−1232, 1979
57. Health, United States, 1979. Hyattsville, Md., DHEW (PHS) Publication No. 80−1232, 1980
58. Healthy People: The Surgeon General's Report on Health Promotion and Disease Prevention. Washington, D.C., DHEW (PHS) Publication No. 79−55071, 1979
59. Hecht A: Tranquilizers: use, abuse and dependency. FDA Consumer pp 21−23, October 1978
60. Herzog MA, Wilson AS: Personality characteristics of the female alcoholic. J Clin Psychol 34:1002−1004, 1978
61. Hicks DJ: Rape: sexual assault. Am J Obstet Gynecol 137:931−935, 1980
62. Hilberman E: The Rape Victim. New York, Basic Books, Inc., 1976
63. Hinds MW: Maternal smoking and cancer risk to offspring. Lancet 2(8196):703, 1980
64. Holmes KK, Puziss M: Recommendations of the study group for research and training in sexually transmitted diseases. J Infect Dis 142:639−642, 1980
65. Ipema DK: Rape: the process of recovery. Nurs Res 28:272−275, 1979
66. Jensen MD, Benson RC, Bobak IM (eds): Maternity Care. The Nurse and the Family (ed 2). St. Louis, CV Mosby Co, 1981
67. Johnson F, Johnson CR: Role strain in high-commitment career women. J Am Acad Psychoanal 4:13−36, 1976
68. Kannel WB, Castilli WP: The Framingham study of coronary disease in women. Med Times 100:173−184, May 1978
69. Kerr MG: The problems of the overweight patient in pregnancy. Br J Obstet Gynaecol 69:988−990, 1962
70. Kessner DM: Infant Death: An Analysis by Maternal Risk and Health Care. Washington, D.C., National Academy of Sciences, 1973
71. Kilpatrick DG, Veronen LJ, Resick PA: The aftermath of rape: recent empirical findings. Am J Orthopsychiatry 49:658−669, 1979
72. Kramer A (ed): Woman's Body. New York, Simon & Schuster, 1981
73. Krause MV, Himscher MV: Food, Nutrition and Diet Therapy. Philadelphia, WB Saunders Co, 1972
74. Krauthamar C: The personality of alcoholic middle-class women: a comparative study with the MMPI. J Clin Psychol 35:442−448, 1979
75. Kretzchmar RM: Smoking and health: the role of the obstetrician gynecologist. Obstet Gynecol 55:403−406, 1980

76. Kushner R: Breast Cancer: A Personal History and Investigative Report. New York, Harcourt Brace Jovanovich, Inc, 1975

77. Lowdermilk DL: Reproductive malignancies, in Fogel CI, Woods NF (eds): Health Care of Women. St. Louis, CV Mosby Co, 1981, pp 301−333

78. Lubchenco LO, Searls DT, Brazie JV: Neonatal mortality rate: relationship to birth weight and gestational age. J Pediatr 81:814−820, 1972

79. Lystad MH: Violence at home: a review of the literature. Am J Orthopsychiatry 45:328−345, 1975

80. Mackenzie M: Obesity as failure in the American culture. Obesity/Bariat Med 5(4):132−133, 1976

81. MacMahon B, Kovar MG, Feldman JJ: Infant Mortality Rates: Socioeconomic Factor, United States. Washington, D.C., Vital and Health Statistics, Series 22, No. 14, 1972

82. MacMahon B, Kovar MG, Feldman JJ: Infant Mortality Rates: Relationships with Mother's Reproductive History, United States. Washington, D.C., Vital and Health Statistics, Series 22, No. 15, 1973

83. Manual of the International Classification of Diseases, Injuries, and Causes of Death, 1975. Geneva, World Health Organization, 1977

84. Marieskind HI: Women in the Health Care System: Patients, Providers and Programs. St. Louis, CV Mosby Co, 1980

85. Martin L: Health Care of Women. Philadelphia, JB Lippincott Co, 1978

86. Mayer J: Obesity. Prog Food Nutr Sci 1:115−122, 1975

87. McIntosh HD: Hypertension—a potent risk factor. Heart Lung 7:137−140, 1978

88. McLachlan JFC, Walderman RL, Birchmore DF, et al: Self-evaluation, role satisfaction, and anxiety in the woman alcoholic. Int J Addict 14:809−832, 1979

89. Mechanic D: Sex, illness, illness behavior, and the use of health services. J Human Stress 2:29−40, 1976

90. Meyer MN, Tonascia JA: Maternal smoking and pregnancy complications and perinatal mortality. Am J Obstet Gynecol 128:494−502, 1977

91. Moore EC: Women and health in the United States, 1980. Public Health Rep, 1980 Supplement

92. Moulton R: Some effects of the new feminism. Am J Psychiatry 134:1−6, 1977

93. Naeye RL: Effects of maternal cigarette smoking on the fetus and placenta. Br J Obstet Gynaecol 85:732−737, 1978

94. Naeye RL: Influence of maternal cigarette smoking during pregnancy on fetal childhood and growth. Obstet Gynecol 57:18−21, 1981

95. Naeye RL, Blanc WA: Relation of poverty and race to antenatal infection. N Engl J Med 283:555−560, 1970

96. Naeye RL, Blanc WA: Unfavorable outcome of pregnancy: repeated losses. Am J Obstet Gynecol 116:1133−1137, 1973

97. Naeye RL, Blanc WA: Influences of pregnancy risk factors on fetal and newborn disorders. Clin Perinatology 1:187−195, 1974

98. Nahmias AJ: Herpes simplex virus infection—present status of diagnosis and management. South Med J 68:1191−1194, 1975

99. National Center for Health Statistics: Births, marriages, divorces, and deaths for February 1981. Washington, D.C., Monthly Vital Statistics Report 30(2):1−11, May 1981

100. Niswander KR, Gordon M: The Women and their Pregnancies. Philadelphia, WB Saunders Co, 1972
101. Niswander KR, Singer J, Westphal M, et al: Weight gain during pregnancy and prepregnancy weight: association with birth weight of term gestation. Obstet Gynecol 33:482−491, 1969
102. Noble E: Alcohol and Health. Rockville, Md., DHEW Publication No. (ADM) 78−569, 1978
103. Office on Smoking and Health: Smoking and Health. Rockville, Md., DHEW Publication No. (PHS) 79−50066, 1979
104. Oken B, Hartz A, Giefer E, et al: Relation between socioeconomic status and obesity changes in 9046 women. Prev Med 6:447−453, 1977
105. Owen AL, Owen GM: Maternal nutrition, in Jensen MD, Benson RC, Bobak IM (eds): Maternity Care. The Nurse and the Family (ed 2). St. Louis, CV Mosby Co, 1981, pp 238−263
106. Petry JA: Obesity with pregnancy. Obstet Gynecol 7:299−303, 1956
107. Pitkins RM: Nutritional influences during pregnancy. Med Clin North Am 61:3−15, 1977
108. Powell B, Reznikoff M: Role conflict and symptoms of psychological distress in college-educated women. J Consult Clin Psychol 44:475−479, 1976
109. Prather JE, Fidell LS: Drug use and abuse among women: an overview. Int J Addict 13:863−885, 1978
110. President's Commission on Mental Health: Mental Health of Women. Washington, D.C., 1978
111. Rooks JP: The women's movement and its effect on women's health care, in McNall L (ed): Current Obstetrics and Gynecological Nursing. St. Louis, CV Mosby Co, 1980, pp 3−26
112. Romney SL, Gray MJ, Little AB, et al: Gynecology and Obstetrics: The Health Care of Women. New York, McGraw-Hill, Book Co, 1975
113. Rubin G, McCarthy B, Shelton J, et al: The risk of childbearing re-evaluated. Am J Public Health 71:712−716, 1981
114. Sandmaier M: Alcohol Programs for Women: Issues, Strategies, and Resources. Washington, D.C., Government Printing Office No. 241−186/1132, 1977
115. Sandmaier M: Women helping women. Alcohol Health Res World 2:17−23,1977
116. Sandmaier M: The Invisible Alcoholics—Women and Alcohol Abuse in America. New York, McGraw-Hill Book Co, 1980
117. Schlesinger ER, Mazundar SM, Logrillo VM: Long-term trends in perinatal death among offspring of mothers with previous child losses. Am J Epidemiol 96:255−262, 1972
118. Schuckit MA: Sexual disturbances in the woman alcoholic. Med Aspects Human Sexuality 6:44−65, 1972
119. Schuckit MA, Morrisey ER: Drug abuse among alcoholic women. Am J Psychiatry 136:607−611,1979
120. Seiden A: Overview: research on the psychology of women. Part II. Women in families, work, and psychotherapy. Am J Psychiatry 133:1111−1123, 1976
121. Sexually transmitted diseases affect 1 in 20 Americans. Public Health Rep 95:496, 1980
122. Shapiro S, Schlesinger ER, Nesbitt REL: Infant, Perinatal, Maternal, and

Childhood Mortality in the United States. Cambridge, Harvard University Press, 1968

123. Straus MA: Social stress and marital violence in a national sample of American families. Ann NY Acad Sci 347:229–250, 1980

124. Streissguth AP: Maternal drinking and the outcome of pregnancy. Am J Orthopsychiatry 47:422–430, 1977

125. Stunkard AJ: From explanation to action in psychosomatic medicine: the case of obesity. Psychosom Med 37:195–236, 1975

126. Suffet F, Brotman R: Female drug use: some observations. Int J Addict 11:19–23, 1976

127. Tavris C, Offin C: Longest War. New York, Harcourt Brace Jovanovich, Inc, 1977

128. The Health Consequences of Smoking. Washington, D.C., DHEW Publication No. (HSM) 73–8704, 1973

129. Tietze C: New estimates of mortality associated with fertility control. Fam Plann Perspect 9:74–76, 1977

130. Tracy TA, Miller GL: Obstetric problems of the massively obese. Obstet Gynecol 33:204–208, 1969

131. Travers CK: Obesity and pregnancy: a review. Obesity/Bariatr Med 5(5):172–177, 1976

132. Urquhart J: Effect of the venereal diseases epidemic on the incidence of ectopic pregnancy—implications for the evaluation of contraceptives. Contraception 19:455–485, 1979

133. US Department of Labor: Women and Work. Washington, D.C., Monograph No. 46, 1977

134. Vavra HM, Querec LJ: A Study of Infant Mortality from Linked Records: by Age of Mother, Total-Birth Order, and Other Variables, United States, 1960 Live-Birth Cohort. Washington, D.C., Vital and Health Statistics, Series 20, No. 14, 1973

135. Vital Statistics of the United States, 1977. Volume I—Natality. Hyattsville, Md., DHHS Publication No. (PHS) 81–1113, 1981

136. Vital Statistics of the United States, 1977. Volume II—Mortality, Part A. Hyattsville, Md., DHHS Publication No. (PHS) 81–1101, 1981

137. Vital Statistics of the United States, 1977. Volume II—Mortality, Part B. Hyattsville, Md., DHHS Publication No. (PHS) 80–1102, 1980

138. Weissman M, Klerman G: Sex differences and the epidemiology of depression. Arch Gen Psychiatry 34:98–111, 1977

139. Weissman MM, Myers JK: Clinical depression in alcoholism. Am J Psychiatry 137:372–373, 1980

140. Williams J (ed): Psychology of Women: Selected Readings. New York, WW Norton and Co, 1979

141. Wilsnack SC: Sex role identity in female alcoholism. J Abnorm Psychol 82:253–261, 1973

142. Wolf CR, Zamel N: The respiratory effects of regular cigarette smoking in women. Chest 78:707–713, 1980

143. Woods NF: Women and their health, in Fogel CI, Woods NF (eds): Health Care of Women. St. Louis, CV Mosby Co, 1981, pp 3–26

144. Woods NF, Hulka BS: Symptom reporting and illness behaviors among married mothers: a comparison of employed women and homemakers. J. Community Health 5:36–45, 1979

145. Women critique medical profession: the prognosis is grim. Chicago Tribune, October 19, 1980, Section 12, p 10

146. Yerushalmy J: The classification of newborn infants by birth weight and gestational age. J Pediatr 71:170–172, 1967

147. Zelnick M, Kantner JF: Sexual and contraceptive experience of young unmarried women in the United States, 1976 and 1971. Fam Plann Perspect 9:55–71, 1977

148. Zelnick M, Kim YJ, Kantner JF: Probabilities of intercourse and contraception among U.S. teenage women, 1971 and 1976. Fam Plann Perspect 11:177–183, 1979

Ann M. Koontz

2

Providers of Women's Health Care Services

An array of health professionals provide health care services for women. Over the past 25 years the types of providers involved and their scope of practice have shifted and expanded. Multiple factors impacting on the health care delivery system have brought about these changes and influenced women's health care utilization.

PATTERNS OF HEALTH CARE UTILIZATION

Information on women's utilization of health care services and usual sources of care currently must be drawn from multiple data sets. Several national surveys carried out by the National Center for Health Statistics provide data on the use of medical care.[41] Findings from the 1974 Health Interview Survey indicate that the family practice physician or general practitioner was most often identified (61.2%) as the usual physician seen among all women having an ongoing source of care.[41] Obstetrician-gynecologists were reported as the general source of care for 16.6 percent of those women aged 20–44 years and for 5.3 percent of those aged 45–64 years.[37] Findings from the 1977 National Ambulatory Medical Care Survey (NAMCS) are similar. Of all office visits to physicians made by women 15 years old and over, 39.7 percent were to the general or family practice physician, 16.5 percent were to obstetrician-gynecologists, and 12.7 percent were to internists.[41]

Acknowledgment: All views expressed in this chapter are those of the author and are not necessarily those of the U.S. Department of Health and Human Services.

An in-depth look at the NAMCS data on the three most frequently visited specialties provides information on the type of physician the women selected when faced with a new condition. Data on visits to the obstetrician-gynecologist (OBG) group were compared to data on visits to the group of general or family practice physicians (GFP) and internists. The OBGs were selected for 67 percent of the special examinations, most of which were prenatal or gynecological, for 62.3 percent of the family planning visits, and for 40.8 percent of the visits for genitourinary symptoms. Additionally, the OBGs were selected for small percentages of the visits for digestive or musculoskeletal complaints, general symptoms, general examinations, and diagnostic tests, while the GFPs and internists handled over 60 percent of the visits for these same conditions. The amount of care provided by the GFPs and internists for genitourinary problems was comparable to that provided by the OBGs. Even though the OBGs were the predominant care provider for family planning, the GFPs and internists were selected for 36.6 percent of these visits.[41]

Data on utilization of other types of health care providers are harder to obtain. It is frequently necessary to infer utilization from encounter statistics or surveys of these providers. National natality statistics collected from all birth certificates through the Vital Statistics Cooperative Program classify live births by attendant and place of delivery. Before 1978 the categories for attendant at birth included physician in hospital, physician not in hospital, and midwife or other not in hospital.[39] Due to changing trends among attendants, the natality data from 1978 on have been cross-tabulated according to attendant (physician, midwife, and other) and place of birth (in hospital or not in hospital). This cross tabulation provides data on the number of hospital deliveries being carried out by midwives.[40] The category of midwife is not delineated further in this reporting system due to variability in information required by states.[40] In general, hospital deliveries would be attended by nurse-midwives, while those not-in-hospital births attended by midwives could be attributed either to nurse-midwives or lay midwives.

Data from a 1976–1977 survey of nurse-midwives by the American College of Nurse-Midwives indicate that 521 nurse-midwives reported doing 33,613 deliveries in the 12 months before the survey (approximately 1% of all live births in the United States at that time).[11] Estimates of the proportions of live births now delivered by nurse-midwives in the United States vary from 1–4 percent.[32] Data reported for maternity services provided in the 1980 fiscal year by state Maternal and Child Health agencies (excluding Maternity and Infant Care Projects) reveal that 3.5 percent of all patients were seen by certified nurse-midwives.[23] Indication of utilization of the physician's assistant is available from a 1978 national survey of physician's assistants. Of the 3416 respondents, 1.9 percent reported working primarily in the specialty area of obstetrics and gynecology.[44]

From the mixture of data available, it is not possible to infer the extent to which each type of health care provider serves as the usual source of care for women or as the primary care provider. The primary care provider affords the contact or entry to the health care system, carries a longitudinal responsibility for the patient, and coordinates the range of health care services needed.[35]

In 1975, 1881 counties out of 3084 in the United States (61%) had no obstetrician-gynecologist.[45] It is known that the distribution of providers varies widely by geographic location, with physician specialists more likely to be located in urban areas. In 1977 the percentage of communities of a designated size served by board-certified obstetrician-gynecologists rose from 5 in communities with a population of 5000 or less to 80 or more for communities with a population greater than 20,000. In the same year, while board-certified family practice physicians also were serving at least 80 percent of the larger communities, they were found practicing in 37 percent of the very small communities.[24] A study of physician-delivered births in Washington state in 1978 showed that the proportion of births delivered by medical doctors in obstetrics-gynecology decreased with the increase in the rurality of a county; a reverse trend was seen for births delivered by medical doctors in family or general practice.[49]

Primary care providers other than physicians are more likely than physicians to be found in smaller communities. Of the nurse-midwives in clinical practice in 1976−77, 10 percent were located in communities of less than 10,000 persons and 18.5 percent were found in communities ranging in size from 10,000 to 49,999 persons.[11] Among the physician's assistants responding to their 1978 survey, 25 percent of those in practice were in communities with populations under 10,000.[44] Data from the Area Resource File indicate that fewer than 1 percent of all physicians practice in these very small communities.[4]

HEALTH CARE PROVIDERS

Success in meeting the health care needs of women at the health care system level depends on the collaborative efforts of many health care professionals. Recognition should be given to the expertise of each type of professional and to the complementary nature of their special areas of knowledge. The view of health care service delivery as a team approach does not imply that every woman should have her health care needs attended to by multiple providers. Rather, it implies that the primary care provider will be cognizant of other health care resources and will utilize support systems or refer to other health personnel when necessary.[24]

The following descriptions of health care providers include primary care providers of women's reproductive health care and nurses working in women's health care who are not primary care providers. The important contribution of others, such as social workers, nutritionists, and health educators, is not overlooked but is beyond the scope of this discussion.

Certified Nurse-Midwife (CNM)

Nurse-midwives have been caring for women in the United States since 1925. In that year the first nursing center in what is now known as the Frontier Nursing Service was opened in Kentucky by Mrs. Mary Breckenridge. American nurses who had studied midwifery in England were employed to provide care to mothers and young children where there were no resident physicians.[48]

Between 1931 and 1932 the Association for the Promotion and Standardization of Midwifery (later renamed the Maternity Center Association) opened the Lobenstine Midwifery Clinic and the first school for nurse-midwives in New York City. These activities were initiated to study situations where obstetricians delegated the responsibility of care of maternity patients to nurse-midwives and to train a limited number of public health nurses who would subsequently work as instructors and supervisors of untrained midwives and of nurses with minimal obstetrical nursing.[31,48] It was recognized then that nurse-midwives could contribute their expertise to the health care system in more than one role.

Growth of the profession and changes in existing nurse organizations led to the incorporation in 1955 of the American College of Nurse-Midwifery, as the professional organization. By 1962 this group of professionals had accepted the definitions that follow for nurse-midwife and nurse-midwifery.

The nurse-midwife is a Registered Nurse who by virtue of added knowledge and skill gained through an organized program of study and clinical experience recognized by the American College of Nurse-Midwifery, has extended the limits (legal limits in jurisdictions where they obtain) of her practice into the area of management of care of mothers and babies throughout the maternity cycle so long as progress meets criteria accepted as normal.

Nurse midwifery is an extension of nursing practice into the area of management of care of mothers and babies throughout the maternity cycle so long as progress meets criteria accepted as normal.[5]

These definitions remained for 16 years. In 1969 the American College of Nurse-Midwifery merged with a Kentucky originated group, the American Association of Nurse-Midwives, to become the American College of Nurse-Midwives (ACNM). Educational preparation and clinical practice were examined extensively, and credentialing procedures for accreditation and certification were initiated. To reflect trends within the profession and the health care system, the definitions were revised in 1978. A certified nurse-midwife is now defined as follows:

A certified nurse-midwife (CNM) is an individual educated in the two disciplines of nursing and midwifery, who possesses evidence of certification according to the requirements of the American College of Nurse-Midwives (ACNM).[16]

The professional practice is characterized in a separate definition:

Nurse-midwifery practice is the independent management of care of essentially normal newborns and women, antepartally, intrapartally, postpartally and/or gynecologically. This occurs within a health care system which provides for medical consultation, collaborative management, and referral and is in accord with the "Functions, Standards and Qualifications for Nurse-Midwifery Practice" as defined by the ACNM.[16]

The revised definition of nurse-midwifery practice describes more precisely the functional capability of nurse-midwives and establishes the general limits of practice. It conveys that the nurse-midwife is a primary care provider for women who are healthy or medically uncomplicated. If at any time a patient develops a medical complication, the nurse-midwife implements her health services coordination responsibility by seeking medical consultation or initiating a referral. Depending on the nature of the problem, the patient may remain under the management of the nurse-midwife or may transfer to the care of a physician. Nurse-midwives care for women seeking routine gynecologic services as well as those seeking care throughout pregnancy. Given their breadth of practice, nurse-midwives are able to move back and forth between ambulatory and inpatient or birthing settings.

By mid-1982 the ACNM had certified almost 2600 nurse-midwives, 1663 of whom were members of the ACNM. These members were located throughout the United States, although unevenly distributed. Forty percent lived in the states on the East Coast while 16 percent lived on the West Coast or in Hawaii. Almost 20 percent lived in the East Central states and the rest were scattered among the Mountain and West Central states.[17]

Selected information on nurse-midwives has been retrieved from several surveys of all known nurse-midwives in the United States carried out periodically since 1963. Another survey will be completed during 1983.[17] The percentage of respondents who were in clinical practice in 1971 was 36.9 percent; this proportion increased to 50.7 percent by 1976−1977.[11] Findings in the 1976−1977 survey indicate that nurse-midwives were most likely to be practicing clinically in the Southwest, Southeast, and in Southern Appalacia, all locales with substantial rural or poverty stricken areas.[11] Practice options have expanded in subsequent years, and it is expected that the overall proportion of nurse-midwives in clinical practice will be greater in the future. We may see, also, that higher percentages of nurse-midwives have entered clinical practice in more urban states.

Nurse-midwives must successfully complete an accredited education program and must pass the ACNM National Certification Examination in order to be a certified nurse-midwife. Education programs vary in length from 9 months to 2 years depending on whether graduate work in an associated area is included in the curriculum. At the time the American College of Nurse-Midwifery was incorporated in 1955, there were three certificate and two master's degree programs.[11] The number of programs has fluctuated over the years but by mid-1982 these numbers had expanded to 11 certificate and 14 master's degree programs located throughout the United States. Foreign trained nurse-midwives must successfully complete either a basic or a refresher program (generally 3−4 months in length) to be eligible for national certification.

Accreditation of nurse-midwifery education programs is carried out by the Division of Accreditation (ACNM), a semi-autonomous body affiliated with the ACNM. Before 1980 this credentialing process was labeled approval rather than accreditation, and older documents as well as some licensure statutes or regulations refer to ACNM approved programs. The Division sets guidelines to assure development of a quality education program and awards preaccreditation status to new nurse-midwifery education programs that demonstrate that their planning is within the Division's guidelines. Evaluation for full-accreditation status occurs following completion of the program by the first class of students.[16]

All accredited nurse-midwifery programs are designed to prepare a safe, beginning practitioner.[9] Expected competencies of new graduates are identified in the ACNM document, *Core Competencies in Nurse-Midwifery: Expected Outcomes of Nurse-Midwifery Education*.[10] The ACNM National Certification Examination, developed and administered by the Division of Examiners of the ACNM, is an entry level examination designed to test individuals for safe practice. Content areas covered by the examination include: management of antepartum, intrapartum, postpartum, neonatal, and family planning/gynecological care, as well as professional issues. Candidates are tested for knowledge and judgment abilities related to normal phenomena and to deviations from normal phenomena in all clinical areas.[15] It is assumed that the education programs have approved the candidates' technical and interpersonal skills.

All certified nurse-midwives have similar basic competencies; however, their scope of practice or services provided may vary depending on type of position held, practice setting, legislative or regulatory authorization in the jurisdiction of practice, and individual philosophy and competence. The profession has established general standards and functions for practice, and guidelines for evaluating new functions for inclusion in practice.[7,8]

Statements have been issued by the ACNM on two specific areas of practice. One allows the CNM to practice in a variety of settings including hospital, home, and birth center.[12] The second statement prohibits the performance of an abortion by a CNM.[6] Certified nurse-midwives are expected to practice in a manner consistent with the official policies of the ACNM. Disciplinary action may be taken by the ACNM through a formal mechanism of peer review in instances of noncompliance.[14]

Nurses

Multiple types of nurses participate in the health care of women. Distinguishing one type of nurse from another is often difficult for patients and health care providers alike. Roles and functions of nurses have evolved as a result of major forces in society and changes in the health care system. Concern about potential manpower shortages in obstetrics and pediatrics following the so-called baby boom in the mid-1950s led to the recommendation that nurses be utilized in expanded roles. Consumerism, the women's movement, advances in technology and our knowledge base, and greater emphasis in prevention have impacted on the manner in which nurses participate in the health care system.

Nurses moved into primary health care in 1965 when the first nurse practitioner program (in pediatrics) was started in Colorado. At the same time clinical specialization options were increasing in graduate nursing programs. Current titles for nurses vary based on preparation, area of concentration, work setting, and function. Definitions for nursing titles adopted by the Nurses Association of the American College of Obstetricians and Gynecologists (NAACOG) reflect generally accepted characteristics and are as follows:

Professional Nurses

Qualifications: Graduated from an accredited basic nursing program and licensed to practice nursing.

Role/Function: Professional nurses provide direct care to patients utilizing the nursing process in arriving at decisions. They work in a collegial and collaborative relationship with other health professionals to determine health care needs and assume responsibility for nursing care. In the course of their practice, they identify and carry out systematic investigations of clinical problems, assess the effectiveness of actions taken, and engage in periodic review of their contributions to health care and those of their professional peers.

On entry into the profession of nursing, it is recognized that the new graduate needs an extensive orientation period or internship to provide an opportunity for assimilation of knowledge and application of clinical skills.

Nurse Clinicians

Qualifications: Professional nurses who demonstrate expertise in nursing practice and ensure ongoing development of expertise through clinical experience and continuing education. This role can be recognized by means of certification for special knowledge.

Role/Function: Nurse clinicians have well-developed competencies in utilizing the nursing process for both direct and indirect nursing care. Knowledge and clinical expertise is utilized to provide care aimed at returning the patient to the highest level of health in the shortest period of time. Nurse clinicians coordinate actions of other health team members to provide continuous physical care and emotional support for the patient.

Nurse Practitioners

Qualifications: Professional nurses prepared in a specialized education program with emphasis on certain medical diagnostic and therapeutic knowledge and skills, and able to function in an expanded role. This preparation shall be in the context of a formal nurse practitioner educational program. This role can be recognized by means of certification for special knowledge.

Role/Function: Nurse practitioners provide primary health care in a variety of settings. As primary care providers, nurse practitioners assess the physical and psychosocial status of patients by means of health history, physical examination, and diagnostic tests. The nurse practitioners interpret data, develop and implement plans of management, and follow through on the continuum of care of the patient. The

practitioners implement these plans through independent action, appropriate referrals, health counseling, and collaboration with other members of the health care team.
Clinical Nurse Specialists

Qualifications: Professional nurses with advanced knowledge, skill, and competence in a specialized area of nursing. Clinical nurse specialists are prepared at the master's degree level with emphasis in specific areas of clinical nursing. This role can be recognized by means of certification for special knowledge.

Role/Function: The role of clinical nurse specialists is defined by the needs of a select patient population, the expectations of society, and the clinical expertise of the nurse. By exercising judgements and demonstrating leadership ability, clinical nurse specialists function within a field of practice that focuses on the needs of the patient and system, and encompasses interactions with others in the nursing and health care systems serving the patient.

Clinical nurse specialists effect change directly by nursing care and indirectly by planning and guiding care with other health care team members and promoting and utilizing research. Their roles include ... [participating] in activities designed to continue self-development, ... [advancing] the goals of the nursing profession, and ... [promoting] effective collaborative relationships with members of the health care disciplines.*

Title usage is not as precise as implied by these definitions. Once employed, the nurse generally takes on a title which describes her practice rather than her preparation. Thus, a clinical nurse specialist with assessment skills may be filling a nurse-practitioner position. It is less likely, however, that graduates of nurse practitioner programs are employed as clinical nurse specialists. Specialty areas are designated in the titles, and those titles related to women's health care are numerous. Some examples are obstetrics-gynecology, maternal-child, family planning, women's health, and maternal-infant.[28] These specialty areas are further refined by the various certification programs (see Table 2-1). Nurses other than those with maternal and child health-associated titles providing primary care to women are the family nurse practitioner and the adult nurse practitioner.

Complete counts of nurses in the various categories are not available. Data gathered by the Nonphysician Health Care Provider (NPHCP) Technical Panel for the Graduate Medical Education National Advisory Committee (GMENAC) indicated that, as of the end of 1979, approximately 16,000 nurses had been graduated from programs training them for primary care. It was estimated that 10 percent of this group specialized in maternity or family planning areas and that there are 210 new graduates in this specialty each year.[46] Early in 1982 NAACOG had a membership of 16,560 nurses. Of the 16,340 who indicated their job setting, 10,175 (62.3%) were working in

---

*Reprinted with permission from Nurses Association of the American College of Obstetricians and Gynecologists: Standards for Obstetric, Gynecologic, and Neonatal Nursing. Washington, D.C., NAACOG, 1981.

Table 2-1

Number of Nurses Certified in Women's Health Care Related Specialties by Specialty Area and Certifying Agency, June 1983

Certifying Agency and Specialty Area	No. of Nurses*
ANA-MCH/NCC Joint Certification Program	
Ambulatory Care Nursing	61
Labor and Delivery	184
Maternal/Newborn Nursing	22
Neonatal Nursing	29
Postpartum Nursing	23
Women's Health Care I	93
Women's Health Care II	2
NAACOG Certification Corporation	
Inpatient Obstetric Nurse	865
Ob/Gyn Nurse Practitioner	2284
Neonatal Intensive Care Nurse	405
American Nurses' Association	
High Risk Perinatal Nurse	45
Maternal and Child Health Nurse	59

*Data from American Nurses' Association, personal communication, 1983 and NAACOG Certification Corporation, personal communication, 1983.

hospital inpatient units, 2521 (15.4%) were in hospital outpatient or office settings, 1394 (8.5%) were teaching in schools of nursing, and 797 (4.9%) were in government or community health positions.[42]

Organized programs of study that prepare nurses for expanded roles are classified broadly into certificate and master's level programs. Guidelines for the nurse-practitioner certificate programs are available from several sources including the U.S. Department of Health and Human Services* and the American Nurses' Association (ANA).[51] Accreditation is not required but may be requested through the ANA. No specific guidelines have been developed for curricula in master's level programs. Accreditation of graduate programs of nursing is carried out by the National League for Nursing (NLN) according to their criteria. Accreditation status applies to the total graduate program, indicating overall quality of a composite of speciality areas. The NLN does not purport to accredit individual specialty programs within the graduate school.

*U.S. Department of Health and Human Services, Health Resources and Services Administration, Bureau of Health Professions, Division of Nursing. Personal Communication, 1982.

Certification for nurses interested in women's health was offered beginning in 1976 by the ANA-MCH/NCC Joint Certification Program. This program was operational through 1978, certifying a total of 414 nurses for excellence in practice in maternal-gynecological-neonatal nursing[20] (also NAACOG, personal communication 1983). Subsequently, the ANA and the NAACOG Certification Corporation each developed their own programs to test for special knowledge.[51] A list of the specialty areas and the number of nurses certified in each appears in Table 2-1. Eligibility requirements vary according to program and specialty area but relate to education and experience. As of 1980 four states required national certification for practice in the extended role and six states recognized certification in place of an approved course of study.[52]

Collectively, these nurses provide nursing care and primary health care services in all phases of the woman's reproductive cycle except for managing the delivery of the infant. Typically, however, an individual nurse's scope of practice does not span the continuum but focuses on care related to a setting, such as ambulatory obstetrical and gynecologic services or inpatient obstetric nursing, or to a particular area of practice, such as family planning or high risk perinatal nursing. Functions allowed for the nurse functioning as a primary care provider can be limited by specifics of the nurse practice act of the state within which he or she practices, other regulations in the pertinent jurisdiction, and by practice protocols. Basing practice on preparation is not adhered to perfectly as evidenced by data from a longitudinal study of nurse practitioners. Of those reporting that they provided maternity care/family planning services, only 20 percent of the pediatric nurse practitioners and 45.5 percent of the adult nurse practitioners indicated that they had formal preparation to provide these services.[36] Monitoring quality of practice is more difficult given the multiple combinations of role and specialty area that exist. In addition to the general provisions for disciplinary activities in nurse practice acts, many work settings or employers establish standards and programs of review.

Physicians

Obstetrician-Gynecologist

Obstetrician-gynecologists specialize in caring for conditions related to the female reproductive system. Specialty preparation is attained through a residency training program accredited by the Liaison Committee on Graduate Medical Examination (LCGME) and its Residency Review Committee on Obstetrics and Gynecology. Physicians beginning medical education after 1976 must have a minimum of four years of approved clinically-oriented graduate medical education of which three years must be in obstetrics-gynecology. Outpatient and operative experience must be included in the training.[27]

Certification of the obstetrician-gynecologist is offered by the American Board of Obstetrics and Gynecology, Inc. To be eligible, candidates must have a Doctor of Medicine or equivalent degree, an unrestricted license to practice medicine in one of the states or territories of the United States or provinces of Canada, and four years graduate education in an accredited program which demonstrates progressive responsibility including being Chief Resident. The examination is in two parts. A written examination which tests eight knowledge areas and application of knowledge to the management of clinical problems is taken in the last year of residency. Following a two year period of practice, which encompasses inpatient and outpatient care and surgical procedures, an oral examination is taken. Candidates must demonstrate basic knowledge of obstetrics and gynecology and patient management problems, as well as the ability to manage complications, and to perform independently major gynecologic operations and spontaneous and operative obstetrical deliveries.[26] Upon successful completion, obstetrician-gynecologists are referred to as board certified. A recertification procedure has been initiated but is not required.

Data on the numbers of obstetrician-gynecologists are collected by their professional organization, The American College of Obstetricians and Gynecologists (ACOG) and by the American Medical Association (AMA). The AMA master file of physicians enumerates all licensed physicians in the United States expressing an emphasis on or a practice limited to obstetrics-gynecology. This may include those who are not board certified or those only partially trained in the specialty. ACOG excludes these categories of physicians in their counts but does include physicians in active process of board certification. According to recent AMA data there were 23,591 obstetrician-gynecologists in the United States in 1978 and 25,617 in 1980, a change of 8.6 percent. ACOG identified 18,798 specialists in 1980 and 19,719 in 1982, a 4.9 percent rise in the two year period.[21] Between 1970 and 1980, the AMA reported a 38.5 percent increase in the number of obstetrician-gynecologists.[30,54]

Subspecialization in obstetrics-gynecology is a relatively new phenomenon. The three subspecialty areas certified and numbers of members by mid-1982 were: fetal-maternal medicine (223), reproductive endocrinology (135), and gynecologic oncology (202). Growth in these subspecialties has been dramatic. From 1978 to mid-1982, maternal-fetal medicine increased by 105 percent, reproductive endocrinology changed 111 percent, and gynecologic oncology grew 55 percent. The number of physicians in process of subspecialty certification in 1982 in each category was greater than those certified at that time. In the three-year period between 1979 and 1982, the percentage of certified subspecialists among all certified obstetrician-gynecologists rose from 2.6–3.7 percent.[22]

Family Physicians

Family physicians are specialists in Family Practice. The definition of Family Practice adopted by the American Academy of Family Physicians (AAFP) and the American Board of Family Practice follows:

Family Practice is comprehensive medical care with particular emphasis on the family unit, in which the physician's continuing responsibility for health care is not limited by the patient's age or sex nor by a particular organ system or disease entity. Family Practice is the specialty in breadth which builds upon a core knowledge derived from other disciplines — drawing most heavily on internal medicine, pediatrics, obstetrics and gynecology, surgery and psychiatry — and which establishes a cohesive unit combining the behavioral sciences with the traditional biological and clinical sciences. The core of knowledge encompassed by the discipline of Family Practice prepares the Family Physician for a unique role in patient management, problem solving, counseling, and as a personal physician who coordinates total health care delivery.[27]

The AAFP also states that the Family Physician "serves as the patient's or family's advocate in health related matters, including the appropriate use of consultants and community resources."[27]

Residency training in Family Practice, accredited by the LCGME, includes a component on obstetrics and gynecology.[27] A joint ad hoc committee of the AAFP, the ACOG, the Council on Resident Education in Obstetrics and Gynecology, and the Association of Professors of Gynecology and Obstetrics developed a recommended core curriculum in obstetrics-gynecology for family physicians. The minimum experience required is three months in a structured obstetric-gynecologic educational program, with an additional three months of structured experience recommended for family practice residents planning to make obstetrics and gynecology a substantial part of their practice. Longitudinal experience in obstetrics-gynecology is obtained throughout the residency program in the family practice centers. Generally, the family physician is prepared to manage uncomplicated obstetrics and gynecology, to identify risk factors, and to attend some variants from normal. The residents who expect to practice in communities without readily available obstetric-gynecologic consultation are strongly advised to obtain further intensified experience with emphasis on acquiring skills necessary to perform cesarean sections, tubal ligations, abortions, and amniocenteses.[2] Family physicians are certified by the American Board of Family Practice and are required to be recertified every six years.[4]

Data on the supply and distribution of family practitioners frequently have been combined with that on general practitioners due to similarities in practice. A downward trend in the number of physicians in this joint category was apparent until the late 1970s when the trend reversed.[54] This reversal is attributed to the rapid growth of the relatively new family practice specialty despite a continued decline in the number of general practitioners.[50] By 1979 the AMA data indicated there were 24,924 family physicians and 33,206 general practitioners.[54] The American Board of Family Practice reported that 26,358 family physicians had been certified by the end of 1981.[4]

Distribution of family and general practitioners varies regionally, with physician–population ratios being highest in the West and North Central areas of the United States. Generally speaking, the higher the physician–population ratio for obstetrician-gynecologists (as well as some other specialists), the lower the ratio of family and general practitioners.[50] The extent to which obstetrics-gynecology is incorporated into the family physician's practice depends on availability of hospital privileges for this component. In some regions of the country, such as the Northeast, obstetric privileges are heavily restricted for family physicians, a factor which also limits the amount of obstetrics-gynecologic training available in the residency programs in those regions.[4]

Other Health Care Providers

Smaller proportions of women's health care are contributed by other providers such as physician's assistants and lay midwives. Physician's assistants work dependently under the supervision of a licensed physician, according to the definition adopted by the American Academy of Physician Assistants.[3] Lay midwives are a diverse group comprised of trained and untrained individuals. The few training programs for lay midwives in operation are not currently subject to standardization through a formal accreditation procedure. Requirements for licensure and scope of practice are governed by state and jurisdictional statutes and regulations.

INFLUENCES ON PROVIDERS' PRACTICE AND QUALITY

Membership in professional associations and a variety of credentialing procedures exert direct influence on health professionals' practice and activities. Additionally, they serve as mechanisms to assure the quality of health care providers.

Health Professional Associations

In general, health professional associations assume responsibility for maintaining and improving professional competence. Customary activities include defining the profession; establishing and promoting standards of practice and care; setting requirements for education and professional recognition; determining qualifications for membership; publishing professional journals or educational materials; identifying members through directories or registries; providing a means of communication among members; and informing the public and other professional groups of their purposes and actions.[29,38] Interprofessional activities have resulted in the issuance of several joint position statements related to women's health care services. In 1978 a statement promoting the development of family-centered maternity/newborn care in hospitals was released.[33] Several years later the ACNM and the ACOG issued a *Joint Statement of Practice Relationships Between Obstetrician/Gynecolo-*

gists and Certified Nurse-Midwives. This document advances the idea that certified nurse-midwives and obstetrician/gynecologists have individual, collaborative, and interdependent responsibilities within the maternity care team, and quality of care is enhanced by working in a relationship of mutual respect, trust, and professional responsibility.[18]

Increasingly, professional associations are appointing individuals to oversee government affairs and to represent the association on issues of concern or when called upon by legislators or administrators. Legislative bodies and health agencies rely on the expertise of health professionals when laws are being considered or policies are being formulated. Acknowledgment of professional standards of care or practice is apparent in many health-related statutes and regulations and in health programs guidelines.[17,43]

Credentialing Processes

Credentialing acknowledges competence and professional capability. Credentialing processes may be concerned with the institutional level, as in accreditation, or with the individual health professional, as in licensure and certification. Credentialing is regarded generally as a means to benefit and protect the public. Responsibility for the various processes lies either with government or private agencies. States have the legal right and responsibility to protect the public, whereas health professions assume a general accountability for services rendered and responsiveness to consumer needs.[25,29]

Accreditation

Accreditation is the process whereby a nongovernmental agency or organization publicly recognizes an institution or program of study as having met established qualifications or criteria.[25,29] Evaluations are carried out on a periodic basis. The accreditation process provides the opportunity for both internal and external assessment. Self-evaluation by the institution and faculty promotes improvement in the program, and review by experts provides a judgment of program quality.

Typical steps in the accreditation process include the following:

1. The institution or program requests initiation of accreditation process.
2. Faculty members prepare a self-evaluation report addressing accrediting agency's review criteria.
3. Accrediting agency visits the program site.
4. A review board determines accreditation status from materials submitted by the program and site visitors.

Reaccreditation is carried out according to timetables set by each accrediting body. Agencies maintain lists of currently accredited programs and periodically publicize this information.

Accreditation has a significant influence on the supply of health professionals and the quality of health care. Accreditation frequently is tied to professional certification and licensure. In many instances eligibility for these other credentialing processes depends on the professional having completed an accredited program of study. Thus, the setting and monitoring of educational standards impacts on subsequent credentialing processes.

Certification

Certification is the process whereby a nongovernmental agency or association grants recognition to an individual who has met certain predetermined qualifications cited by the agency or association.[25] Within many health professions there are specialty boards and certification bodies established to distinguish the quality of personnel. Applicants for certification may be required to have completed an accredited educational program and to have acquired particular types of experience, and most are required to pass an examination given by the certifying agency. In some instances, it may be possible for an applicant to substitute experience for a formal program of study. Rosters of certified individuals generally are maintained by the certifying body.

Licensure

Licensure of health personnel in the United States is the process by which a governmental agency grants permission to persons meeting specified qualifications to practice a given occupation within the agency's legal jurisdiction. It may also allow the use of a particular title.[29] Some licensing statutes make it unlawful to practice the designated occupation without a license. States, in exercising their authority to regulate health personnel, must be cognizant of maintaining an equitable balance between individual rights and public needs.[34]

State legislative bodies are empowered to enact laws. Statutes which control health care providers generally include the definition of the given professional practice, requirements for licensing, penalties for infractions, and a designation of the administrative agency to whom the implementation and enforcement of the particular statute is delegated.[34] Rules and regulations promulagated by administrative agencies, such as Boards of Nurse-Midwifery or Boards of Medical Examiners, elaborate on the statute with further delineation of professional functions, mechanisms for obtaining licenses, and conditions for practice and renewal of licensure. In an attempt to ensure continued competence of the practitioners, some states require that health professionals obtain specified amounts of continuing education for relicensure. Provisions for monitoring individual practice may be defined in some statutes or regulations. Other peer review mechanisms are developed through professional organizations or societies.

Physicians and nurses currently are required to be licensed in all states and the District of Columbia.[29] Since 1971 the legislative thrust in nursing licensure has been to authorize an expanded and more independent role for qualified registered nurses.[47] By 1980, 45 states either permitted or did not prohibit the expanded scope of practice for nurses, for example, allowing nurses to provide family planning services to clients.[47,52] Statutes covering the physician's assistant either authorize delegation of functions to be performed under supervision of a physician or require licensure.[19]

Other licensure laws pertinent to the delivery of women's health care are those regulating nurse-midwives and lay midwives. At the end of 1981 nurse-midwives could legally function in all states and the District of Columbia under a variety of legislative or regulatory arrangements.[17] Data published by The American College of Obstetricians and Gynecologists in 1981 indicate that lay midwives are recognized by statute in 17 states. In an additional 21 states the laws are subject to interpretation by the state, and may provide for the occasional attendance at birth by an unlicensed individual under emergency or inadvertent circumstances.[19]

FUTURE ISSUES FACING WOMEN'S HEALTH CARE PROVIDERS

It is evident from the foregoing the extent to which credentialing mechanisms and health professional associations can control which professionals are allowed to provide health services to women and can shape the practice of those allowed. The current system of health care services for women reflects the impact of numerous factors. Looking ahead, many of these elements will continue to be influential. Brief descriptions of some of the immediate issues facing women's health care providers follow.

Overlapping Spheres of Practice

One of the substantive issues to be faced is that the spheres of practice of the various health professionals serving women are not mutually exclusive. Overlap in function has led to increasing competition. A health professional's access to practice is constrained if he or she is unable to obtain either hospital privileges, malpractice insurance, and/or direct third-party reimbursement. Despite statutory definitions of practice domains, health care providers are often reluctant to acknowledge the competency of other groups of providers. The caregiver should be able to act independently within his or her identified sphere of practice yet feel comfortable referring patients to other providers. Operationalizing this premise would help resolve some of the thorny issues confronting health professionals, such as liability of one professional for another, and differentiating consultation and supervision. It also would facilitate separating the concepts of practice organization and practice domain which are used interchangeably in a confusing manner. Professional responsibilities and functions (domain) differ from the business arrangements (organization) of a professional's practice and should be so distinguished.

Responsiveness to Consumers

The notion of patients as consumers has stimulated the health care industry to look carefully at its procedures and make alterations when feasible. Being responsive to consumer demands is an issue extending beyond the unique wishes of an individual patient. Within the patient—provider relationship consideration is given to specific requests. A broader responsibility lies in noting whether particular demands reflect the interests of a larger population of women. Health professionals should determine if the need or demand is sufficient and if the resources are adequate and appropriate to institute new or revised practices within the health care delivery system. Adopting this approach to care and recognizing the impact of changes on the system will be an ongoing challenge.

A side effect of women's health consumerism has been the attention drawn to stereotypic differences in practices and the promotion of competition among the various types of health professionals. The overlap in functions is increasing as providers try to attract patients.

Need For and Availability of Providers

Estimates of future requirements for health personnel in obstetrics and gynecology have been developed by governmental agencies and task forces and by professional societies.[1,22,45,46] To date there has been no attempt to determine personnel needs for women's health services that extend beyond the scope of obstetrics and gynecology. In the data that are available, requirement figures differ based on the varying assumptions employed in the estimation models. No one model satisfies all professional groups and interests.

The Graduate Medical Education National Advisory Committee (GMENAC) study on physician supply and requirements for 1990, completed in 1980 for the U.S. Department of Health and Human Services, provides recent manpower estimates. Among the factors considered in making these projections was the potential impact of nonphysician providers. It was felt that although there is a one-to-one equivalency between physicians and nonphysician providers for selected types of medical visits, each provider type performs unique services and a simple inverse relationship was not sufficient to project needs. Other factors in the model included: incidence and prevalence rates of diseases, levels of preventive care, amounts or norms of care, and productivity estimates.[45,46]

According to GMENAC methodology, the supply of obstetrician-gynecologists projected for 1990 is 34,450 and the number required is 24,000, resulting in a surplus of 10,450. The supply of nurse-midwives expected in 1990 is 4000—5000 with 2800 in clinical practice. Of an anticipated total supply of 3900 obstetrics-gynecologic nurse practitioners, there are to be 2900 in active practice. In addition 400 physician's assistants are estimated to be providing women's health services. Initial recommendations for nonphysician provider input were adjusted downward to reflect the constraint imposed by the projected excess of obstetrician-gynecologists and the productivity of the expected supply of nonphysician providers. Ultimately, GMENAC recommended that for 1990 nurse-midwives care for 5 percent of the uncomplicated deliveries, and that the three groups of nonphysician providers would be responsible for 20 percent of the ambulatory obstetrics visits and 18 percent of the ambulatory gynecologic visits.[45,46]

Estimates of the demand for subspecialists in obstetrics-gynecology have been published by The American College of Obstetricians and Gynecologists. By 1990 the presumed demand for gynecologic oncologists and reproductive endocrinologists will be met. The needed supply of maternal-fetal medicine specialists is greater but is expected to be reached in the year 2002.[22]

It is apparent from these projections that a surplus of obstetrician-gynecologists is likely in the next few decades. This impending excess will heighten attention to the issues already surfacing about and among providers of women's health care. Because the issues are so complex, it is difficult to predict their outcome. Whatever the responses or attempts at resolutions, health professionals must continue to meet the challenge of providing high-quality health care services to women.

REFERENCES

1. A Report to the President and Congress on the Status of Health Professions Personnel in the United States. Washington, D.C., DHEW Publication No. (HRA) 80−93, 1980
2. ACOG-AAFP Recommended Core Curriculum and Hospital Practice Privileges in Obstetrics-Gynecology for Family Physicians. Kansas City, MO, American Academy of Family Physicians, Reprint No. 261
3. American Academy of Physician Assistants: The Professional Role of the Physician Assistant. Arlington, VA, AAPA
4. American Board of Family Practice: Personal communication, 1982
5. American College of Nurse-Midwives: Definitions. Washington, D.C., ACNM, 1962
6. American College of Nurse-Midwives: Statement on Abortion. Washington, D.C., ACNM, 1971
7. American College of Nurse-Midwives: Functions, Standards and Qualifications. Washington, D.C., ACNM, 1975
8. American College of Nurse-Midwives: Guidelines for Evaluation of Nurse-Midwifery Procedural Functions. Washington, D.C., ACNM, 1977
9. American College of Nurse-Midwives: Statement on Nurse-Midwifery Education. Washington, D.C., ACNM, 1977
10. American College of Nurse-Midwives: Core Competencies in Nurse-Midwifery: Expected Outcomes of Nurse-Midwifery Education. Washington, D.C., ACNM, 1978
11. American College of Nurse-Midwives; Nurse-Midwifery in the United States: 1976−1977. Washington D.C., ACNM, 1978

12. American College of Nurse-Midwives: Statement on Practice Settings. Washington, D.C., ACNM, 1980
13. American College of Nurse-Midwives: Survey of Legislation Pertaining to the Practice of Nurse-Midwifery and Update Tables. Washington, D.C., ACNM, 1980
14. American College of Nurse-Midwives: Grievance Procedures. Washington, D.C., ACNM, 1981
15. American College of Nurse-Midwives: Information for Candidates for the National Certification Examination in Nurse-Midwifery. Washington, D.C., ACNM, 1981
16. American College of Nurse-Midwives: What is a Nurse-Midwife? Washington, D.C., ACNM, 1981
17. American College of Nurse-Midwives: Personal communication, 1982
18. American College of Nurse-Midwives, American College of Obstetricians and Gynecologists: Joint Statement of Practice Relationships Between Obstetrician/Gynecologists and Certified Nurse-Midwives. Washington, D.C., ACNM and ACOG, 1982
19. American College of Obstetricians and Gynecologists: Entry constraints imposed by federal legislature or manpower policy actions, in Manpower Planning in Obstetrics and Gynecology. Washington, D.C., ACOG, 1981
20. American College of Obstetricians and Gynecologists: Nurses Association of The American College of Obstetricians and Gynecologists, in Manpower Planning in Obstetrics and Gynecology. Washington, D.C., ACOG, 1981
21. American College of Obstetricians and Gynecologists: Comparison of ACOG fellowship with AMA physician data, in Manpower Planning in Obstetrics and Gynecology. Washington, D.C., ACOG, 1982
22. American College of Obstetricians and Gynecologists: Subspecialization in obstetrics and gynecology, in Manpower Planning in Obstetrics and Gynecology. Washington, D.C., ACOG, 1982
23. Association of State and Territorial Health Officials: Selected Title V Maternal and Child Health Services, 1980. Silver Spring, Md, ASTHO Publication No. 59, 1980
24. Better Health for Our Children: A National Strategy, The Report of the Select Panel for the Promotion of Child Health, Volume 1, Major Findings and Recommendations. Washington, D.C., DHHS (PHS) Publication No. 79−55071, 1981
25. Certification in Allied Health Professions. Washington, D.C., DHEW Publication No. (NIH) 73−246, 1973
26. Directory of Medical Specialists, Volume 1, Chicago, Marquis Who's Who, Inc., 1981−1982
27. '81/'82 Directory of Residency Training Programs Accredited by the Accreditation Council for Graduate Medical Education. Chicago, American Medical Association, 1981
28. Division of Nursing: A Directory of Expanded Role Programs for Registered Nurses: 1980. Hyattsville, MD: Health Resources Administration, DHHS, 1980
29. Health Resources Statistics: Health Manpower and Health Facilities, 1976−77 Edition. Hyattsville, MD, National Center for Health Statistics, 1977
30. Health, United States, 1980. Washington, D.C., DHHS Publication No. (PHS) 81−1232, 1981

31. Hemschemeyer H: Midwifery in United States: how shall we care for million mothers whose babies are born at home? Am J Nurs 39:1181–1187, 1939
32. Institute of Medicine, Commission on Life Sciences: Research Issues in the Assessment of Birth Settings. Washington, D.C., National Academy Press, 1982
33. Interprofessional Task Force on Health Care of Women and Children: Joint Position Statement on the Development of Family-Centered Maternity/Newborn Care in Hospitals. Washington, D.C., American College of Nurse-Midwives, 1978
34. Kinkela GG, Kinkela RV: Licensure: what's it all about? J Nurs Adm 4(2):18–19, 1974
35. Kotthoff ME: Current trends and issues in nursing in the United States: the primary health care nurse practitioners. Int Nurs Rev 28:24–28, 1981
36. Longitudinal Study of Nurse Practitioners, Phase II. Hyattsville, MD, DHEW Publication No. 78–92, 1978
37. Marieskind HI: Women in the Health System. St. Louis, CV Mosby Co, 1980
38. Moore WE: The Professions: Roles and Rules. New York, Russell Sage Foundation, 1970
39. National Center for Health Statistics: Monthly Vital Statistics Report, Advance Report, Final Natality Statistics, 1977. Hyattsville, MD: DHHS Publication No. (PHS) 79–1120, 1979
40. National Center for Health Statistics: Monthly Vital Statistics Report, Advance Report, Final Natality Statistics, 1978. Hyattsville, MD: DHHS Publication No. (PHS) 80–1120, 1980
41. National Center for Health Statistics: Office Visits by Women: The National Ambulatory Medical Care Survey, United States, 1977. Hyattsville, Md, DHEW Publication No. (PHS) 80–1796, 1980
42. Nurses Association of The American College of Obstetricians and Gynecologists: Membership Profile for NAACOG as of 1/29/82. Washington, D.C., NAACOG, 1982
43. Omnibus Reconciliation Act of 1980, P.L. 96–499, Sec. 965 (42 CFR 405.2401 and 42 CFR 440.165)
44. Perry HB, Fisher DW: The physician's assistant profession: results of a 1978 survey of graduates. J Med Educ 56:839–845, 1981
45. Report of the Graduate Medical Education National Advisory Committee, Volume I, GMENAC Summary Report. Washington, D.C., DHHS Publication No. (HRA) 81–651, 1981
46. Report of the Graduate Medical Education National Advisory Committee, Volume VI, Nonphysician Health Care Provider Technical Panel. Washington, D.C., DHHS Publication No. (HRA) 81–656, 1981
47. Roemer R: The nurse practitioner in family planning services: law and practice. Fam Plann/Pop Reporter 6:28–34, 1977
48. Shoemaker MT: History of Nurse-Midwifery in the United States. Washington, D.C., The Catholic University of America Press, 1947
49. Starzyk PM: Physician-delivered births in Washington state, 1978: geographic patterns. Am J Public Health 71:1063–1065, 1981
50. Supply and Characteristics of Selected Health Personnel. Washington, D.C., DHHS Publication No. (HRA) 81–20, 1981

51. Take the Extra Step ... Become a Certified Nurse. Kansas City, MO, American Nurses' Association, 1982
52. Trandel-Korenchuk DM, Trandel-Korenchuk KM: Current legal issues facing nursing practice. Nurs Adm Q 5:37–55, 1980
53. Twenty Years of Nurse-Midwifery, 1933–1953. New York, Maternity Center Association, 1955
54. Wunderman LE: Physician Distribution and Medical Licensure in the U.S., 1979. Monroe, WI, American Medical Association, 1980

PART II

Clinical Management

Certain goals are of paramount importance for nurse-midwifery management of women's health care. These goals include the following:

- Focus on reproduction as a normal process
- Maintenance of optimal health
- Facilitation of the developmental process in the mother, fetus-newborn, and family
- Family-centered care with integration of the mother and family in decision making about health care
- Continuity of care
- Continuous monitoring and updating of a data base with evaluation and alteration in the plan of management as indicated
- Early identification of deviations, or potential deviations, from the expected
- Deletion of unnecessary interventions in the childbearing process
- Facilitation of appropriate utilization of available resources for meeting the needs of individual women and members of their families

Nurse-midwifery management takes place in an orderly fashion during all phases of the reproductive cycle whether a woman is pregnant or not. The major components of this process are outlined below:

- Systematic and thorough assessment of maternal and/or fetal health status, as applicable, through interview of the woman, physical examination, and the use of laboratory tests
- Interpretation of findings
- Formulation of an individualized and relevant list of problems and needs
- Development of a plan for nurse-midwifery intervention, consultation, or referral for identified problems and needs
- Preparation of a comprehensive plan for management of health care
- Effective implementation of the management plan
- Continuous evaluation of management effectiveness with alterations in the plan as indicated

This management takes place in a health care system that provides for appropriate medical consultation and collaborative management.

Constance J. Adams

3

Pregnancy

Pregnancy is a major event not only in the life of a woman, but also in the lives of her relatives and friends. Issues which must be faced by pregnant women and their families, as well as by the nurse-midwives who supervise their health care, are addressed in this chapter in the context of the mother and fetus as an integral unit within the family. The impact of these issues on the family and topics requiring special consideration during pregnancy are also discussed.

ASSESSMENT OF MATERNAL AND FETAL HEALTH STATUS

Responsibility for the supervision and management of health care during pregnancy requires an astute assessment of maternal and fetal health status during initial and follow-up prenatal visits. This assessment must include all pertinent information about the physical and psychosocial parameters of maternal well-being and all pertinent information about fetal well-being. Information obtained from each assessment of maternal and fetal health status is needed to develop an appropriate plan for health care supervision and to identify high-risk, or potential high-risk, situations.

All pregnant women should obtain a complete history and physical examination early in pregnancy and these are usually completed during an initial prenatal visit. The same basic protocol should be followed as that recommended for all adults and comprehensive protocols for an adult history and physical examination have been published in several text books. Careful attention especially should be given to the information in Tables 3-1 and 3-2, which is obtained as a result of a complete history and physical examination during pregnancy.[21,108,175,193]

Table 3-1
Complete Medical History of the Pregnant Woman

Age
Race
Marital status
Parity
Past obstetrical history, including:
    Date of each delivery
    Duration of each gestation
    Significant problems
    Spontaneous or induced onset of labor
    Length of each labor
    Complications of labor
    Presentation of each infant at delivery
    Vaginal or cesarean section delivery
    Type of anesthesia used at each delivery
    Condition of each infant at birth
    Birth weight of each infant
    Postpartum problems, including:
      Infection
      Hemorrhage
      Depression
    Problems of each infant, including:
      Jaundice
      Respiratory distress
      Infection
      Congenital anomalies
    Type of infant feeding
    Current health status of each child
Present obstetrical history, including:
    Date last normal menstrual period began (LMP)
    Bleeding since last normal menstrual period
    Symptoms of pregnancy
    Date when fetal movements were first felt
    Feelings about pregnancy
Medical history, including:
    Infections
    Allergies

Diabetes mellitus
Renal disease
Heart disease
Pulmonary disease
Endocrine disorders
Liver disease
Spastic conditions
Cancer
Hypertension
Sickle cell disease
Mental illness
Anemia
Exposure to x-ray
Medication history
Habitual use of alcohol, tobacco, and mood-altering drugs

Gynecological history, including:
Genital tract anomaly
Cervical incompetence
Myomas
Contracted pelvis
Ovarian mass
Vaginal infection
Endometriosis
Venereal disease
Abnormal Pap smear results
Surgery
Menstrual history
Sexual history
Contraceptive history

Family history, including:
Infections
Allergies
Diabetes mellitus
Renal disease
Heart disease
Pulmonary disease
Endocrine disorders
Liver disease
Spastic conditions
Cancer
Hypertension
Mental illness
Anemia
Medication history
Habitual use of alcohol, tobacco, and mood-altering drugs

Socioeconomic Status

Table 3-2
Complete Physical Examination of Pregnant Woman

Blood pressure
Height
Weight
Breasts, including:
    Nodularity, tenseness, and enlargement
    Discharge
    Skin pigmentation
Abdomen, including:
    Pigmentation and striae
    Fetal lie, presentation, position, and attitude
    Fundal height
    Fetal heart tones
    Estimated fetal weight
    Fetal movement
Extremities, including:
    Edema
    Varicosities
    Homan's sign
    Deep tendon reflexes
Pelvic examination, including:
    Discharge
    Fissures, lesions, cysts, or tumors
    Uterine enlargement
    Hegar's sign
    Piskacek's sign
    Chadwick's sign
    Goodell's sign
    Internal ballottment
    Clinical pelvimetry

In order to obtain a complete picture of maternal health status and its impact on the developing fetus, several laboratory tests are done routinely in most settings during the initial prenatal visit, and results are then evaluated in conjunction with findings from the history and physical examination. These tests include those cited in Table 3-3.

Continued assessments of maternal and fetal well-being are made at each follow-up prenatal visit. It is imperative that the maternal record be reviewed before each visit so that the nurse-midwife can become reacquainted with the findings, problems, concerns, and unique needs of the mother and so that a complete data base can be established. Review of the record is also necessary to ensure continuity in the plan for management of care.

Table 3-3
Routine Laboratory Tests Conducted During an Initial Prenatal Visit

Pap smear
Gonococcal culture (GC)
Blood type (ABO)
Rh factor
Rubella titer
Sickle cell prep or hemoglobin electrophoresis
Tuberculin test
Venereal Disease Research Laboratory test (VDRL) or Rapid Plasma Reagin test (RPR)
Hemoglobin or hematocrit
Urinalysis for albumin, glucose, and microscopic examination

During each prenatal visit the mother should be interviewed so that information can be obtained about the subjects listed in Table 3-4.[193] A modified physical examination should also be done in order to assist in the detection of problems or potential problems that may be a threat to maternal or fetal well-being. Table 3-5 is a list of what this examination should include, but not necessarily be confined to.[108,175,176,193] Routine laboratory tests for venereal disease and the hematocrit or hemoglobin are frequently repeated during the third trimester of pregnancy.

Table 3-4
Subjects to Include in each Prenatal Interview

Concerns, complaints, questions, or problems
Headaches
Visual disturbances
Dizziness
Fever and/or chills
Nausea and/or vomiting
Fetal movement
Abdominal pain
Back pain
Dysuria
Vaginal discharge and/or bleeding
Bowel irregularities
Hemorrhoids
Leg aches or cramps
Edema
Exposure to infectious disease
Medications being taken
Medical care needed since last visit

Table 3-5
Physical Examination for each Prenatal Visit

Weight

Blood pressure

Abdominal evaluation, including:
    Presentation and position of the fetus
    Engagement
    Location and rate of the fetal heart tones
    Fundal height
    Estimated fetal weight
    Estimated gestational age

Presence of edema

Urinalysis for albumin and glucose

IMPLICATIONS OF FINDINGS FROM THE HISTORY AND PHYSICAL EXAMINATION

Careful use of all findings obtained during a history and physical examination is necessary in developing an appropriate plan for management of care, obtaining additional information when needed, and making alterations in the management plan as indicated. A discussion of the major factors to be considered in formulation of a plan for health care management and supervision during pregnancy follows.

Sociodemographic Factors

Sociodemographic factors include maternal age, race, marital status, and socioeconomic classification. All of these factors are interrelated when considered with respect to pregnancy and pregnancy outcome. See Chapter 1 for a discussion of the sociodemographic variance of birthrates.

Rates of illegitimate live birth are over 80 percent higher among women from other than white races than they are among white women.[197] The state of illegitimacy as a moral issue should not be the focus of concern; pregnancy among unmarried women becomes of particular concern for women who have only unstable support systems available to them.[52,123,186] Several investigators have noted that stress resulting from unique needs experienced by individual women during pregnancy is often mediated when there is strong support from networks of family members and friends.[49,144]

Illegitimate pregnancy forces many women to live in poverty, and their children therefore must live in poverty. During 1977 one in three households headed by females and one in two of those headed by black females had annual incomes lower than the federally designated poverty level.[122]

Although advances in the practice of medicine have been credited with the prevention of some pregnancy losses[97]—which include death of a fetus before birth or death of a live-born infant—many mothers are still plagued with the problems resulting from pregnancy loss.[199] Women in the United States at greatest risk of pregnancy loss include those less than 20 years old or more than 34 years old,[27,29,194] members of other than white racial groups,[27,29,86,105] and/or women with low socioeconomic status.[27,86,105]

Past Obstetrical History

Data from several studies indicate that women are exposed to greater than average risks of pregnancy loss when the present pregnancy is a fourth or greater pregnancy,[6,27,29,194] when there is a positive history of pregnancy loss,[29,106,133,172] or when the interval between onset of the present pregnancy and delivery of the immediately prior conceptus is less than one year.[48,86] Infants of plural births are at a particularly high risk of early infant death because of the greater incidence of low birth weight in this group of babies compared with those from single gestations (see also Chapter 1).[6,27,28]

Single offspring of the same parents tend to be of similar birth weights and this often holds true for low birth weight babies.[53,181] Babies with a birth weight of less than 2500 g, and particularly those with a birth weight of less than 1500 g, are at greater risk of encountering major threats to health and well-being than babies with a weight of at least 2500 g at birth.[89,181] This is true whether the babies are appropriate (in weight)-for gestational-age (AGA), small-for-gestational-age (SGA), or large-for-gestational-age (LGA). These threats often include not only death, either before birth or early in infancy, but also neonatal asphyxia, hypoglycemia, polycythemia, problems with thermal regulation, congenital malformations, poor growth and development, cerebral palsy, epilepsy, or mental retardation.[54,181] Problems experienced by low birth weight babies later in childhood are often exhibited in difficulties with learning, visual or hearing disabilities, or frequent hospitalizations for illness.[89]

Major factors thought to be associated with the birth of low birth weight babies include maternal malnutrition, intrauterine infection, maternal hypertension, multiple gestation, high altitudes during pregnancy, smoking during pregnancy, maternal alcoholism, maternal drug abuse, and exposure to ionizing irradiation.

First-born infants are often of a lower birth weight than their siblings and birth weight tends to increase with each subsequent pregnancy.[53,89,181] A birth weight of greater than 4000 g may indicate maternal diabetes mellitus, and this possibility must be considered carefully during evaluation of maternal health status.

Excessive weight at birth (over 4000 g) may also be due to genetic predisposition of the fetus since large women tend to bear large babies.[89] Risks of early death and exposure to selected types of morbidity are higher for heavy babies born at or near term than they are for babies with a birth weight of between 2500 and 4000 g. Some of these casualties are thought to be due to difficulties encountered during delivery such as shoulder dystocia or due to the use of midforceps. Brachial plexus palsy, facial paralysis, a fractured clavicle, or a depressed skull fracture are frequently associated with shoulder dystocia or the use of midforceps. Cesarean sections are frequently used in instances of cephalopelvic disproportion. Low Apgar scores have been noted to occur more frequently among babies weighing 4000 g or more at birth than among babies weighing between 2500 and 4000 g.

Accurate anticipation of the birth of an excessive size infant should allow planning for management of labor and delivery with a focus on prevention of unnecessary trauma to the mother or baby.

Many conditions associated with pregnancy tend to recur in a present pregnancy. These conditions may be physical, psychological, or sociocultural.[53,54,71] It is important to understand that spontaneous abortion, unexplained stillbirth, toxemia, premature rupture of the membranes, hemorrhage, multiple pregnancy, malpresentation of the fetus (particularly breech presentation), dystocia, and mastitis are among the pregnancy-related conditions which do tend to recur. Hemorrhage and toxemia, along with infection, are the major causes of maternal mortality in the United States.[198] Repeated spontaneous abortions during the second trimester may be indicative of an incompetent cervix. A woman who has experienced precipitate labor, often associated with neurologic damage to the fetus, may be at risk of experiencing rapid cervical dilatation and rapid delivery again.

An obstetrical history of special delivery measures may indicate the potential for recurring problems. For example, induced labor may be required for reasons similar to those impacting its prior use. Having had a prior cesarean section may or may not mandate its use for the present pregnancy.[14] Use of forceps for delivery of previous children may have been due to cephalopelvic disproportion, and there is potential that this problem will recur.

Knowledge of the neonatal and present health of all children previously born to the mother, including congenital malformations, infection, birth trauma, and developmental or learning problems, can provide important clues to potential problems which may be encountered by offspring from the present pregnancy.

Psychological attitudes or problems, as well as sociocultural conditions, may not change substantially from one pregnancy to another.[89] It is important to gain as much information as possible about a woman's other pregnancy experiences and their impact, as well as the impact of family needs and desires, on her hopes and expectations for the present pregnancy. Is she pregnant against her will? Are there children in the family who are now subject to deprivation, abuse, or neglect? What are her attitudes toward analgesia or anesthesia before delivery? What means of infant feeding and care has she experienced and how successful were they? The approach of each woman to a new pregnancy is based on a complex combination of experiences and needs.

Present Obstetrical History

Accurate information about the present pregnancy is essential for determining whether the progress of pregnancy is normal. The date on which the last normal menstrual period (LMP) began is used as a basis for estimating the date of confinement (EDC) or, in lay terms, the due date. One easy method for calculating the EDC is to subtract three months and add seven days to the reported first day of the LMP. It is important to note that this "rule of thumb" is based on an average 27-day menstrual cycle. Since ovulation usually occurs 14 days before the next menstrual period, a woman with a 35-day cycle would most likely ovulate on day 21 of the cycle rather than on day 14 which is when a woman with a 27-day cycle would most likely ovulate.[159] The number of days a woman's menstrual cycle is longer than 27 days should be added to the EDC and the number of days a woman's cycle is shorter than 27 days should be subtracted from the EDC for accuracy.

Vaginal bleeding during pregnancy is a sign of abnormality and must be evaluated carefully. The most common causes of bleeding during the first and second trimesters include spontaneous abortion, ectopic pregnancy, and hydatidiform mole.[19,40,56] During the latter part of pregnancy, bleeding may be due to placenta previa, abruptio placentae, or impending labor. Bleeding due to cervical erosion or vaginal infection can occur at any time throughout pregnancy. Amounts of bleeding during pregnancy vary from minor spotting to hemorrhage and may or may not be accompanied by pain or cramping. Nausea, breast fullness, abdominal bloating, and edema are frequently noted in conjunction with pregnancy related bleeding.

Evaluation of the symptoms, or signs, of pregnancy is important not only for the diagnosis of early pregnancy, but also for ruling out possible disease states and establishing a data base which will be useful in monitoring the progress of pregnancy. Due to great variability in the expression of subjective and objective signs among individual women, the signs of pregnancy have been classified as presumptive, probable, or positive.[79,108,193] Presumptive signs are those resulting from physiologic changes noted by the mother and include the signs listed in Table 3-6. Probable signs of pregnancy are those resulting from physiologic and anatomic changes in the mother which can be identified during physical examination and are other than the presumptive signs. They are termed "probable" because there are clinical conditions other than pregnancy which can cause each of the signs. The probable signs of pregnancy include those shown in Table 3-6. Authorities disagree about whether the signs shown in the third column in Table 3-6 should be classified as presumptive or probable. Positive signs of pregnancy are those which substantiate the presence of at least one fetus. They include auditory evidence of a fetal heart beat and radiologic or ultrasonographic evidence of the fetus. Authorities

Table 3-6
Signs of Pregnancy

Presumptive	Probable	Presumptive or Probable (Authorities Disagree)	Positive
Amenorrhea 10 or more days after the expected onset of menstruation	Asymmetrical enlargement of one uterine cornu (Piskacek's sign)	Progressive abdominal or uterine enlargement	Auditory evidence of fetal heart beat
Nausea	Internal ballottement	Softening of the uterine isthmus (Hegar's sign)	Radiologic evidence of fetus
Appetite changes	Uterine souffle	Bluish or cyanotic color of the cervix and upper vagina (Chadwick's sign)	Ultrasonographic evidence of fetus
Weight gain	Palpation of fetal parts	Softening of the junction between the uterus and cervix (McDonald's sign)	
Constipation	Positive test results for human chorionic gonadotropin (HCG) in the urine or serum	Softening of the cervix (Goodell's sign)	
Excessive salivation		Palpation of Braxton-Hicks' contractions	
Fatigue			
Increased frequency of urination			
Fingernail changes			
Tingling, soreness, and enlargement of the breasts and nipples			
Expression of colostrum from the nipples			
Color changes of the breasts with darkening of the nipples and primary or secondary areolar changes			
Skin pigmentation such as chloasma, breast and abdominal striae, linea nigra, vascular spiders, or palmar erythema			
Appearance of Montgomery's tubercles or follicles			
Elevation of the basal body temperature in the absence of infection			
Quickening			

differ in their views about whether palpation of active fetal movements should be classified as a probable sign or as a positive sign of pregnancy.

Noting the approximate date of quickening, or the first time a mother notices fetal movement, may be helpful in dating the duration of her pregnancy. Initially, it may be difficult for a mother to differentiate fetal movements from the movement of gas through her intestines but many women, particularly multigravidas, can make this differentiation as early as the 14th−16th week of pregnancy.[79,193] Primigravidas may not be able to do so until the 18th−20th week of pregnancy.

Assessment of a woman's feelings about her pregnancy is essential if the nurse-midwife is to be effective in the management of her health care. Every woman experiences some anxiety about being pregnant no matter how much the pregnancy was desired. Pregnancy brings with it a sense of dependence resulting from a state of irreversible biologic change which, in itself, is cause for anxiety.[33] Concerns about maternal and fetal well-being, as well as the potential impact of the pregnancy and baby on personal and family life-styles, are inevitable to some degree.[53]

Many of the anxieties experienced by pregnant women are predictable in that the psychological processes of pregnancy often seem to be correlated with the biological changes taking place in the mother as pregnancy progresses.[193] During the first trimester the woman must accept her pregnancy as a reality and resolve negative or ambivalent feelings about it. A decision should be made about her desire to carry the pregnancy to term. Quickening occurs during the second trimester which usually verifies the pregnancy in her mind and allows her to conceptualize the baby as an individual. Many of her thoughts and concerns are apt to be focused on the role and responsibilities of a caregiver. This period in pregnancy is usually relatively free of physical discomforts and most women experience noticeable improvements in their sexual desires and sexual relationships. During the third trimester there often seems to be great impatience to have the delivery over with yet uneasy concern that the baby could arrive at any time. Fears of loss of her own life or the baby's, of having an abnormal baby, and of pain and loss of control during labor and delivery are very common during this time. During this period the mother actively prepares for the baby with anticipation, but experiences increased physical and psychological discomfort.

It has been suggested by Barclay and Barclay[13] that characterization of pregnancy as a major source of psychic stress falsely dramatizes a basic physiologic function of women. Although they admit that pregnancy produces fears and concerns in women, they suggest that similar findings are typical at many times in life and that pregnant women bring to pregnancy a set of normative systems for dealing with life events. As a result, they strongly suggest that emphasis be placed on the normal and developmentally appropriate feelings and attitudes that pregnant women express, as opposed to the pathologic aspects of pregnancy concerns and attitudes.

Medical and Family History

It is helpful to obtain information about a woman's family history while eliciting information about her medical history since many disease conditions, or conditions which jeopardize a state of health, are passed from generation to generation. Conditions which have a direct impact on pregnancy may be familial or they may be related to lifestyle and personal exposure. Their identification is essential because of potential hazardous effects on the mother, the baby, or both, and because many of the potential hazardous effects can be alleviated with proper medical care. Presence of the following most prominent conditions should be identified during an initial interview with the mother. Physical examination and laboratory testing will be useful adjuncts for substantiating and monitoring some of these conditions throughout pregnancy.

Infections

Before the widespread use of vaccines and antibiotics for the treatment of viral and bacterial infections, it was well documented that pregnant women did not tolerate infectious conditions as well as women who were not pregnant.[96] There are still several infectious conditions, including some sexually transmitted diseases, which are of concern during pregnancy. These include, but are not limited to, rubella (German Measles), urinary tract infections, gonorrhea, nongonococcal urethritis, genital herpes, syphilis, cytomegalovirus infection, and toxoplasmosis. Other infectious conditions which are of concern when they do occur during pregnancy but which are relatively rare among pregnant women in the United States include pneumonia, poliomyelitis, group B coxsackievirus infection, variola (smallpox), herpes gestationis, and malaria.[79,167,193]

Although maternal symptoms of rubella are frequently so mild that the condition is not recognized, the effects of the rubella virus on the fetus can be devastating. Maternal infection during the first trimester of pregnancy is associated with the highest incidence of fetal congenital malformations compared to infection during the second and third trimesters, however, intrauterine infection after the first trimester in pregnancy also usually results in compromised fetal outcome.[167] The most common problems experienced by babies who were infected with the rubella virus while in utero include growth retardation, deafness or impaired hearing, cardiovascular lesions, eye lesions, and hepatosplenomegaly.[169,181] If rubella infection should occur in the fetus during the period of eye formation, the incidence of congenital eye defects—ranging from cloudiness of the cornea to total blindness—has been reported to be as high as 75 percent.[167] Because of the potential teratogenic effects of attenuated rubella virus vaccine, vaccination during pregnancy is contraindicated. Women who are not immune to the rubella virus and who contract a rubella infection during the first 12−14 weeks of pregnancy are usually informed of the fetal risks involved and advised that a therapeutic abortion is the treatment of choice.

It has been estimated that as many as one out of 10 pregnant women will have significant amounts of bacteria in the urine and that as many as 37 percent of these women will develop pyelonephritis during pregnancy.[200] Asymptomatic bacteriuric pregnant women have a much higher risk of developing pyelonephritis during pregnancy than pregnant women without bacteriuria. Predisposition to urinary tract infections during pregnancy is thought to be due to dilatation of the renal pelvis, ureter, and bladder, as well as to a decrease in ureteral peristalsis and a slowing of urine passage from the kidney to the bladder. Urinary stasis resulting from these conditions provides an excellent culture medium for the growth of microorganisms. Woman with symptoms of pyelonephritis during pregnancy deliver premature infants twice as frequently as asymptomatic bacteriuric women or as nonbacteriuric women. It is not clear whether asymptomatic bacteriuric women are more likely to deliver premature infants than nonbacteriuric women.

Sexually transmissible diseases represent a major health problem among young adults in the United States and have potential for effecting grave outcomes in the offspring of these individuals. Each year in this country there are an estimated 2.5 million cases of gonorrhea; 2.5 million cases of nongonococcal urethritis; 500,000 cases of genital herpes; and 80,000 new cases of syphilis.[73] Close to 90 percent of these diseases occur in individuals 15−29 years old. There is no vaccine available to combat these infections although intensive efforts are being made to develop a vaccine against gonorrhea.

Neonatal gonorrheal opthalmia, which sometimes results in blindness, is the major result of untreated maternal gonorrhea during pregnancy.[167] Nongonococcal ureteritis is usually transmitted to the baby directly from the birth canal and frequently results in neonatal conjunctivitis or pneumonia.

To date there is no satisfactory treatment for genital herpes. Once the infection is contracted it may become active at any time.[56] The frequency of genital herpes infection is about three times greater in pregnant women than in nonpregnant women and infections seem to be more severe during pregnancy than at other times.[45] The risk of spontaneous abortion as a result of primary infection during the first trimester of pregnancy has been reported to be greater than 50 percent[140] and as high as 30 percent for women with a recurrent infection.[56] When conception occurs immediately after the development of infection, the risk of spontaneous abortion increases markedly.[51] Primary genital herpes infection after 20 weeks of gestation is associated with a prematurity rate of 35 percent, and recurrent infection after 20 weeks of gestation is associated with a prematurity rate of about 14 percent.[167] Major problems encountered by infants who were infected in utero with the herpes simplex virus include marked microencephaly, severe mental retardation, retinal dysplasia, patent ductus arteriosus, intracranial calcification, and vesicles filled with yellow purulent discharge.[139]

Invasion of the fetus by spirochetes occurs after 16−18 weeks of gestation in pregnant women with an untreated primary syphilitic infection.[77,167]

Approximately 25 percent of the fetuses who contract a luetic infection in utero die before birth and an equal number die in the early neonatal period. Of the infected babies who live, about 40 percent will eventually develop symptomatic syphilis involving mucous membrane, skin, and skeletal lesions. Treatment of the mother during pregnancy will cure the fetal infection but fetal damage incurred before treatment cannot be corrected.

Cytomegaloviruses can be found in the cervix or urine of about 3−5 percent of pregnant women and account for the most frequent cause of congenital infection in the United States.[75] Unfortunately, infected women are usually asymptomatic and the disease is not suspected until after delivery. Congenital infection occurs in 0.5−1.5 percent of all births.[167] Short-term effects on infected infants include hepatomegaly, splenomegaly, jaundice, and purpura. The two major long-term effects are cerebral palsy and microencephaly. Other long-term effects include intracerebral calcifications, hyperactivity, conduction deafness, epilepsy, visual defects, sensorineural defects, speech defects, and nonspecific mental retardation. Multiple defects among these children are not uncommon.

Toxoplasmosis is most likely contracted through eating infected raw or partially cooked meat or through contact with infected cat feces.[79,167,193] Acute primary infections are thought to occur in about 2/1000 pregnant women in the United States, and about 30 percent of these women are thought to transmit the infection to their offspring. Severe congenital toxoplasmosis is associated with growth retardation, microcephaly, hydrocephalus, microphthalmia, chorioretinitis, central nervous system calcification, thrombocytopenia, and jaundice.

Allergies

Information about maternal allergies during pregnancy is necessary for correct interpretation of clinical symptoms, provision of appropriate nutrition and health care counseling, and judicious use of medications.

Diabetes

Diabetes mellitus is a familial disease which, if not already present, may be precipitated by the endocrinological and hormonal changes of pregnancy. It is a complicating factor in about 2 percent of all pregnancies.[167] Since the advent of insulin the maternal mortality rate among diabetic mothers has declined from 25 percent to less than 1 percent. Diabetes mellitus continues, however, to have a deleterious effect on pregnancy.[30,35] Toxemia occurs concomitantly with diabetes mellitus in about one out of four diabetic pregnancies.[30,35]

Rates of perinatal loss among the offspring of diabetic mothers have been estimated to be as high as 20 percent and tend to increase as the severity of maternal disease increases. Most fetal deaths occur during the last month of pregnancy and neonatal deaths tend to be due to respiratory distress or congenital anomalies. Infants of diabetic mothers have a three times greater risk of incurring major congenital anomalies than infants of mothers who do not have diabetes and this relative risk increases with the severity of maternal diabetes.[148] Infants with birth weights of 10 pounds or more are the products of almost 30 percent of all diabetic pregnancies and these infants experience particularly high rates of respiratory distress and hypoglycemia.

Renal Disease

Renal blood flow and the glomerular filtration rate are increased during pregnancy in order to facilitate the clearance of maternal and fetal waste products. Disease conditions of the kidney require medical attention in order to prevent maternal deterioration with implications for the well-being of the fetus. Symptoms of kidney disease, such as hypertension, edema, and proteinuria, must be differentiated from the development of toxemia during pregnancy.[167]

Heart Disease

With reductions in maternal mortality due to toxemia, hemorrhage, and infection, heart disease has become one of the major causes of maternal death, and congenital heart disease is being encountered with greater frequency. Mortality rates may be as high as 20 percent for pregnant women with severe cardiac complications; however, under optimal conditions for diagnosis and medical treatment, this risk of maternal death is greatly reduced.[167]

Pulmonary Disease

Fewer than 1 percent of all pregnant women in the United States suffer from bronchial asthma.[79] Of those who do, about 50 percent of them report a family history of allergy. The effects of pregnancy on asthma are unpredictable, however, severe asthma may be life threatening during pregnancy. Women with bronchial asthma do experience higher rates of spontaneous abortion and premature labor than women without asthma. Due to the physiological changes in the vascular system which accompany pregnancy, pulmonary embolism and aspiration pneumonia are occasionally experienced by pregnant women.

Endocrine Disorders

Endocrine disorders that may be present during pregnancy include diabetes mellitus and disorders of the thyroid, parathyroid, pituitary and adrenal glands, and the ovary. Pregnant women with severe hypothyroidism experience high rates of spontaneous abortion, premature labor, and toxemia.[156] Although hypothyroidism is rare among pregnant women because it usually develops after the reproductive ages,[167] children born to mothers with hypothyroidism experience high rates of mental retardation.[117] Disorders of the parathyroid, pituitary, and adrenal glands are uncommon among pregnant women. However, when they do occur they are associated with undesirable fetal outcomes. Ovarian tumors complicate only about 0.1 percent of all pregnancies; the major complications associated with ovarian tumors are torsion and hemorrhage.[167]

Liver Disease

Due to the metabolic load of pregnancy, women who are decompensated cirrhotics with jaundice, ascites, esophageal varices, and laboratory evidence of impaired liver function are at high risk of developing hepatic coma.

Therapeutic abortion is usually recommended as the treatment of choice under such severe circumstances.[167] Maternal and fetal prognosis is improved greatly in instances where there is laboratory evidence of adequate liver function. Efforts should be made, however, to avoid additional liver insults such as drugs, toxins, or infections. Hepatitis complicates fewer than 3/10,000 pregnancies in the United States but is associated with high rates of spontaneous abortion, premature labor, and perinatal death.[34,167]

Spastic Conditions

Epilepsy is a serious complication in only about 1/1000 pregnancies but seizures may be more frequent or severe in association with other pregnancy complications such as edema, alkylosis, fluid-electrolyte imbalance, cerebral hypoxia, hypoglycemia, or hypocalcemia.[79] Women are at higher risk for developing multiple sclerosis (MS) after pregnancy, but MS can complicate pregnancy for women who develop MS before becoming pregnant. Remissions and exacerbations are unrelated to the state of pregnancy. Pregnancy among women with myasthenia gravis is usually carried through to safe delivery as long as precautions are taken for protection of the mother from accidental injury.

Cancer

The coexistence of cancer with pregnancy occurs in about 1/1000 pregnancies.[150] There is limited evidence suggesting that neoplastic disease is occasionally transmitted from the mother to the fetus through the placenta, particularly in instances of malignant melanoma or leukemia-lymphoma.[166] This does not seem to be a universal phenomenon. Most types of maternal carcinoma are not potentiated by pregnancy. Management of care must be planned on an individual basis with the knowledge that both chemotherapy and radiologic treatment of malignant disease within a pregnant woman are potentially harmful to her fetus.

Hypertension

Data in the literature pertaining to hypertensive disorders of pregnancy are somewhat difficult to interpret because different classification systems have been used and the various disorders are often hard to distinguish clinically. Depending upon the nature and cause of hypertension during pregnancy, it may be present prior to pregnancy, during pregnancy, or it may not appear until early in the postpartum period.

Preeclampsia usually develops after the 20th week in pregnancy but may develop earlier in the presence of hydatidiform mole or choriocarcinoma.[79] It occurs in about 5 percent of all pregnant women in the United States. The incidence is three to five times greater, however, among some groups of women from low socioeconomic populations. A major concern for preeclamptic women is the potential development of eclampsia which exposes them to a 3–5 percent risk of maternal mortality and a 17–20 percent risk of fetal death.[71] Predisposition to preeclampsia includes multiple pregnancy, hydatidiform mole, dietary deficiency, comparatively young or old maternal age within the childbearing years, and a family history of preeclampsia or eclampsia.[31] Primigravidas and women with chronic cardiovascular or renal disease seem to be particularly prone to the development of preeclampsia.

Hypertension prior to pregnancy is frequently a manifestation of cardiovascular or renal disease. Women with definite hypertension before 20 weeks of gestation and with superimposed preeclampsia tend to be older, multiparous, and to have a strong family history of hypertension.[71] Although the risk of maternal death among these women is not as high as it is among women with eclampsia, the risk of fetal death has been reported to be as high as 60 percent and, among individual women, tends to increase with each succeeding pregnancy.

Sickle Cell Disease

Sickle cell disease is a recessive, hereditary, hemolytic anemia found primarily in individuals of black or Mediterranean ancestry. It occurs in less than one out of 3000 pregnancies among black women in the United States. It is associated, however, with high risks of maternal death, spontaneous abortion, stillbirth, and neonatal death. Risk of maternal death has been reported to be as high as 10 percent and fetal wastage has been noted in about one out of three such pregnancies.[121,167]

Mental Illness

The type and severity of mental disorders among pregnant women have implications for the abilities of these women to cope with the stresses of pregnancy and eventually to assume responsibility for childrearing.

Anemia

Anemia is the most common complication of pregnancy and occurs in approximately 8 out of 10 pregnant women in the United States.[167] Iron-deficiency anemia accounts for about 95 percent of all diagnosed pregnancy anemias.[79] Increased risks of abortion, premature labor, infection, toxemia of pregnancy, intrauterine growth retardation, perinatal mortality, and perinatal morbidity have been associated with anemia during pregnancy.[79,167]

Exposure to X-Ray

Maternal exposure to large doses of ionizing radiation (more than 150 rads) during pregnancy has been associated with a high incidence of spontaneous abortion, congenital anomalies, and the development of leukemia or other cancers in live-born children.[1,54,205] It has been suggested that no avoidable radiation exposure during pregnancy be considered ''safe''.[54]

Medication History

Many drugs taken during pregnancy, particularly certain antibiotics, steroids, and mood altering drugs, are known to have potentially adverse effects on the developing fetus. Extreme effects result in congenital malformations, chemical and metabolic disturbances, and disturbances of the central nervous system.[1,54] Pregnant women addicted to mood-altering drugs are at much greater risk of spontaneous abortions, stillbirths, or delivery of babies who experience a variety of complications during the first month of life than pregnant women who are not addicted to these drugs.[122]

Habitual Use of Alcohol

The most common problem noted in children of alcoholic mothers is mental retardation,[54] however, risks of stillbirth, low birth weight, and defects of the brain and central nervous system in the newborn have been found to be higher among mothers who consume alcoholic beverages during pregnancy than among those who do not consume any alcohol during pregnancy.[122,179] A high incidence of heart valve defects, brain cell abnormalities, and various facial abnormalities has also been noted in infants of mothers who consume large amounts of alcohol consistently during pregnancy.

Habitual Use of Tobacco

It has been estimated that about one-half of all pregnant women in the United States smoke cigarettes.[90] These women experience placenta previa, abruptio placentae, bleeding during pregnancy, and premature or prolonged rupture of the membranes significantly more often than mothers who do not smoke during pregnancy.[5,54] The mean birth weight of babies born to mothers who smoke during pregnancy is less than that for babies of mothers who do not smoke during pregnancy. Mothers who smoke while pregnant have been found to deliver babies with a birth weight of less than 2500 g almost twice as frequently as mothers who do not smoke while pregnant.[5,39,70,127,131] Growth retardation is the major fetal complication of maternal smoking during pregnancy and it often results in spontaneous abortion, fetal death, or neonatal death. Many live-born children of these mothers survive the first month of life without apparent difficulties but eventually develop measurable deficiencies in physical, intellectual, or emotional growth.[5,146] It appears that the risks of undesirable pregnancy outcome among women who smoke during pregnancy are heightened when these women are from population groups of low socioeconomic status, are poorly nourished, or have poor obstetrical histories.[39,118]

Gynecologic History

Genital tract anomalies or a contracted pelvis have potential for obstructing the fetus in its successful passage through the birth canal during labor and delivery. It seems likely that large uterine myomas or fibroids could interfere with the growth and development of a fetus since they often grow rapidly during pregnancy.[163] They are found most frequently in nulliparas and occur five times more often in black women than in white women. Infertility and spontaneous abortion are more common among women with leimyomas (myomas or fibroids) than in women without them. Cervical leimyomas are extremely rare.[41] Cervical incompetence is highly associated with spontaneous abortion during the second trimester of pregnancy. It can usually be corrected, however, before or during pregnancy.[79] Ovarian masses may obstruct an enlarging uterus and have implications for medical diagnosis and treatment.[124] Prior gynecologic surgery may result in obstructive or problematic scar tissue and sometimes requires planning for a surgical delivery. The presence of endometriosis during pregnancy has been found to have variable effects on pregnancy. Regression of the condition has been noted only in some pregnant women.[115]

Of all pregnant women, as many as one in three harbor the protozoan *trichomonas vaginalis* and symptoms of vaginal infection may appear or become more severe during pregnancy due to alterations in the composition of the vaginal flora.[79,113] *Candida albicans*, a fungus, has been noted in as many as one out of two healthy adults[113] and in one out of four pregnant women at term.[79] Symptoms of vaginal infection due to this fungus are frequently noted during pregnancy—particularly in association with diabetes mellitus, antibiotic therapy, or steroid therapy—because of changes in the vaginal flora or lowered host resistance. Babies born to mothers with an active infection of candidiasis sometimes develop oral thrush due to direct contact with the infection during delivery. Simple vaginitis due to *Hemophilus vaginalis, escherichia coli*, staphylococci, or streptococci, all of which affect the normal acidity of the vagina, is also commonly apparent during pregnancy.[79,85] All of these infections are sexually transmitted.

Abnormal Papanicolaou smear results at any time, whether during pregnancy or otherwise, have implications for medical diagnosis and treatment of possible malignancy.[41] Accurate information about menstruation is important for determining the correct estimated date of confinement (EDC) and for use as baseline information while monitoring fetal growth and development during pregnancy.

A careful sexual history will be useful in providing the information necessary for appropriate sexuality counseling during pregnancy and in planning for the future. Information about the woman's use of contraceptives is important for determining what problems she may have encountered with contraception and whether her contraceptive may have implications for the present pregnancy. Concerns pertaining to a present pregnancy may include an intrauterine device in situ, withdrawal bleeding after discontinuing the use of oral contraceptives, or an unplanned, and possibly unwanted, pregnancy due to contraceptive failure.[158]

Physical Examination and Laboratory Tests

Every woman should receive a careful and thorough physical examination early in pregnancy. Findings of this examination should clarify information obtained during history taking, provide a tentative diagnosis of pregnancy, including the point in gestation, and make the nurse-midwife aware of any potential health-related problems which may be encountered by the mother or her offspring. The results of selected laboratory tests should also be used to confirm findings about the maternal history and from the physical examination, as well as to identify other potential problems such as cervical cancer, venereal disease, ABO blood type or Rh factor incompatibility with the fetus, rubella, sickle cell disease, tuberculosis, anemia, albuminuria, glycosuria, or urinary tract infection. Direction in conducting a thorough physical examination, interpreting the examination findings, and interpreting laboratory results is beyond the scope of this chapter.

Periodic assessment throughout pregnancy of both maternal health status and fetal health status is important so that problems or potential problems can be resolved. Although it has not been clearly documented that the amount of prenatal care is associated with the quality of pregnancy outcome,[86,143] it seems logical that the earlier in pregnancy one initiates prenatal care the more opportunity there is to identify and resolve problems. The difficulty that some investigators have encountered in trying to clarify any association between the amount of prenatal care and resulting pregnancy outcome may be due to the fact that many women known to have medical problems purposely initiate early prenatal care.[159] A recommended guide to follow in scheduling prenatal visits subsequent to the initial visit is:

- Once each month through the 6th month of pregnancy
- Every other week during the 7th and 8th months of pregnancy
- Each week after the 8th month of pregnancy

Some women need to be seen by a health care professional more frequently than this guide suggests.

The nurse-midwife must differentiate the signs and symptoms of potentially pathologic conditions from the many common complaints and discomforts of pregnancy. Among some groups of women certain conditions including hypertension, anemia, diabetes mellitus, urinary tract infection, and vaginitis are quite common. Basic criteria have been established to assist the caregiver with clinical assessment and early identification of these problems.

Assessing the Symptoms of Pathologic Conditions in Pregnancy

Hypertension. The Committee on Terminology of the American College of Obstetricians and Gynecologists has recommended that the term "pregnancy toxemias" no longer be used and that the hypertensive states of pregnancy be classified as shown in Table 3-7.[71]

Anemia. There are many anemias and hemoglobinopathies which complicate pregnancy. Initial identification of a problem is usually based on a hemoglobin of less than $10.0-11.0$ g/100 ml of blood during pregnancy.[159,193]

Iron deficiency anemia is the most common anemic condition found among pregnant women[79,167] but it can usually be treated effectively with the

Table 3-7
The Hypertensive States of Pregnancy*

Disorders	Classification
Mild:	
Gestational edema	Accumulation of fluid resulting in $> +1$ edema after 12 h of bed rest or a weight gain of 5 lbs or more within 1 wk
Gestational proteinuria	Presence of protein in the urine in the absence of hypertension, edema, renal infection, or intrinsic renovascular disease
Gestational hypertension	Development of hypertension during pregnancy, or within the first 24 h postpartum, in previously normotensive women. Hypertension is identified by a blood pressure reading of 140/90 mm Hg. or a rise of 30 mm Hg. in the systolic blood pressure and/or a rise of 15 mm Hg. in the diastolic blood pressure over the baseline blood pressure. [193]
Acute:	
Preeclampsia or eclampsia	Development of hypertension during pregnancy in conjunction with proteinuria, edema, or both, after about 20th wk gestation. Sometimes found before 20th wk in cases of hydatidiform mole or choriocarcinoma
Severe preeclampsia	Systolic blood pressure is 160 mm Hg. or more or the diastolic blood pressure is 110 mm Hg. or more on two occasions at least 6 h apart while the mother is on bed rest. Proteinuria of 5 or more in 24 h (3 + or 4 + quantitative). Oliguria of 500 ml or less in 24 h. Cerebral or visual disturbances. Epigastric pain. Pulmonary edema with or without cyanosis
Eclampsia Convulsion	
Chronic hypertension with superimposed preeclampsia or eclampsia	Exhibition of definite hypertension before pregnancy and development of even higher blood pressure and proteinuria after 20th wk gestation
Chronic hypertensive disease of whatever cause	
Unclassified hypertensive disorders with insufficient information to classify the hypertensive state	

*Adapted from the American College of Obstetricians and Gynecologists, cited in Hayashi T: Disease specific to pregnancy, in Romney SL, Gray MJ, Little AB et al (eds): The Health Care of Women (ed 2). New York, McGraw-Hill Book Co., 1981, pp 661−695 administration of iron. Oral iron supplementation of 30−60 mg daily is the usual route of administration because of its simplicity and relative safety.[55,159] Some women, however, experience nausea, vomiting, abdominal cramping, diarrhea, or constipation due to gastrointestinal irritation while on oral therapy. Alternative options for developing and maintaining adequate iron reserves during pregnancy need to be considered for these women.

Some clinicians recommend that 200−400 μg of supplemental folic acid be ingested daily.[55] The absorption of folic acid is thought to be decreased during pregnancy when there are increased demands for tissue synthesis. Dietary intake of folic acid also is frequently insufficient to meet the requirements of pregnancy, particularly among women with limited economic resources.

Diabetes. Since the endocrinologic and hormonal changes of pregnancy have potential for precipitating the development of diabetes mellitus, pregnancy is a time when women not known to have diabetes should be observed carefully for the signs, symptoms, and conditions often associated with it. Particular factors which need to be taken into account include obesity, glycosuria, recurrent monilial infection, familial history of diabetes, unexplained prior stillbirths or spontaneous abortions, prior delivery of an infant with a birth weight of 4000 g or more, or prior delivery of an infant with multiple congenital anomalies.[167,193] Occasionally symptoms of diabetes, such as excessive urine output, excessive thirst, or excessive eating, as well as weight loss or weakness, may be noted.[193] Women presenting with any of these characteristics should be screened for diabetes mellitus.

The use of blood sugar level determination 2 hours after the patient has ingested 100 g of glucose has been found effective for initial screening of pregnant women for the presence of diabetes.[167] Fasting blood sugar levels are often normal in early or latent diabetes and, therefore, are not sufficiently reliable for initial screening. In instances where a woman does not tolerate oral glucose well, a blood sugar level determination can be done on blood drawn 2 hours after she has eaten a meal. If a 2-hour blood sugar level is found to be questionable, a glucose tolerance test (GTT) should be done.

Urinary Tract Infection. Infection of the urinary tract may involve the urethra (urethritis), bladder (cystitis), or kidney (pyelonephritis) and may be symptomatic or asymptomatic. Since as many as one out of four women with asymptomatic bacteriuria early in pregnancy will develop a symptomatic urinary tract infection during pregnancy, clean-catch urine specimens are often obtained for culture and sensitivity routinely during initial prenatal visits.[96,121,193,200] Urine cultures should also be done when symptoms of urgency, frequency, dysuria, hematuria, fever, malaise, back and flank pain, or nausea and vomiting are present.[56,121]

Bacteria colony counts of more than 100,000/mg of urine are considered diagnostic of infection when a clean-catch voided specimen has been analyzed.[56,121] This manner of obtaining urine specimens has been recommended as the method of choice since catheterization risks introduction of infectious organisms into the bladder.[56,121] In addition, clean-catch specimens infrequently give false-positive indications of infection.[121]

Treatment of urinary tract infection—including advice about proper hygiene, recommendation that large quantities of fluid be ingested daily, and antibacterial medication—is often initiated before culture and sensitivity results are available because of the symptoms of infection. Some clinicians find it helpful to use dipsticks, slide tests, microscopic examination of urine sediment for leukocyte clumps, and examination of gram-stained urine drops to confirm symptomatic findings. These tests can be conducted with relative ease in an office setting, provide immediate information, and usually result in information which correlates well with culture findings.[121]

Vaginitis. Increased amounts of vaginal discharge are normal during pregnancy. The acidic properties of vaginal secretions at this time should protect the mother and fetus from harmful infection, however, a medium which fosters the development of vaginitis often results. The most common causes of vaginitis during pregnancy are *Hemophilus vaginalis, trichomonas vaginalis*, and *Candida albicans*.[56,81,85,97,193] Excessive vaginal discharge may also be due to other organisms including those responsible for venereal disease, mechanical irritants, or contact allergens.

It is now believed that the "nonspecific vaginitis" diagnosed by clinicians in the past was, for the most part, due to *Hemophilus vaginalis*.[85] Vaginitis due to this bacillus is characterized by a grayish-white, foul-smelling, discharge. Usually little itching, burning, or soreness is found to accompany the discharge. *Hemophilus vaginalis* can be identified on a smear treated with physiologic saline by the characteristic "clue cells".[61] Clinical identification of the organism is important since the success of identification by laboratory culture has been highly variable.[85] Treatment of the mother and her sexual partner with an oral antibiotic or metronidazole (Flagyl, Searle & Co., Chicago, Il) is usually effective in resolving the infection, however, caution must be exercised in the use of these drugs during pregnancy. Concerns have been expressed about the oncologic effect in animals and the mutagenic effect of metronidazole in bacteria.[96] It has been recommended, therefore, that metronidazole be used only during the second or third trimester of pregnancy for women in whom local palliative treatment has been inadequate for control of the symptoms of infection.[11]

The signs and symptoms of vaginitis due to *trichomonas vaginalis* include a yellowish to greenish, frothy and copius, purulent discharge with a foul odor and identification of the one-celled flagellate trichomonads on a saline wet smear.[56,79,113,193] Characteristic "strawberry spots" may be noted on the cervix or vaginal walls and, in severe infections, acute inflammation of these structures is not uncommon. Women tend to complain of burning, itching, dysuria, or dyspareunia with severe infection. The treatment of choice is usually metronidazole (Flagyl) for both the mother (as appropriate during pregnancy) and her sexual partner. This medication should not be given to the mother during the first trimester of pregnancy.[11]

Monilial infection caused by *Candida albicans* is characterized by whitish, cottage cheese-like, patches, or plaques of discharge which adhere to the vaginal walls, cervix, and labia.[56,79,113,193] When scraped or removed from the site of attachment, bleeding usually results. Both the vagina and cervix often look red and swollen, and infected women tend to complain of vulvular itching. The spores of *Candida albicans* can be readily identified upon microscopy of slides smeared with vaginal discharge and treated with potassium hydroxide. Effective treatment often results from the use of antifungal agents such as Monostat cream or Nystatin suppositories. Control of reinfection, particularly among women with diabetes mellitus or women who are taking large doses of oral antibiotics, is a major problem of this monilial infection.

It is not uncommon for women who have vaginitis to be infected with more than one organism at the same time. For this reason, it is recommended that physiologic saline and potassium hydroxide slides be made for all diagnostic vaginal smears.[56] These smears are indicated when symptoms of infection are present and when the patient has not douched or used any medication so that the specimens will accurately reflect the composition of the vaginal flora.

Instruction about good habits for personal hygiene should accompany all prescriptive treatments for vaginitis. The perineal area should be washed and patted dry frequently with clean linens which have not been shared with another individual.[56] Wiping the perineum from front to back prevents the introduction of bacteria from the rectum into the vagina or urethra. Clothing, such as underpants and pantyhose, that contacts the perineum should be clean and made of a fabric such as cotton that allows free airflow. Douching should be avoided, or at least infrequent, since it can strip the vagina of its natural flora, introduce new bacteria, or aggravate inflammation.

Diagnostic Measures to Identify Fetal Problems

Monitoring fetal well-being during pregnancy begins with careful determination of the estimated date of confinement (EDC) and assessment of fetal size. When the fetus is large enough, an assessment is also made of fetal heart tones, movement, lie, presentation, position, and attitude. Conditions such as multiple pregnancy, polyhydramnios, and the possibility of hydatidiform mole should be ruled out during physical examination of the mother. Progression of fetal growth is estimated through measurement of the fundal height at each prenatal visit. Most accurate estimates are obtained when the mother empties her bladder just prior to the examination,[206] when the same technique for measuring fundal height is used at each visit, and when the measurement is done consistently by one individual.

A variety of diagnostic measures can be used to assist the clinician with identification of fetal problems during pregnancy. Their use should be considered when the possibility of certain problems is indicated by the maternal history, physical examination, or from laboratory tests. These diagnostic measures include amniocentesis, radiography, ultrasonography, fetoscopy, amnioscopy, estriol level determination, the oxytocin challenge test (OCT), and the nonstress test (NST).

Amniocentesis. Amniocentesis is a transabdominal procedure to obtain samples of amniotic fluid from the gestational sac. Technologic advances in the methods available for analyzing amniotic fluid have made it possible to diagnose essentially every chromosomal defect and more than 130 metabolic defects while the fetus is still in utero.[62] The procedure is usually indicated for a pregnant woman who is more than 35 years old or one who has previously delivered a child with a chromosomal abnormality, and when there is a familial history of cytogenetic disease, X-linked disease, neural tube defect, or metabolic disease.[180] Although the sex of the fetus can be determined upon examination of the amniotic fluid, amniocentesis is not recommended for the identification of fetal sex alone because of the risk of potential complications.

Since the number of cells in the amniotic fluid which have shed from the fetus needs to be sufficient for analysis and since the uterus needs to be large enough to be readily accessible during the procedure, amniocentesis is usually done between the 14th and 18th week of pregnancy.[62,193] The risk of fetal loss, in the form of spontaneous abortion or fetal death, due to amniocentesis has been estimated to be no higher than 0.5 percent. Maternal problems associated with the procedure, such as amniotic fluid leakage, transient vaginal bleeding, or transient uterine contractions, have been found to be mild and to be experienced by only about 2 percent of all women having amniocentesis.[142]

Conflicting evidence has been found in the literature about whether or not preamniocentesis ultrasonography for identification of placental location reduces the likelihood of bloody taps, feto–maternal transfusion, or multiple uterine punctures.[142] This may be due partially to the fact that, in many of the studies reviewed, the same obstetrician did not conduct amniocentesis with ultrasound and amniocentesis without ultrasound. This inconsistency makes comparison of data from experimental and control groups inappropriate.[62,193]

Based on evidence in support of preamniocentesis ultrasonography, as well as the relative safety of amniocentesis for the mother and fetus, the Task Force on Predictors of Hereditary Disease or Congenital Defects, of the National Institute of Child Health and Human Development, has recommended that ultrasonography be used before amniocentesis in order to guide proper insertion of the needle.[183] Since it has been documented that the placenta can shift its contour and therefore its position with the passage of time or with patient movement,[74] some authorities have suggested that preamniocentesis ultrasound is effective only if it is done immediately prior to amniocentesis.[74,83]

No information is available on whether a bloody tap is more frequently associated with spontaneous abortion, fetal damage, prematurity, abruptio placentae, or culture failure than a nonbloody tap.[83]

It has been estimated that amniocentesis needs to be repeated in only about 2 percent of all cases because of failure to obtain fluid or to cultivate an adequate number of cells for analysis.[62] The reliability of obtaining a diagnosis following amniocentesis, including those cases with multiple taps, has been reported to be from about 97 percent to almost 100 percent.[62,180]

The suggestion has been made that commitment to have an elective abortion if fetal abnormality is diagnosed not be a prerequisite for amniocentesis.[149] More and more alternatives to abortion are becoming available for certain conditions[50,84] and parental reaction to knowledge of a specific condition may be very different than initial reaction to an unsubstantiated but potential abnormality.

Radiography. It has been estimated that in utero exposure to x-ray doubles a child's risk of developing cancer during the first 15 years of life and that such exposure also increases the risk of developing other disease conditions.[122] Some authorities, however, feel that these risks are minimal during the third trimester of pregnancy if the lowest possible doses of x-ray are used.[62,155] As a result, radiography continues to be used in some settings to diagnose a variety of congenital malformations, including anencephaly, hydrocephalus, microcephaly, encephalocele, myelomeningocele, and cleft palate,[62] and to confirm multiple pregnancy. Radiography is also used during the latter part of pregnancy to diagnose cephalopelvic disproportion.[155]

The Food and Drug Administration (FDA) is continuing its efforts to prevent the inappropriate use of x-ray during pregnancy.[122] A recommendation has been made to the medical community that pregnancy status be ascertained before ordering abdominal x-rays for women who are of reproductive age; patient-oriented posters and pamphlets, which advise women who are pregnant or who may be pregnant that they should provide their physicians with this information before undergoing x-ray, have been widely distributed to health facilities where x-rays are ordered or conducted; and the Food and Drug Administration, the American College of Obstetricians and Gynecologists, and the American College of Radiology are developing a joint statement which will advise physicians against the routine use of x-ray pelvimetry to determine the need for cesarean section.

Ultrasonography. This technique uses low-intensity pulses of high-frequency soundwaves to reflect the contents of the uterus as a two-dimensional picture on a screen.[54] The many uses of ultrasonography include the early diagnosis of pregnancy, determination of gestational age, localization of the site of placental implantation, diagnosis of multiple pregnancy, identification of hydatidiform mole, and diagnosis of congenital malformations such as hydrocephalus, anencephaly, or Siamese twins.[54,81,162,193] Information from a series of ultrasonic scans taken over a period of one week or more has been useful in the diagnosis of intrauterine growth retardation, impending abortion, and fetal death.

The use of ultrasonography has become so extensive since some of its benefits in monitoring pregnancy were realized in the early 1970s[180] that more than 50 percent of all pregnant women in the United States are thought to be exposed to it. Clinicians seem to have assumed this technology to be safe because of its noninvasive nature and the absence of ionizing irradiation.[62] Only recently have questions been raised about potential long-term effects on the fetus. Ultrasonography has been found to damage tissue[184] and to fragment mammalian DNA molecules[60,152] but the implications of these findings are not yet understood. In response to questions being raised about the effects of ultrasonography on the human fetus, the Food and Drug Administration is conducting and supporting biological research which is pertinent to the issue.[122]

Findings from a recent study of women exposed to ultrasonography indicate that most women are anxious about the procedure.[119] Almost all of the women studied wanted to know the baby's age and size but feared that there would be some abnormality present. Most of them were unclear about what kind of image they would see and more than one-half of them feared that their babies were being subjected to harm even though their physicians had stressed the contrary.

In another study of women's reactions to the fetal image resulting from ultrasonography, it was found that some of the women reacted positively to the image while others had negative reactions.[192] During postpartum follow-up of these women, the investigator felt that the process of maternal-infant bonding had been initiated at the time of ultrasonography among those women who reacted positively to the fetal image.

Fetoscopy. This relatively new procedure permits direct visualization of the fetus and placenta through an endoscope which has been inserted through a small abdominal incision.[62,107,193] In addition to the prenatal diagnosis of congenital anomalies, fetoscopy provides the capability for drawing blood samples from the placental veins and for obtaining small skin biopsies from the fetus. This procedure is still considered to be highly experimental since both the mother and the fetus are put at risk of induced tissue damage and potential hemorrhage.[62]

Amnioscopy. This procedure permits direct visualization of the amniotic fluid through the fetal membranes at the cervical os and is useful in the identification of meconium-staining.[193] It has several drawbacks in that the cervix must be sufficiently dilated for visualization and the membranes may be ruptured inadvertently during the procedure. In addition, the procedure often is uncomfortable for the mother, and the internal manipulations may predispose her to genital tract bleeding or infection.

Estriol level determination. The measurement of estriol synthesis is a useful indicator of the status of fetoplacental functioning since optimal functioning depends upon the fetal adrenal glands, the fetal liver, and an intact placenta all functioning in an integral relationship.[54,100,101,193] Secretions from both the mother and the fetus reach the placenta through the circulatory system and eventually are converted to estriol. Almost all estriol produced by the fetoplacental unit enters the maternal circulation in unconjugated form but is excreted in the urine in almost entirely conjugated form. Estriol production and excretion tend to increase throughout pregnancy, particularly during the third trimester, and to peak at term gestation.

Estriol assays done in series have been found useful in the diagnosis of intrauterine growth retardation and prolonged gestation. Until recently, most assays were done on 24 hour urine specimens to determine the level of urinary estriol. Due to wide variations in normal levels of urinary estriol during pregnancy, the fact that many conditions in the mother unrelated to fetal well-being will decrease the level of urinary estriol, and the inconvenience inherent in the collection of 24-hour urine specimens, many clinicians have questioned the validity of urinary estriol determinations.

A rapid, sensitive, and convenient radioimmunoassay has now been developed which makes it possible to measure either total or unconjugated plasma estriol.[100] The major advantage of plasma estriol determination is that there is control over the timing and accuracy in collecting blood samples. In addition, serum unconjugated estriol is derived almost exclusively from the fetal liver and adrenal glands, as opposed to both maternal and fetal, and it is cleared by the maternal liver instead of the maternal kidney. The maternal liver is rarely affected in problem pregnancies while the kidney is often affected.

Occasionally false-positive findings are obtained as the result of plasma estriol level determination. This factor should be taken into account when considering management options and the risks involved.[100]

Oxytocin challenge test (OCT). The OCT, or stress test, is a mechanism for testing fetoplacental respiratory reserve during uterine contractions.[100,193] It is usually indicated for patients suspected of being at high risk for placental insufficiency such as in instances of pregnancy that is known or suspected to be more than 42 weeks in gestation, intrauterine growth retardation, hypertension, diabetes mellitus, renal disease, Rh sensitization, previous unexplained stillbirth, or homozygous hemoglobinopathies. An OCT is also indicated when the results of other examinations, such as a low or falling estriol level, a nonreactive nonstress test, or meconium stained amniotic fluid, suggest fetal compromise.

The fetal respiratory reserve is determined by observations of the fetal heart rate during uterine contractions. Uterine blood flow is slowed by uterine contractions which results in reduced intervillous space perfusion and placental exchange. The normally oxyenated fetus does not react to periodic decreases in its PO_2 during contractions but a fetus with low basal oxygenation will usually exhibit the fetal heart rate pattern of late deceleration.

Oxytocin challenge tests can be done when contractions have started naturally or when they have been induced with oxytocin. The fetal heart rate is recorded simultaneously with each contraction using external fetal monitoring equipment. The clinician must always keep in mind the fact that an OCT has potential for initiating premature labor.

The results of an OCT are considered to be negative when no late decelerations occur during at least 3 adequate contractions within a period of 10 minutes. The term "adequate" has not been defined in a standardized manner. The definition for contractions considered to be adequate may therefore differ from setting to setting or from clinician to clinician. Chances of fetal death occurring during the 7 days subsequent to a negative OCT are less than 1/100 tests. Fetal deaths that have occurred during the first week after OCTs have been due primarily to cord accidents or abruptio placentae.[100] These conditions cannot be identified with an OCT. The primary value of negative results from an oxytocin challenge test therefore is the prevention of inappropriate premature interventions in situations where the risk of clinical misdiagnosis is high such as in cases of intrauterine growth retardation or postdate pregnancy.

Unequivocal late decelerations occurring with every contraction in a period of 10 minutes indicate positive findings from an OCT. Although it has been documented that positive results of an OCT are associated with increased risks of stillbirth, intrauterine growth retardation, and neonatal morbidity, it must be remembered that the incidence of false-positive results from OCTs has been reported to be as high as 50 percent.[100] Pregnancy should not be terminated in the presence of positive OCT findings unless there are other clinical signs which support them. The OCT is usually repeated weekly until delivery.

Nonstress Test (NST). The NST is a mechanism for obtaining information about fetal well-being through the observation of fetal heart rate responses to fetal movement. It is noninvasive and there are no contraindications to, or complications associated with, this procedure. It often provides useful information in instances where an OCT is contraindicated such as in cases of previous cesarean section, placenta previa, or threatened premature labor.[193]

The fetal heart rate and fetal movement are monitored during an NST for a period of about 40 minutes using external fetal-monitoring equipment. This period is usually sufficient for monitoring a fetus during sleep-wake cycles which tend to last from 20–40 minutes.[100]

Findings from an NST should be used only to determine whether or not further testing is indicated. According to the classification system developed by Schifrin and his colleagues,[171] tracings from the fetal monitor are read as reactive, nonreactive, or unsatisfactory. A reactive tracing shows at least two accelerations (15 beats per minute, minimum amplitude; 15 seconds, minimum duration) associated with fetal movement or contractions of the uterus in 10 minutes. If accelerations are insufficient at the end of 40 minutes, the test is considered to be nonreactive. The test is classified as unsatisfactory when the fetal heart rate cannot be satisfactorily recorded.

SPECIAL CONSIDERATIONS DURING PREGNANCY

There are a variety of needs and circumstances which deserve special consideration during pregnancy. They include, but are not limited to, nutritional needs, informational needs, unique needs, and selecting the place of birth.

Nutritional Needs

Normal growth and development of the fetus during pregnancy are dependent upon receipt of an adequate supply of essential nutrients from the mother. The influence of pregnancy-related physiologic and emotional changes on nutritional needs is unclear. In addition, the influence of nutrition on reproductive capacity and outcome is not fully understood.

Studies of relationships between maternal nutritional status and reproductive outcome have become more sophisticated as more has become known about nutrition, reproduction, and human growth. Because little information was available on the nutritional composition of foods during the nineteenth century, nutritional counseling for pregnant women was based only on casual observations. Many of these observations became so widely known that concepts stemming from them are still held by some clinicians. For instance, Prochownick, a German obstetrician, observed that pregnant women on a diet high in protein but severely restricted in carbohydrates and fluids for 6 weeks before delivery had smaller babies and fewer problems during labor and delivery than women who did not follow this regime.[55,195] Although there is strong evidence at this time which suggests that such a diet would be harmful during pregnancy, similar diets are still recommended by some practitioners. It was also believed—and still is among some practitioners—that pregnant women have an innate ability to produce viable offspring regardless of maternal health or nutritional status, that women will eat instinctively during pregnancy so that maternal and fetal needs for nutrients will be met automatically, and that a fetus will get as much nourishment as it needs no matter what or how much food the mother eats as long as she takes plenty of vitamins.[55]

At the beginning of the twentieth century, scientific efforts were made to identify relationships between maternal nutritional status and reproductive outcome. A few of the studies done at this time were classic and the findings had major ramifications for clinical practice which continue to be ascribed to in some settings. Infants born to mothers with nutritionally sound diets were reported to be much healthier than infants born to mothers with poor diets,[24] and mothers who received dietary supplements during pregnancy were reported to experience significantly fewer stillbirths and neonatal deaths among their offspring than mothers who did not receive these supplements.[11,43] The major criticism of these studies was that dietary intake was used as the only measure of nutritional status. Systematic attempts to determine actual nutritional status of the women studied, before and during pregnancy, were not made.[195]

Data conflicting with the scientific information already published began to appear in the literature as a result of studies conducted during the 1950s. Researchers at Vanderbilt University reported the findings of a study designed to determine whether a significant relationship could be found between nutritional status of the mother—according to diet, physical findings, and laboratory test results—and the development of maternal or fetal complications.[112] After study of 2300 pregnancies, however, perinatal deaths, premature births, and the development of toxemia during pregnancy could not be attributed to variations in maternal diet or nutritional status. Women who consumed an average of less than 50 g of protein each day during pregnancy were found to be no more likely to develop toxemia than those with higher intakes of protein, and it could not be shown that women who had taken vitamin and mineral supplements had better pregnancy courses or outcomes than women who had not taken these nutritional supplements.

Due to concerns about the lack of control for the effects of parity on reproductive performance and the dependence on dietary recall inherent in earlier studies, an investigation was conducted during the years 1950–1953 of 489 primigravidas who each kept home-weighed food records for 1 week during the 7th month of pregnancy.[187] Although the nutrient intakes among these women were found to vary considerably, no associations could be found between diet during pregnancy and the length of gestation or the incidence of antepartal hemorrhage, fetal congenital malformation, or perinatal death. After adjustment of the data for maternal height and social class, however, it was noted that women from the upper social classes were taller and heavier than women from the lower social classes. Likewise, women from the upper social classes were found to consume more calories than women from the lower social classes and the mean birth weights of their babies, when standardized for length of gestation and maternal height, were found to be higher than those for the babies born to women from the lower social classes. It was concluded from these findings that the mother's height and weight, as a reflection of life-long nutrition, and social class were more important than dietary intake during pregnancy in affecting the course of pregnancy and its outcome. It was also suggested that women of good nutritional status before conception could tolerate relatively wide variations in both the quantity and the quality of their diets during pregnancy without exhibiting clinically apparent effects among themselves or their offspring.

During the 1960s, women of the Western world generally were considered to be well-nourished.[195] Obesity was much more frequent among these women than leanness. With diminished concern about the direct impact of diet during pregnancy on reproductive outcome, weight restriction became a routine part of prenatal care. It was reasoned that pregnancy was a good time to encourage maternal weight loss because the fetus would serve as a "perfect parasite" that could meet its own nutritional needs by simply drawing from the stored reserves of its well-nourished mother. Some clinicians continue to ascribe to this reasoning.

Much of the nutritional research pertaining to pregnancy has been focused on animals since, for ethical reasons, maternal-fetal relationships operating at cellular and molecular levels in humans cannot be studied directly. Care must be taken in interpreting the findings of these studies because they are not directly applicable to humans, however, several important findings warrant serious consideration and further study. For instance, many prenatal factors have been found to influence fetal growth and, among them, maternal malnutrition has been found to be one cause of growth failure resulting in small offspring of low birth weight.[195] Consequences of maternal malnutrition for the fetus seem to depend on the timing, the severity, and the duration. Baby animals that were malnourished throughout pregnancy due to restrictions in the maternal diet tend to have reduced numbers and sizes of cells in the placenta, reduced numbers of brain cells and head sizes, proportional reductions in the sizes of other organs, and alterations in normal cell constituents and biochemical processes. It seems clear that animal fetuses are not "perfect parasites" that can survive periods of intrauterine insult without adverse effects.

Famine has been imposed periodically on large groups of women during times of war. Data from these "natural experiments"[195] indicate that severe malnutrition during pregnancy is highly associated with fetal death, low birth weight, and congenital malformation.[4,173] Malnutrition during the early months of pregnancy appears to affect development of the embryo and its capacity to survive while malnutrition in the latter part of pregnancy seems to be associated with growth retardation.

Organs of infants who were born alive but died within the first 48 hours of life have been studied to determine whether differences could be found according to socioeconomic status of the mother. Findings from one such study in which instances of multiple gestation, maternal complication, or congenital malformation were excluded, indicated that infants born to women from poor families in the United States tended, according to level of income, to have less adipose tissue and smaller organs than infants born to women from nonpoor families.[136] Small-sized human placentas also have been associated with low socioeconomic status, both in the United States and elsewhere.[94,204] It has been suggested that the prognosis of pregnancy may be related not only to the social class of the woman who is pregnant, but also to the social class of her own mother at the time her mother was pregnant.[9]

The most significant finding of nutritional research pertaining to pregnancy to date is that both maternal body size (according to height and prepregnancy weight) and maternal weight gain during pregnancy have shown consistent associations with infant birth weight.[64,132] These factors appear to be independent but have cumulative effects on birth weight; babies of taller and heavier mothers tend to be larger than babies of shorter and lighter mothers,[187] and mean birth weight increases as the amount of weight gain during pregnancy increases.[42] In addition, the largest babies, in terms of body size and organ weight, are born to mothers who were overweight before pregnancy and who also gained a large amount of weight during pregnancy; the smallest babies are born to mothers who were underweight before pregnancy and either lost weight during pregnancy or had a minimal amount of weight gain.[134]

The average amount of weight gained during pregnancy among healthy women is usually between 22 and 28 pounds.[32] Young women and primigravidas often gain more weight than older women and multigravidas.[196] It is frequently recommended that women gain at least 2.2 pounds in any one month during the second and third trimesters of pregnancy but not more than 7 pounds in any month during pregnancy.[55] Best obstetrical outcomes have been reported to occur among women of normal weight for height who gain between 22 and 32 pounds and among underweight women who gain at least 30 pounds during pregnancy.[130] The suggestion has been made that guidelines for appropriate weight gain during pregnancy be developed according to units of prepregnant body weight.[82]

Obesity has been associated with a sevenfold increase in the risk of experiencing hypertension while pregnant[190] and with increased risks of experiencing diabetes mellitus, pyelonephritis, prolonged labor, delivery of an infant with a birth weight of 4000 g or more, or even maternal death.[25,66,69,190] Clinically, women are usually considered to be high risk if prepregnancy weight is 20 percent or more above standard weight for height and age recommendations.[55] Inadequate weight gain during pregnancy has also been identified as a phenomenon among obese women. In a prospective study of 327 single gestation, diabetes free pregnancies which were 38−42 weeks in duration, pregnancy weight gain was compared with prepregnancy weight.[69] The incidence of inadequate weight gain, defined as a gain of 12 pounds or less, was found to be much higher in the obese women than in the nonobese women. Three out of four of the massively obese women (women whose weight prior to conception was more than 150 percent of the median weight for height according to Metropolitan Life Insurance tables) were found to have net weight losses during pregnancy.

Women who do not gain any weight during pregnancy and those who lose weight are at serious risk of delivering low birth weight infants.[55,127] These infants experience particularly high rates of prematurity and perinatal death. Disorders found most frequently in undernourished gestations include maternal anemia, amniotic fluid infection, placental growth retardation, abruptio placentae, and fetal congenital malformation. These poor outcomes are thought to be associated with undernourished gestation.[44,92,116,126,137,138]

It appears that adequate weight gain during pregnancy is a critical factor for women who are underweight at the time of conception. In a recent study of 654 pregnancies, it was found that prepregnant weight was not associated with the amount of weight gained during pregnancy and that more than 50 percent of the infants born to women who did not gain more than 9 k (just under 20 pounds) during pregnancy weighed less than 2500 g at birth.[22]

Acetonuria is found most frequently in undernourished gestations and has been associated with the undesirable pregnancy outcomes often experienced by these mothers.[55,135] There is recent evidence, however, which suggests that damage to infants who survive such gestations may not be as permanent as originally thought. Data from the Collaborative Perinatal Project of the National Institutte of Neurological and Communicative Disorders and Stroke were reanalyzed to determine if children had an excess of psychomotor or intelligence impairment when their mothers had acetonuria, weight loss, or low weight gain during pregnancy.[135] These data pertained to 53,518 pregnancies in the United States during the years 1959–1966. The children of these pregnancies had been followed prospectively from birth through 7 years of age, and a variety of mental and motor tests had been used to determine whether these maternal factors had any effect on child development. During this reanalysis the data were controlled for a number of non-nutritional factors that influence psychomotor and intellectual development such as major congenital anomalies, Down's syndrome, inborn errors of metabolism, head trauma during or after birth, lead intoxication during childhood, mental retardation in either parent, hyperthyroidism in the mother, convulsive disorders in the mother, maternal alcoholism, and maternal diabetes. No consistent impairments were found at any age among the remaining children studied.

Caloric restriction during pregnancy, a common practice, has not been based on scientific fact. At one time it was thought that dietary restrictions limiting the intake of calories would not only decrease the incidence of dystocia due to cephalopelvic disproportion, but would also reduce the incidence of toxemia. However, as mentioned earlier in this chapter, it has been determined that infant birth weight in uncomplicated pregnancies is related predominantly to maternal height and prepregnant weight.[132] Large amounts of maternal weight gain during pregnancy are often associated with delivery of large infants but, in most instances, the increase in infant size due to the amount of maternal weight gain is not sufficient to cause mechanical difficulties during labor and delivery.[55] Furthermore, a relationship has not been found between excessive maternal weight gain during pregnancy, based on the amount of fat accumulation, and toxemia of pregnancy.[151] Toxemia continues to be a prevalent disease of unknown etiology among certain groups of women. Although a variety of dietary approaches are used in the management of toxemia, caloric restriction is not appropriate.[32,55]

Dietary restriction of sodium during pregnancy has been a common clinical recommendation for many years.[32,55,203] It was thought that this restriction would be useful in reducing the risk of toxemia, however, it has never been shown that the use of sodium restriction or diuretics has any influence on the incidence of toxemia. It is now strongly recommended that sodium restriction no longer be encouraged during pregnancy. In light of recent research findings, there is realization that healthy pregnancy normally results in sodium retention.[145,151] This is necessary in order for the body to accommodate to tissue and fluid expansion. Dietary restriction of sodium can result in sodium depletion which, it appears, can stress the physiologic system of sodium conservation severely. This stress may result in reduced blood volume expansion and hyponatremia. Such circumstances place the mother and fetus at a particular disadvantage and unnecessary risk of poor pregnancy outcome.[203]

There is continuing controversy about whether women should receive vitamin and mineral supplements routinely during pregnancy.[196] Some clinicians feel that the profound conception-related physiologic changes which occur in the mother and the impact of these changes on measures of nutritional status are normal. They suggest that healthy pregnant women are in no need of nutritional supplements. Other clinicians believe that normal serum concentrations of essential nutrients cannot be achieved or maintained during pregnancy without an inordinate increase in total calories consumed and, therefore, that oral supplements must be offered. No one argues with the fact that increased levels of most nutrients are required during pregnancy. The problem is the difficulty in determining what total amounts of each nutrient for each 100 ml of blood are most conducive to optimal well-being for the mother and the fetus and what degree of variation can be allowed without compromising optimal health.

The Food and Nutrition Board of the National Research Council has published Recommended Dietary Allowances (RDA) for pregnancy.[57] These recommended allowances are based only on available evidence from metabolic balance studies and indirect estimates of appropriate nutrient values. Because values used as a basis for the development of recommendations are usually derived from experimental subjects, actual recommendations are often adjusted upward to assure that amounts will cover variations in individual needs within the general population.[196]

Caloric supplements, both with and without high levels of dietary protein, have been recommended for select population groups. For the most part, caloric supplementation has been associated with increased mean birth weight among infants born to mothers who received the supplements.[93,154] Limited evidence, however, suggests that there may be some adverse effects on fetal growth and development in instances where the mother consumed large amounts of protein during pregnancy as the result of dietary supplementation.[168] These adverse effects include prematurity, low birth weight, neonatal death, and inadequate psychological performance at one year of age. It appears that the controversy about routine supplementation during pregnancy will not be resolved until further research findings are available concerning maternal metabolism and its effects on nutritional requirements during pregnancy.

In summary, it is clear that women have increased nutritional needs during pregnancy that must be met to maintain good health and to support an intrauterine environment which will promote optimal fetal growth and development. Daily consumption of a well-balanced diet including a wide variety of foods is the preferred method of ensuring intake of all necessary nutrients whether or not additional supplements are taken for selected nutrients. Factors that place a woman at risk of undesirable pregnancy outcome, such as poverty, poor education, a deprived environment, or poor health, generally have operated over the span of her lifetime and most likely will continue. However, data regarding the effects of maternal height, prepregnancy weight, and maternal weight gain during pregnancy on the size of term infants indicate that improvement in maternal nutrition before and during pregnancy possibly can have positive effects on maternal and fetal health.

Informational Needs

Informational needs seem, to many women, to become paramount during pregnancy as these women are forced to struggle with new anxieties. The ways in which these needs are most frequently met include information from family members, friends, or health care professionals and through reading, class attendance for prenatal education and preparation for childbirth, or exposure to the public media. Nurse-midwives usually find that much of their time is spent in helping women obtain the information that will be helpful to them and their families during pregnancy and during the early months of parenthood.

Prenatal anxiety has been described as a composite of concerns that pregnant women have about themselves, their unborn children, and their anticipated roles as mothers.[177] Many studies have attempted to determine whether maternal anxiety during pregnancy is associated with undesirable pregnancy outcome and, more specifically, whether participation in prenatal classes is associated with the progress of labor or the condition of the infant at birth. In one recent study of 32 primiparous women who had been interviewed prenatally, it was found that those who expressed conflict in accepting pregnancy experienced significantly more anxiety during labor, as measured by plasma epinephrine levels, than the women having expressed no such conflict.[95] High epinephrine levels during labor had previously been associated with low Apgar scores at 1 and 5 minutes after birth[36,37] and, in this study,[95] were associated with abnormal fetal heart rate patterns during active labor as well as low Apgar scores. Several investigators have found participation in prenatal education classes to be associated with shorter lengths of labor, decreased perception of pain, decreased use of medication during labor, decreased use of obstetrical interventions, and better condition of the infant at birth.[16,36,37,95,188] Based on these findings it has been implied that education during pregnancy reduces maternal anxiety with resulting improvements in pregnancy outcome.

Care must be taken in generalizing the findings of these studies to individual pregnant women. Not only have inconsistent findings been reported as the result of similar studies,[17] but concern has been expressed about the insufficient attention given to certain methodologic errors which affect the validity of findings.[16] Several issues need to be addressed more carefully in these studies, including the use of random assignment to treatment or control groups, the possibility that women's reactions to interview or to labor may have been altered by the knowledge that they were being included in a study (Hawthorn effect), and the use of appropriate tests for measuring pain or anxiety. The need for much more thorough information about treatment procedures, such as content included in prenatal classes and its manner of presentation, is also apparent.

No one has documented any harmful effects on pregnancy or its outcome due to prenatal education or counseling. It is now recognized that behavior is an important determinant of pregnancy outcome since the health of the infant can be influenced by the degree to which its mother uses tobacco, alcohol, or drugs, and by the quality of her diet. Prenatal education has been strongly recommended as a most important mechanism for altering maternal behaviors which have potential for poor prognosis in the mother or the infant.[125] Suggestions for the type of information which should be provided to women and their families during pregnancy can be found in many publications, however, suggested content varies widely.

In 1978, due to the lack of documentation about information concerning childbirth offered to prospective parents during pregnancy, the Nurses' Association of the American College of Obstetricians and Gynecologists (NAACOG) developed an ad hoc committee to investigate the status of childbirth education in the United States.[170] Based on a stratified random sample of childbirth educators, 776 questionnaires were mailed to childbirth educators throughout the country. Although information from only 238 questionnaires was sufficiently complete to utilize in analyses of the data, the findings provide enlightening information about the importance of selected areas of content as perceived by the respondents. Table 3-8 shows the content areas included on the questionnaire in descending order according to the percentage of respondents who reported always including that particular area of content in a series of childbirth education sessions.

Table 3-8

NAACOG Questionnaire for Childbirth Educators: Information Offered to Parents During Pregnancy

Content	Respondents who always include content %
Signs and symptoms of labor	95.8
Stages and phases of labor and delivery	95.4
Admission to labor and delivery room	95.4
Episiotomies	91.2
Correct posture	87.8
Relationship of placenta, uterus, and fetus	87.0
Kegel exercise	87.0
Role of father	87.0
Finding a comfortable position	86.6
Medications used in labor and delivery	86.6
Transition breathing	86.6
Anatomical changes during pregnancy	85.3
Pelvic rock	85.3
Slow chest breathing	84.9
Expulsion breathing	84.9
Explanations of cesarean birth	84.9
Vaginal bleeding	84.5
Urinary frequency	83.6
Shallow breathing	83.2
Bonding/attachment	83.2
Selective muscular relaxation contraction/relaxation	80.3
Postpartum feelings of mother	80.3
Tailor sitting	79.4
Fetal positions/presentations	78.6
Breathing; relax on exhalation/work on inhalation	73.5
Emotional lability	73.5
Postpartum change in husband—wife relationship	71.8
Correction of "old wives' tales"	71.4
Comparison of client expectations of labor and delivery with reality	70.2
Parents' ambivalent feelings about newborn	68.9
Use of nonprescription drugs	68.1
Postcesarean-section care	68.1
Circulatory problems such as swelling, numbness, or dizziness	67.2
Comparison of client expectations for the new baby with reality	66.8
Edema of hands and face	66.8
Intercourse after delivery	65.5
Normal fetal development	64.3
Problems with sleep	63.0
Tailor press	62.2
Restricted freedom due to infant	61.8

Newborn's state of awareness	60.5
Conception and reproduction process	59.7
Working mothers and breastfeeding	59.2
Consequences of smoking	59.2
Father's conflicting feelings about newborn including jealousy	58.8
Circumcision	58.8
Headaches and/or seeing spots	58.0
Gastrointestinal discomfort	57.6
Alternative birthing methods	57.1
Skeletal problems/changes	55.5
Slow, deep abdominal breathing	55.0
Growth and development of infant	54.2
Urinary tract problems/changes	53.8
Consequences of alcohol consumption	52.9
Cord care	52.5
Leg lift	50.4
Continued use of previously prescribed drugs	50.4
Individual differences in infants	47.5
Large weight gain within short time	47.1
Strategies for remembering questions to ask their health care provider	46.6
Daily requirements of the basic food groups for pregnant mothers	46.2
Types of antenatal tests for fetal well-being	46.2
Hazards for the infant	45.8
Tailor reach	45.0
Methods of contraception	44.5
Daily requirements of the basic food groups for lactating mothers	43.7
Excessive nausea and vomiting	42.4
Caloric requirements for lactating mothers	41.6
Arm extension	41.6
Use of x-rays	41.6
Acceptable weight gain for low-, medium-, and high-weight mothers	39.5
Interpretation/discussion of instructions given by their health care provider	39.5
Expectations of work for pregnant mother	38.7
Caloric requirements for pregnant women	37.0
Signs of respiratory difficulty	37.0
Appropriate methods of seeking desired changes in the health care delivery system	36.6
Layette baby bath	35.7
Problems with siblings	35.7
Community resources available before and after delivery	34.9
Relationship with extended family	34.5
Menstrual cycle	32.4
Emotional development of the infant	31.5
Comparison of client expectations for birth control with reality	31.5
Social development of infant	29.8

(continued)

Table 3-8 (continued)

Content	Respondents who always include content %
Comfortable positions for intercourse	26.9
Possible complications due to German measles and sexually transmitted diseases	21.8
Birth defects	19.3
Child spacing expectations	16.8
Instructing siblings for attendance at birth	13.9
Personal finance and budgeting	11.8
Insurance: resources, desirability, and benefits	10.5
Special problems of single parent	10.1
Preparation for home birth	9.7
Special problems of handicapped parent	3.4

Adapted from Sasmor JL, Grossman E: Childbirth education in 1980. JOGN Nurs 10:155–160, 1981.

Respondents in the NAACOG study[170] were also asked to indicate which areas of content would be ideal. Little difference was noted between perceived ideal content and the content actually taught. A majority of the respondents felt that there is a need for national guidelines pertaining to the preparation of childbirth educators and the content of parents' childbirth education.

Evidence from a recent study of 91 pregnant women indicates that these women found information provided to them during pregnancy by their physicians to be most helpful.[153] They also found information obtained through hospital tours, reading, and prenatal classes to be helpful. The areas in which almost 50 percent of these women felt they received inadequate information from any source included adjusting to changes in marriage due to pregnancy, preparing other children for the new baby, adjusting sexual activity to pregnancy, and helping the baby's father prepare for parenthood. Many women have reported that they received limited information, or even conflicting advice, about alcohol consumption, cigarette smoking, sexuality, or nutrition during pregnancy. This has occurred in spite of the fact that all of these potential areas of concern are known to be important influences on the physiologic and psychosocial well-being of the mother and the fetus.

The harmful effects of maternal alcoholism during pregnancy on growth and development of the offspring have been well documented.[54] Even one ounce of absolute alcohol daily during pregnancy has been associated with significant reductions in newborn birth weight.[103] No level of alcohol ingestion is known to be safe during pregnancy[122,179] yet, in a recent survey of 189 women who were each 8 months pregnant, 43 percent indicated that they did not receive any information about drinking alcoholic beverages during pregnancy.[38] Of the women who received some information about consumption of alcohol during pregnancy, 64 percent were told that drinking in moderation is permissible.

An association between smoking during pregnancy and fetal growth retardation, resulting in high rates of fetal loss or low birth weight infants, has also been well documented.[5,39,70,127,131,146] In the same survey of 189 pregnant women mentioned above,[38] 32 percent indicated that they did not receive any information about smoking during pregnancy. Of the women who did receive some information about smoking during pregnancy, however, only 10 percent were told that some smoking is permissible.

Pregnancy is a time of maturational crisis with sexually related changes in roles, functions, and expectations between a man and a woman.[46,99] The stress resulting from these changes has potential for causing major disruptions in a marital relationship.[110] Although sexual counseling during pregnancy is thought to be beneficial in helping couples cope effectively with such stress,[99] there is evidence that as many as two out of three women may not receive the advice they need from health care professionals.[153,160] It is not known whether this lack of sexual counseling during pregnancy is due to health care professionals' personal discomfort in discussing sexual issues or to inconsistent recommendations in the literature.

Until recently, most physicians recommended abstinence from intercourse for 6 weeks before the anticipated date of delivery, and for 6 weeks after delivery.[99] This recommendation was based on tradition, passed on by obstetricians from generation to generation, rather than on scientific fact. The findings vary even in recent scientific reports on the effects of coitus during the latter part of pregnancy on pregnancy outcome. Several investigators have reported increased risks of ruptured membranes and amniotic fluid infections as a result of coitus late in pregnancy[63,128] while others have concluded that coitus late in pregnancy has no causal relationship to these complications.[110,128,129,157]

To assist in clarifying whether a relationship exists between coitus and amniotic fluid infection, data from 28,886 single-gestation pregnancies were analyzed thoroughly. These pregnancies resulted in delivery during the years 1959–1966, and the placentas had been saved for pathologic examination as part of the United States Collaborative Perinatal Project.[143] It was found that amniotic fluid infection occurred at a frequency of 156/1000 births when the mothers reported having had coitus more than once each week during the month prior to delivery and at a frequency of 117/1000 births to mothers who reported having had no coitus during the month prior to delivery.[129] Among infected infants, 11 percent of those born to mothers with reported coitus died while 2.4 percent of those born to mothers with reported abstinence died. The frequency of low Apgar scores, neonatal respiratory distress, and hyperbilirubinemia was also found to be two times higher among infants from coitus births than among infants from births preceded by one month of abstinence.

Associations between coitus and amniotic fluid infections, low Apgar scores, neonatal respiratory distress, and hyperbilirubinemia were more notable in infants born before term than in those of term gestations. These findings indicate only that there may be a relationship between coitus and amniotic fluid infections since the study was done retrospectively, subjects were not randomized into treatment and control groups, and there was limited control over collection of data.[79] The investigator did not recommend abstinence from intercourse late in pregnancy except in women with a poor reproductive history or with clinically diagnosed premature ripening of the cervix.[129] It has also been suggested that abstinence be adhered to in the presence of ruptured membranes, uterine bleeding, or pain associated with coitus.[99]

Although a well-balanced diet consisting of a wide variety of foods is known to be important during pregnancy, there are many factors affecting the nutrients any particular woman consumes. Health behaviors often are based on individual feelings and beliefs rather than on facts[164] so nutritional counseling must be tailored to meet the needs of each individual woman. Particular emphasis should be given to positively reinforcing good eating habits and continuing evaluation of nutritional status. Nutrition counseling must take into account not only actual consumption of calories and nutrients, but also individual and cultural food preferences and available resources for purchasing foods.

Individual food habits vary widely within each cultural or ethnic group but nutrient needs can be met by eating appropriate combinations of a variety of foods preferred by each group. Experienced clinicians, however, have noted that variations in diet within each of these groups often result in less than optimal nutrition during pregnancy. Findings reported by these clinicians include the following:[55,79,202]

1. Black women tend to fry many foods, using fats such as salt pork, lard, and fat back extensively, and to have a high carbohydrate intake. Vegetables are often overcooked and intake of citrus fruits, enriched breads, or milk is frequently insufficient.

2. Spanish-American or Mexican women tend to use lard and sugar in excessive amounts while intakes of meat, vegetables, and milk are often limited.

3. Rice is a staple food among oriental women and should be of an enriched variety. Large assortments of fruits and vegetables are usually eaten but meats and fish are usually eaten only in small quantities. Milk is seldom used.

4. Women of American Indian heritage frequently have diets which are inadequate in all nutrients due to poverty. Alcoholism, obesity, dental caries, and iron deficiency anemia are not uncommon among these women.

It seems that variations in economic status would be associated with variations in cultural or ethnic food habits.

Vegetarian diets are becoming more common in the United States for a variety of socioeconomic, cultural, religious, and personal reasons.[55] In order to ensure an adequate diet during pregnancy, milk, milk products, and eggs should be used for intake of vitamin B_{12}, vitamin D, riboflavin, calcium, and iron, protein, and calories. Vegetarian diets should include generous amounts of legumes, nuts, and meat analogues made from wheat and soy products.

The foods pregnant women most need, such as fresh or frozen foods containing large amounts of protein, vitamins, and minerals, are frequently the most expensive.[55] Good compromises are nonfat dry milk, cheese, which is high in nutrition with no waste, and fish, which is high in protein and relatively inexpensive.

All pregnancy counseling should be individualized to best meet the needs of each woman and her family. Information about certain danger signs of pregnancy, including persistent nausea and vomiting, headache and dizziness, puffiness of the face and hands, leakage of fluid from the vagina, and vaginal bleeding, should be reviewed periodically so that each mother will understand the importance of reporting them. Only when the pregnant woman promptly reports symptoms can impending problems be alleviated as soon and as much as possible.

Unique Needs

Each pregnant woman has unique needs. Women in a variety of circumstances, including those having a first child (particularly at an older age), those who already have several children, those with negative attitudes about pregnancy or with an unwanted pregnancy, adolescents, those who work outside of the home during pregnancy, and those representing certain cultural and ethnic groups all have some common and predictable needs and concerns.

First child

The woman expecting her first child is faced with many unknowns. Transition to the responsibilities of parenthood usually requires major changes in one's thinking and life-style.[165] As the time for labor and delivery approaches, there is usually a heightened sense of vulnerability, or a sense of impending disaster such as loss of control over one's body due to pain and fatigue, loss of bodily intactness, and loss of the baby.[189]

First child at an older age

More and more women are choosing to have their first babies while in their thirties.[78] In 1970 the rate of first births to women between 30 and 34 years of age was 7.3/1000 live births. By 1976 the rate of first births had increased to almost 9/1000 live births to women between 30 and 34 years of age in the United States.[141] The needs of these women vary according to individual circumstances. A woman may have been attempting to become pregnant for many years. Pregnancy will be considered a miracle by some women but regretted by others. The woman who has her first child while in her thirties most typically has delayed childbearing for a career and a certain lifestyle.[141] Maturity seems to give many women an advantage in assuming the responsibilities of parenthood, however, some women consider pregnancy an interruption in attaining career goals or in maintaining a desired lifestyle. Some women also fear they will be too old to relate normally to a child.[78]

Pregnancy for Women with Several Children

Women who already have several children may have mixed emotions during pregnancy even if the pregnancy was planned. A recent report about the adaptation of a multigravida to pregnancy suggests that mothers must have quite a bit of knowledge about child development, nurturance and protection, the culinary and domestic arts, economics, planning, and group dynamics, as well as skill in using this knowledge.[161] Most women have had little or no formal education in any of these areas.

Negative Attitudes Toward Pregnancy

Data from a prospective study of 8000 gravidas indicate that women with negative attitudes toward pregnancy experience significantly more psychological stress than women with strongly favorable or even ambivalent attitudes toward pregnancy.[91] The measures of psychological stress used in this study—the number of outpatient visits to a physician during pregnancy for accidental injury and three or more doses of analgesia for pain during labor—are open to question since they could be attributable to many factors.

Unwanted Pregnancy

There is some evidence indicating that children from unwanted pregnancies experience more problems during childhood than children from wanted pregnancies.[21] A recent study was conducted to identify differences in the number and types of problems children experienced according to whether the pregnancy was wanted or unwanted initially. Data were obtained from hospital delivery, school, and public records for 122 pairs of children assigned to study and control groups. Children in the study group had been born to women whose applications for a legal abortion in 1960 were denied by the National Board of Health and Welfare in Great Britain. Children in the control group were matched, on a one-to-one basis, with children in the study group according to immediate subsequent delivery in the same delivery ward, sex, maternal age, maternal parity, and maternal social class. The initially unwanted children were found to experience more insecurities during childhood, to perform more poorly in school, to display more psychosomatic symptoms, to be registered with social and welfare authorities more often, to need psychiatric treatment more often, and to experience parental divorce more frequently than the initially wanted children.

Adolescent Pregnancy

Adolescents who become pregnant face a multitude of problems and adolescent pregnancy is not disappearing as a phenomenon in the United States. During 1978 approximately 1,142,000 pregnancies among females less than 20 years old were terminated.[186] Only about one in six of these pregnancies resulted in a birth that had been conceived after marriage and an additional 10 percent resulted in births that were premaritally conceived but legitimized by marriage before delivery. Twenty-two percent of the births were illegitimate. About 38 percent of these pregnancies were terminated with an elective abortion and another 13 percent resulted in spontaneous miscarriage.

The proportion of all adolescent girls in the United States who become pregnant each year is gradually increasing. About 10 percent of these girls became pregnant in 1973 and 11 percent became pregnant in 1978.[186] Among those girls reported to be sexually active, however, the pregnancy rate declined from 27 percent in 1973 to 23 percent in 1978. This decreased pregnancy rate among sexually active adolescent girls is thought to be related to greater and more consistent use of contraceptives by these girls.[58,186,208,210] Yet, it has been estimated that one-fourth of all American adolescent girls at this point in time will have been pregnant at least once by the time they reach 19 years of age.[73,186]

Risks of developing medical complications such as anemia or toxemia during pregnancy are much higher for adolescents than for women in their twenties, particularly when the adolescents are less than 16 years old.[147,185] There are also increased risks of preterm delivery, and of maternal, fetal, neonatal, and postneonatal mortality.[185,209] The risk of delivering a low birth weight baby, or one with a birth weight of less than 2500 g, seems to increase proportionally as the age of the mother decreases.[201] Many children born to adolescent mothers encounter developmental problems during childhood which are thought to be due primarily to having been born at a low birth weight. These undesirable maternal and infant outcomes were once thought to be a function of maternal age but are now believed to be more directly related to low socioeconomic status and inadequate prenatal care.[88]

Several authors continue to debate about whether young adolescent mothers have some biologic predisposition to bear smaller infants than older mothers (even than older adolescent mothers) or whether increased rates of low birth weight births to young adolescent mothers are due to inadequate prenatal care. A more focused debate about why many adolescent mothers bear low birth weight babies is whether or not the growth needs of young mothers for available nutrients may compete with the growth needs of their fetuses for nutrients.[111] Information pertaining to 13,830 babies and their mothers was analyzed to determine whether younger mothers had lower weight babies at term than older mothers when the effects of maternal prepregnancy body size, according to height and weight, and weight gain during pregnancy were controlled for in analysis of the data.[132] These data had been obtained for the Collaborative Perinatal Project[143] but pertained only to black women between the ages of 10 and 32 years who had single gestations that terminated at 38−44 weeks of pregnancy. Subjects from the Collaborative Perinatal Project who exhibited factors that could affect fetal growth, such as diabetes mellitus, placenta previa, polyhydramnios, or congenital malformation, were excluded from this analysis. Results of the analysis indicated that the mothers who were between 10 and 16 years old had significantly smaller babies at term than the older mothers. In addition, 5 percent of the mothers who were between 10 and 14 years old were found to have 2+ or greater urinary acetone while only 2 percent of the mothers between 17 and 30 years of age were found to have 2+ or greater acetonuria. Although the reasons do not seem to be fully understood, acetonuria has been shown to be highly associated with perinatal death, particularly in undernourished pregnancies. Among this particular group of babies, fetal and neonatal deaths were 56 percent more frequent when mothers had 2+ or greater urinary acetone during pregnancy than when the mothers had no acetonuria. No information was available on what effects pregnancy may have had, if any, on growth of the very young mothers.[207]

Not only does pregnancy during adolescence disrupt the life of an immature girl, but the repercussions most likely will have long-lasting effects on her entire life. Although an adolescent may have reached a point of biologic maturity appropriate for childbearing, it is not the biologic aspect of age that is most important in our contemporary American society.[123] Mothers, as well as fathers, need sufficient maturity to support and raise a family in a complex society if they are going to have successful, or relatively problem-free, lives. It has been well documented that, in general, adolescent mothers acquire less education, are more often limited to less prestigious and low-paying jobs, have a higher parity which includes unintended and unwanted pregnancies, and have marital relationships that are less stable than their contemporaries.[26,52,147,186,191] Adolescent mothers also continue to be the subject of moral judgment, as many people openly express concern about the moral attitudes and behaviors of the individuals involved in adolescent pregnancy, particularly in cases of out-of-wedlock pregnancy.[144]

Although about two-thirds of the births to unmarried adolescents are unintended, essentially all black girls and about 90 percent of all white girls keep their babies.[186] Findings from a prospective study of 481 female and 249 male, urban, black youths between the ages of 13 and 18 years indicate that the terms "unintended" and "unwanted" are not necesssarily synonymous.[58,88] Only 35 percent of the subjects indicated, on a self-administered questionnaire, that having a baby "now" would make life "worse" or "ruined" while 26 percent of them indicated that they hoped to be pregnant, or have a pregnant partner, before the age of 20 years. No significant differences were found between the responses from female and male subjects.

About 1.3 million children in the United States live with 1.1 million adolescent mothers and more than 50 percent of these mothers are unmarried.[186] Adolescent parenthood places substantial demands on society since about one-half of the monies of the Aid to Families with Dependent Children (AFDC) program go to households containing women who had their first children while they were adolescents.[88] Mean family incomes for women who first gave birth during adolescence have been reported to be equal to about one-half of those for mothers who first gave birth during their twenties. Since welfare benefits increase with each child, some adolescents with two or more children find it impossible, due to limited education and experience, to secure employment that will result in an income greater than that received through public assistance.[191]

Pregnant adolescents tend to receive less prenatal care than older women. This may be due to delays in seeking care because of many insecurities and even fright. Most pregnant adolescents, especially the unmarried, have fears about confirming their pregnancy, about the reactions of their parents, and about the cost of medical care.[185] Many of them do not even know where to go to obtain prenatal care.

There is some evidence that comprehensive prenatal care services for pregnant adolescents may be associated with reduced risks of undesirable pregnancy outcome.[2,73,147,185] These services should include high-quality assessment and management of pregnancy, educational services, social services, and family counseling. Day-care services, job counseling, and community education have also been recommended as useful mechanisms for alleviating some of the major problems associated with adolescent pregnancy.[185] The recent report of the Select Panel for the Promotion of Child Health,[20] states that the importance of preventive care has been demonstrated in various well-controlled studies to be a most valuable factor in promoting child health. It also states that, although the precise components of prenatal care leading to dramatic differences in reproductive outcome have not been clearly identified, it is highly likely that counseling of expectant mothers about potential problems is a major contributor to the effectiveness of prenatal care.

Employment during Pregnancy

Many women must work outside the home while pregnant and others choose to do so. The potential hazards involved—including exposure to toxic chemicals, excessive noise, radiation, and stress, among other things,—sometimes lead to degenerative disease, birth defects, or genetic changes that may be transmitted to future generations.[73,205] Some of these hazards also are associated with increased frequencies of stillbirths, spontaneous abortions, reduced fertility, and sterility.

Women predominate in many low-paying occupations where the risks of exposure to health and safety hazards are high.[122] About three-fourths of the workers employed in hospital and health care settings are female. Exposure to infectious diseases, anesthetic gases, radiation, and accidental injury is not uncommon in these settings.[73,122] More than 90 percent of all hairdressers, or beauticians, are female and many of the aerosol sprays and hair dyes they are exposed to daily are potentially carcinogenic. Clerical workers, 80 percent of whom are female, are exposed not only to injuries from poorly designed equipment and to excessive sitting, but also are exposed to noise and chemicals from office machines.[178] Almost two-thirds of the workers in textile plants and laundry or dry cleaning establishments are female.[122,178] These workers are exposed to high levels of certain dusts and chemicals with degenerative and carcinogenic potential.

The stress encountered by many women who work during pregnancy is at least two-fold. Most women in the United States are employed in low-paying and low-prestige jobs where repetitive work and limited opportunity for advancement prevail.[122,178] These conditions are frequently found to be stressful. In addition, women who work continue to be held responsible for almost all housekeeping and childrearing activities.[205] It has been estimated that women employed outside of the home spend an average of 80 hours each week doing employment and household work while their husbands do an average of 50 hours of work during each week.[178] Parents have responsibility for child care 24 hours each day and this responsibility is most frequently that of the woman.

Cultural and Ethnic Considerations

Cultural and ethnic differences in women's life-styles, dietary patterns or habits, and perceptions about their pregnancies should also be considered when planning management of pregnancy health care.[55,67,68] The caregiver must be aware of the culturally patterned beliefs and behaviors of the patient if recommendations and guidance are to be effective.[65,80] When the caregiver does not communicate clearly, a patient is likely to ignore professional recommendations and adhere to familiar methods for resolving problems or discomforts. Effective counseling can best be accomplished through careful listening and determination of whether personal practices are beneficial, harmful, or will have an uncertain impact on the health of the mother or fetus.

Selecting the Place of Birth

Each woman should make plans prenatally for the delivery setting. Since the late 1930s most women in the United States have automatically planned to have physicians assist them with delivery within traditional hospital maternity care settings. In 1977 more than 98 percent of the 3,326,632 births in that year were reportedly conducted in this manner.[198] Just over one percent of these births were reported to have occurred outside of hospital settings and without the assistance of a physician. Some of these births were likely the result of insufficient time to get to a hospital prior to delivery.

During the 1970s many technologic advances were made in the ability to monitor fetal health status during labor. These technologic advances were accompanied by major increases in the numbers of instrument-assisted and cesarean section deliveries.[110] In 1968 only 5 percent of all births in the United States were the result of cesarean sections while in 1977 the rate of cesarean section births had increased to 12.8 percent. Risk of maternal death after cesarean section has been estimated to be three times higher than that for women who deliver vaginally[12] and the morbidity associated with abdominal surgery is well known. Data pertaining to survival benefits for infants as the result of intensive fetal monitoring are, at best, inconsistent.

Many parents are questioning the need for intensive use of medications and invasive procedures during labor and delivery.[98] This has resulted in a desire for active involvement in decisions about the setting for delivery, the health care provider, and the techniques or modalities of care management.[3] Some parents have even elected to disregard the traditional health care system entirely.

Increasing consumer demands for alternative birthing opportunities have raised questions about the safety of alternative settings, whether in the hospital or outside of the hospital, the preparation and role of various care providers, the appropriateness and use of certain chemical, mechanical, electronic, or surgical intervention modalities, the degree of family involvement in the process of labor and delivery, and the effectiveness of mechanisms for assessment of risk status for the mother or the fetus.[3] Data from studies conducted by proponents of home birth and out-of-hospital birthing centers indicate that these settings provide safe alternatives for many pregnant women.[18,103,104,114,202] Others argue, however, that as many as one out of four women who become high-risk intrapartally could not have been identified prenatally on the basis of high-risk criteria presently being used to screen for potential problems.[7,76,174] Limited evidence is available which suggests that some mothers-to-be will elect to deliver in an in-hospital birthing room, as opposed to at home, if such an option is offered to them.[8,87]

Due to the multitude of questions that health care consumers and professionals have raised about the appropriateness of various birthing options, the American Public Health Association (APHA) has taken the position that all women should have access to settings that endorse the philosophy of family-centered maternity care,[3] as defined by the Interprofessional Task Force on Health Care of Women and Children in 1978.[47] This task force consisted of representatives from the American Academy of Pediatrics, the American College of Nurse-Midwives, the American College of Obstetricians and Gynecologists, the American Nurses' Association, and the Nurses' Association of the American College of Obstetricians and Gynecologists. Family-centered maternity care, as interpreted in the APHA's position statement on alternatives in maternity care, provides for full recognition of human rights with particular attention to informed consent, modification of hospital environments to meet the needs of both high-risk and low-risk mothers, and encouragement of increased family participation in birthing experiences according to the desires of individual families and as consistent with optimal maternal and newborn safety. In order to most effectively meet the needs of each childbearing family, the APHA recommended that there be further development and support of a maternity health care team that includes certified nurse-midwives, nurse practitioners, social workers, and nutritionists, and physicians, and that all members of the maternity health care team should conduct reviews of the quality of care in traditional and alternative settings. The APHA further recommended research to validate assessment measures for predicting potential maternal and fetal risk, for identifying short-term and long-term effects of pregnancy-related drugs and procedures on the mother and the newborn, and for evaluating the effectiveness of varying practices used to support parent—child attachment.

In spite of increasing demands for and use of alternative birthing options, many women who express interest in the use of certain alternatives encounter negative reactions from physician and nurse care providers.[23] The emphasis on developing technologies and practices in obstetrical management during the past 50 years has been on increasing levels of maternal and fetal safety, and most professionals who provide maternity care services in the United States were educated during this era. As a result, many of these professionals are unable to comprehend the importance of requests for low-intervention and alternative birthing experiences because they are seen only as compromises to the margin of safety established in obstetrical practice.

Many care providers also seem to believe that the demands for low-intervention and alternative birthing experiences are expressed by only a few individuals who are from young, uneducated, counterculture groups.[15] Data from studies of parents who elected to have home births indicate that this is not true. The demographic profiles of parents studied indicate that these parents were quite average representatives of the American childbearing population.[15,72] In one study of 300 sets of parents residing in California who elected to have home births, it was found that 90 percent of the time the couple lived in a single-family dwelling, the father of the baby was gainfully employed, the couple owned one or two cars, the family was not receiving welfare payments, and the parents were not members of an ethnic minority group.[72] The investigator for this particular study felt that these parents were very willing and able to assume personal responsibility for making critical decisions in their lives.

SUMMARY

Good communication and understanding are needed between prospective parents and their health care providers if optimal safety and satisfaction during childbirth are to be realized. Careful listening and observation by the nurse-midwife, coupled with clear and relevant explanations, can facilitate these processes. It seems only logical that compliance with recommendations for health maintenance or improvement would be best when these recommendations are understood and have been tailored to meet the needs of individuals and their families.

REFERENCES

1. Aase JM: Environmental causes of birth defects. Cont Educ Fam Phys 3(9):39—46, 1975
2. Adams C: Nurse-midwifery management of health care for pregnant adolescents. Issues Health Care Wom 2(2):53—61, 1980

3. American Public Health Association, Position Paper 7924: Alternatives in maternity care. Am J Public Health 70:310−312, 1980

4. Antonov AN: Children born during the siege of Leningrad in 1942. J Pediatr 30:250−259, 1947

5. A Report of the Surgeon General. Washington, D.C., DHEW Publication No. (PHS) 79-50066, 1979

6. Armstrong RJ: A Study of Infant Mortality from Linked Records: by Birth Weight, Period of Gestation, and Other Variables, United States, 1960 Live-Birth Cohort. Washington, D.C., Vital and Health Statistics, Series 20, No. 12, 1972

7. Aubry RH, Pennington JC: Identification and evaluation of high-risk pregnancy: the perinatal concept. Clin Obstet Gynecol 16:3−27, 1973

8. Averitt SS: Adapting the birthing center concept to a traditional hospital setting. JOGN Nurs 9:103−106, 1980

9. Baird D: The Galton lecture 1970: the obstetrician and society. J Biosoc Sci 3(suppl 3):93−111, 1971

10. Baker CE: Physicians' Desk Reference (ed 35). Oradell, New Jersey, Medical Economics Company, 1981

11. Balfour MI: Supplementary feeding in pregnancy. Lancet 1:208−211, 1944

12. Banta D, Thacker S: Costs and Benefits of Electronic Fetal Monitoring: A review of the Literature. Washington, D.C., DHEW Publication No. (PHS) 79-3245, 1979

13. Barclay RL, Barclay ML: Prenatal anxiety [letter]. Am J Obstet Gynecol 136:1084−1085, 1980

14. Barden TP: Prenatal care, in Romney SL, Gray MJ, Little AB, et al (eds): The Health Care of Women (ed 2). New York, McGraw-Hill Book Co, 1981, pp 595−659

15. Bauwens E, Anderson S: Home births: a reaction to hospital environmental stressors, in Bauwens EE (ed): The Anthropology of Health. St. Louis, CV Mosby Co, 1978, pp 56−60

16. Beck NC, Hall D: Natural childbirth: a review and analysis. Obstet Gynecol 52:371−379, 1978

17. Beck NC, Siegel LJ, Davidson NP, et al: The prediction of pregnancy outcome: maternal preparation, anxiety and attitudinal sets. J Psychosom Res 24:343−351, 1980

18. Bennetts AB: Out-of-Hospital Childbearing Centers in the United States. Doctoral dissertation, University of Texas Health Science Center at Houston, 1981

19. Berman ML: Gestational trophoblastic disease, in Romney SL, Gray MJ, Little AB, et al (eds): The Health Care of Women (ed 2). New York, Mcgraw-Hill Book Co, 1981, pp 1093−1102

20. Better Health for Our Children: A National Strategy. Volume I. Major Findings and Recommendations. Washington, D.C., DHHS (PHS) Publication No. 79-55071, 1981

21. Blomberg S: Influence of maternal distress during pregnancy on postnatal development. Acta Psychiatr Scand 62:405−417, 1980

22. Brown JE, Jacobson HN, Askue LH, et al: Influence of pregnancy weight gain on size of infants born to underweight women. Obstet Gynecol 57:13−17, 1981

23. Burchell RC, Gunn J: The new birth experience. JOGN Nurs 9:250−252, 1980

24. Burke BS, Beal VA, Kirkwood SB, et al: The influence of nutrition upon the condition of the infant at birth. J Nutr 26:569−583, 1943

25. Calandra C, Abell DA, Beischer NA: Maternal obesity in pregnancy. Obstet Gynecol 57:8−12, 1981

26. Card JJ, Wise LL: Teenage mothers and teenage fathers: the impact of early childbearing on the parents' personal and professional lives. Fam Plann Perspect 10:199−205, 1978

27. Chase HC: A Study of Infant Mortality from Linked Records: Comparison of Neonatal Mortality from Two Cohort Studies, United States. Washington, D.C., Vital and Health Statistics, Series 20, No. 13, 1972

28. Chase HC, Byrnes ME: Trends in ''Prematurity'', United States: 1950−67. Washington, D.C., Vital and Health Statistics, Series 3, No. 15, 1972

29. Chase HC: A study of risks, medical care, and infant mortality. Am J Public Health 63:1−56, 1973 Supplement

30. Check WA: Diminishing hazards of diabetic pregnancies. JAMA 244:1301−1302, 1307, 1980

31. Chesley LC: Hypertension in pregnancy: definitions, familial factor, and remote prognosis. Kidney Int 18:234−40, 1980

32. Chez RA: Nutrition and reproduction, in Romney SL, Gray MJ, Little AB, et al (eds): The Health Care of Women (ed 2). New York, McGraw-Hill Book Co, 1981, pp 211−226

33. Colman AD, Colman LL: Pregnancy as an altered state of consciousness. Birth Fam J 1:7, 1974

34. Cossart YE: The outcome of hepatitis B virus infection in pregnancy. Postgrad Med J 53:610−613, 1977

35. Coustan DR: Recent advances in the management of diabetic pregnant women. Clin Perinatol 7:299−311, 1980

36. Crandon AJ: Maternal anxiety and neonatal well-being J Psychosom Res 23:113−115, 1979

37. Crandon AJ: Maternal anxiety and obstetric complications. J Psychosom Res 23:109−111, 1979

38. Davidson S: Smoking and alcohol consumption: advice given by health care professionals. JOGN Nurs 10:256−258, 1981

39. Deibel P: Effects of cigarette smoking on maternal nutrition and the fetus. JOGN Nurs 9:333−336, 1980

40. Denniss RG: Vaginal bleeding. Nurs Times 73:998−1000, 1977

41. Disaia PJ: The cervix, in Romney SL, Gray MJ, Little AB, et al (eds): The Health Care of Women (ed 2). New York, McGraw-Hill Book Co, 1981, pp 1017−1052

42. Eastman NJ, Jackson E: Weight relationships in pregnancy. I. The bearing of maternal weight gain and pre-pregnancy weight on birth weight in full term pregnancies. Obstet Gynecol Surv 23:1003−1025, 1968

43. Ebbs JH, Tisdall FF, Scott WA: The influence of prenatal diet on the mother and the child. Milbank Mem Fund Q 20:35−40, 1942

44. Edwards LE, Alton IR, Barrada MI, et al: Pregnancy in the underweight woman: course, outcome, and growth patterns of the infant. Am J Obstet Gynecol 135:297−302, 1979

45. Edwards MS: Venereal herpes: a nursing overview. J Obstet Gynecol Nurs 7(5):7−15, 1978
46. Ellis DJ: Sexual needs and concerns of expectant parents. JOGN Nurs 9:306−308, 1980
47. Family Centered Maternity Care/Newborn Care in Hospitals. Interprofessional Task Force on Health Care of Women and Children (AAP,ACNM,ACOG,AN-A,NAACOG), 1978
48. Fredrick J, Adelstein P: Influence of pregnancy spacing on outcome of pregnancy. Br Med J 4:753−756, 1973
49. Finlayson A: Social networks as coping resources. Soc Sci Med 10:97−103, 1976
50. Fletcher JC: The fetus as patient: ethical issues [editorial]. JAMA 246:772−773, 1981
51. Florman AL, Gershon AA, Blackett PR, et al: Intrauterine infection with herpes simplex virus. Resultant congenital malformations. JAMA 225:129−132, 1973
52. Fogel CI: Adolescent pregnancy, in Fogel CI, Woods NF (eds): Health Care of Women. St. Louis, CV Mosby Co, 1981, pp 192−208
53. Fogel CI: Assessment of health status, in Fogel CI, Woods NF (eds): Health Care of Women. St. Louis, CV Mosby Co, 1981, pp 118−136
54. Fogel CI: High-risk pregnancy, in Fogel CI, Woods NF (eds): Health Care of Women. St. Louis, CV Mosby Co, 1981, pp 171−191
55. Fogel CI: Nutrition, in Fogel CI, Woods NF (eds): Health Care of Women. St. Louis, CV Mosby Co, 1981, pp 450−483
56. Fogel CI: The gynecologic triad: discharge, pain, and bleeding, in Fogel CI, Woods NF (eds): Health Care of Women. St. Louis, CV Mosby Co, 1981, pp 220−256
57. Food and Nutrition Board, Recommended Daily Dietary Allowances. Washington, D.C., National Academy of Sciences—National Research Council, 1974
58. Forrest JD, Hermalin AI, Henshaw SK: The impact of family planning clinic programs on adolescent pregnancy. Fam Plann Perspect 13:109−116, 1981
59. Freeman EW, Rickels K, Huggins GR, et al: Adolescent contraceptive use: comparisons of male and female attitudes and information. Am J Public Health 70:790−797, 1980
60. Galperin-Lemaitre H, Kirsh-Volders M, Levi S: Fragmentation of purified mammalian DNA molecules by ultrasound below human therapeutic doses. Humangenetik 29:61−66, 1975
61. Gardner HL, Dukes CD: *Haemophilus vaginalis vaginitis.* Am J Obstet Gynecol 69:962−976, 1955
62. Gerbie AB, Fiddler MB, Nadler HL: Genetic counseling, in Romney SL, Gray MJ, Little AB, et al (eds): The Health Care of Women (ed 2). New York, McGraw-Hill Book Co, 1981, pp 805−815
63. Goodlin R, Keller D, Raffin M: Orgasm during late pregnancy. Obstet Gynecol 38:916−920, 1971
64. Gormican A, Valentine J, Satter E: Relationships of maternal weight gain, prepregnancy weight, and infant birthweight. Interaction of weight factors in pregnancy. J Am Diet Assoc 77:662−667, 1980
65. Griffith S: Childbearing and the concept of culture. JOGN Nurs 11:181−184, 1982

66. Gross T, Sokol RJ, King KC: Obesity in pregnancy: risks and outcome. Obstet Gynecol 56:446—450, 1980

67. Harris R: Cultural differences in body perception during pregnancy. Br J Med Psychol 52:347—352, 1979

68. Harris R, Good R, Linn MW, et al: Attitudes and perceptions of perinatal concepts during pregnancy in women from three cultures. J Clin Psychol 37:477—483, 1981

69. Harrison GG, Udall JN, Morrow G: Maternal obesity, weight gain in pregnancy, and infant birth weight. Am J Obstet Gynecol 136:411—412, 1980

70. Haworth JC, Ellestad-Sayed JJ, King J, et al: Relation of maternal cigarette smoking, obesity, and energy consumption to infant size. Am J Obstet Gynecol 138:1185—1189, 1980

71. Hayashi T: Diseases specific to pregnancy, in Romney SL, Gray MJ, Little AB, et al (eds): The Health Care of Women (ed 2). New York, McGraw-Hill Book Co, 1981, pp 661—695

72. Hazell L: A study of 300 elective home births. Birth Fam J 2:11—18, 1975

73. Healthy People: The Surgeon General's Report on Health Promotion and Disease Prevention. Washington, D.C., DHEW Publication No. (PHS) 79-55071, 1979

74. Henry G, Robinson A: Changing placental appearance on ultrasound prior to genetic amniocentesis. Am J Hum Genet 31:123A, 1979

75. Hildebrant RJ, Sever JL, Margileth AM, et al: Cytomegalovirus in the normal pregnant female. Am J Obstet Gynecol 98:1125—1128, 1967

76. Hobel CJ, Hyvarinen MA, Okada DM, et al: Prenatal and intrapartum high-risk screening. Am J Obstet Gynecol 117:1—9, 1973

77. Holder WR, Knox JM: Syphilis in pregnancy. Med Clin North Am 56:1151—1160, 1972

78. Howley C: The older primipara. Implications for nurses. JOGN Nurs 10:182—185, 1981

79. Jensen MD, Benson RC, Bobak IM: Maternity Care. The Nurse and the Family. St. Louis, CV Mosby Co, 1981

80. Johnston M: Cultural variations in professional and parenting patterns. JOGN Nurs 9:9—13, 1980

81. Kaback MM: Prenatal diagnosis of hereditary disease and congenital defects. Pediatr Ann 10(2):22—37, 1981

82. Kaiser IH: Physiologic changes in the pregnant woman, in Romney SL, Gray MJ, Little AB, et al (eds): The Health Care of Women (ed 2). New York, McGraw-Hill Book Co, 1981, pp 163—180

83. Karp LE: Prenatal diagnosis: too little control (Part I) [editorial]. Am J Med Genet 6:265—267, 1980

84. Karp LE: Prenatal diagnosis: too little control (Part II) [editorial]. Am J Med Genet 7:1—3, 1980

85. Kaufman RH, Gardner HL: Diseases of the vulva and vagina, in Romney SL, Gray MJ, Little AB, et al (eds): The Health Care of Women (ed 2). New York, McGraw-Hill Book Co, 1981, pp 979—1005

86. Kessner DM: Infant Death: An Analysis by Maternal Risk and Health Care. Washington, D.C., National Academy of Sciences, 1973

87. Kieffer MJ: The birthing room concept at Phoenix Memorial Hospital. Part II: Consumer satisfaction during one year. JOGN Nurs 9:155—159, 1980

88. Klerman LV: Adolescent pregnancy: a new look at a continuing problem. Am J
     Public Health 70:776—778, 1980
89. Korones SB: High-Risk Newborn Infants (ed 3). St. Louis, CV Mosby Co, 1981
90. Kretzchmar RM: Smoking and health: the role of the obstetrician gynecologist.
     Obstet Gynecol 55:403—406, 1980
91. Laukaran VH, van den Berg BJ: The relationship of maternal attitude to
     pregnancy outcomes and obstetric complications. A cohort study of unwanted
     pregnancy. Am J Obstet Gynecol 136:374—379, 1980
92. Laurence KM, James N, Miller M, et al: Increased risk of recurrence of
     pregnancies complicated by fetal neural tube defects in mothers receiving poor
     diets, and possible benefit of dietary counseling. Br Med J 281:1592—1594,
     1980
93. Lechtig A, Habicht JP, Delgado H, et al: Effect of food supplementation during
     pregnancy on birthweight. Pediatrics 56:508—511, 1975
94. Lechtig A, Yarbrough C, Delgado H, et al: Effect of moderate maternal
     malnutrition on the placenta. Am J Obstet Gynecol 123:191—201, 1975
95. Lederman E, Lederman RP, Work B, et al: Maternal psychological and physio-
     logic correlates of fetal newborn health status. Am J Obstet Gynecol
     139:956—958, 1981
96. Ledger WJ: Infection, in Romney SL, Gray MJ, Little AB, et al (eds): The
     Health Care of Women (ed 2). New York, McGraw-Hill Book Co, 1981, pp
     227—261
97. Lee K, Paneth N, Gartner LM, et al: Neonatal mortality: an analysis of the
     recent improvement in the United States. Am J Public Health 70:15—21, 1980
98. L'Esperance CM: Home birth—a manifestation of aggression? JOGN Nurs
     8:227—230, 1979
99. Lief HI: Sexual counseling, in Romney SL, Gray MJ, Little AB, et al (eds): The
     Health Care of Women (ed 2). New York, McGraw-Hill Book Co, 1981, pp
     853—884
100. Lipshitz J: Late pregnancy evaluation of fetal status, in Ryan GM (ed): Ambula-
     tory Care in Obstetrics and Gynecology. New York, Grune & Stratton, 1980, pp
     147—176
101. Little AB, Billiar RB: Endocrinology, in Romney SL, Gray MJ, Little AB, et al
     (eds): The Health Care of Women (ed 2). New York, McGraw-Hill Book Co,
     1981, pp 87—147
102. Little RE, Schultz FA, Mandell W: Drinking during pregnancy. J Stud Alcohol
     37:375—379, 1976
103. Lubic RW: The impact of technology on health care—the childbearing center: a
     case for technology's appropriate use. J Nurse-Midwifery 24:6—10, 1979
104. Lubic RW: Evaluation of an out-of-hospital maternity center for low-risk pa-
     tients, in Aiken LH (ed): Health Policy and Nursing Practice. New York,
     McGraw-Hill Book Co, 1980, pp 90—116
105. MacMahon B, Kovar MG, Feldman JJ: Infant Mortality Rates: Socioeconomic
     Factor, United States. Washington, D.C., Vital and Health Statistics, Series 22,
     No. 14, 1972
106. MacMahon B, Kovar MG, Feldman JJ: Infant Mortality Rates: Relationships
     with Mother's Reproductive History, United States. Washington, D.C., Vital
     and Health Statistics, Series 22, No. 15, 1973

107. Mahoney MJ: Fetoscopy. Pediatr Ann 10:61−68, 1981
108. Malasanos L, Barkauskas V, Moss M, et al: Health Assessment (ed 2). St. Louis, CV Mosby Co, 1981
109. Marieskind HI: An evaluation of Cesarean section in the United States. Final report submitted to the Office of the Assistant Secretary for Planning and Evaluation/Health. DHEW 1979
110. Masters WH, Johnson VE: Human Sexual Response. Boston, Little, Brown, 1966
111. McAnarney ER: Teenaged and pre-teenaged pregnancies: consequences of the fetal-maternal competition for nutrients [letter]. Pediatrics 68:472−473, 1981
112. McGanity WJ, Cannon RO, Bridgforth EB, et al: The Vanderbilt cooperative study of maternal and infant nutrition. VI. Relationship of obstetric performance to nutrition. Am J Obstet Gynecol 67:501−527, 1954
113. McMaster AJ: Sexually transmitted diseases, in Romney SL, Gray MJ, Little AB, et al (eds): The Health Care of Women (ed 2). New York, McGraw-Hill Book Co, 1981, pp 909−929
114. Mehl LE, Peterson GH, Whitt M, et al: Outcomes of elective home births: a series of 1,146 cases. J Reprod Med 19:281−290, 1977
115. Merrill JA: Endometriosis, in Romney SL, Gray MJ, Little AB, et al (eds): The Health Care of Women (ed 2). New York, McGraw-Hill Book Co, 1981, pp 931−945
116. Merritt TA, Lawrence RA, Naeye RL: The infants of adolescent mothers. Pediatr Ann 9:100−107, 1980
117. Mestman JH: Management of thyroid diseases in pregnancy. Clin Perinatol 7:371−385, 1980
118. Meyer MN, Tonascia JA: Maternal smoking and pregnancy complications and perinatal mortality. Am J Obstet Gynecol 128:494−502, 1977
119. Milne LS, Rich OJ: Cognitive and affective aspects of the responses of pregnant women to sonography. Matern Child Nurs J 10:15−39, 1981
120. Milner PF, Jones BR, Dobler J: Outcome of pregnancy in sickle cell-hemoglobin C disease. An analysis of 181 pregnancies in 98 patients, and a review of the literature. Am J Obstet Gynecol 138:239−245, 1980
121. Mitchell GW, Farber M: Gynecologic urology, in Romney SL, Gray MJ, Little AB, et al (eds): The Health Care of Women (ed 2). New York, McGraw-Hill Book Co, 1981, pp 947−962
122. Moore EC: Women and health in the United States, 1980. Public Health Rep, 1980 Supplement
123. Morris NM: The biological advantages and social disadvantages of teenage pregnancy [editorial]. Am J Public Health 71:796, 1981
124. Morrow CP, Hart WR: Ovaries, in Romney SL, Gray MJ, Little AB, et al (eds): The Health Care of Women (ed 2). New York, McGraw-Hill Book Co, 1981, pp 1123−1181
125. Mullen PD: Behavioral aspects of maternal and child health: natural influences and educational intervention, in Better Health for Our Children: A National Strategy. Volume IV. Background Papers. Washington, D.C., DHHS (PHS) Publication No. 79-55071, 1981, pp 127−188
126. Naeye RL: Causes and consequences of placental growth retardation. JAMA 239:1145−1147, 1978

127. Naeye RL: Effects of maternal cigarette smoking on the fetus and placenta. Br J Obstet Gynaecol 85:732−737, 1978

128. Naeye RL: Causes of fetal and neonatal mortality by race in a selected U.S. population. Am J Public Health 69:857−861, 1979

129. Naeye RL: Coitus and associated amniotic fluid infections. N Engl J Med 301:1198−1200, 1979

130. Naeye RL: Weight gain and the outcome of pregnancy. Am J Obstet Gynecol 135:3−7, 1979

131. Naeye RL: Influence of maternal cigarette smoking during pregnancy on fetal childhood and growth. Obstet Gynecol 57:18−21, 1981

132. Naeye RL: Teenaged and pre-teenaged pregnancies: consequences of the fetal-maternal competition for nutrients. Pediatrics 67:146−150, 1981

133. Naeye, RL, Blanc WA: Unfavorable outcome of pregnancy: repeated losses. Am J Obstet Gynecol 116:1133−1137, 1973

134. Naeye RL, Blanc W, Paul C: Effects of maternal nutrition on the human fetus. Pediatrics 52:494−503, 1973

135. Naeye RL, Chez RA: Effects of maternal acetonuria and low pregnancy weight gain on children's psychomotor development. Am J Obstet Gynecol 139:189−193, 1981

136. Naeye RL, Diener MM, Dellinger WS: Urban poverty: effects on prenatal nutrition. Science 166:1026, 1969

137. Naeye RL, Harkness WL, Utts J: Abruptio placentae and perinatal death: a prospective study. Am J Obstet Gynecol 128:740−746, 1977

138. Naeye RL, Peters EC: Amniotic fluid infections with intact membranes leading to perinatal death: a prospective study. Pediatrics 61:171−177, 1978

139. Nahmias AJ: Herpes simplex virus infection—present status of diagnosis and management. South Med J 68:1191−1194, 1975

140. Naib ZM, Nahmias AJ, Josey WE, et al. Association of maternal genital herpes infection with spontaneous abortion. Obstet Gynecol 35:260−263, 1970

141. National Center for Health Statistics: US Census Bureau Digest Feb 1978, p 20

142. NICHD National Registry for Amniocentesis Study Group: Midtrimester amniocentesis for prenatal diagnosis. Safety and accuracy. JAMA 236:1471−1476, 1976

143. Niswander KR, Gordon M: The Women and their Pregnancies. Philadelphia, WB Saunders Co, 1972

144. Nuckolls KB, Cassell J, Kaplan BH: Psychological assets, life crisis and the prognosis of pregnancy. Am J Epidemiol 95:431−441, 1972

145. Oakes GK, Chez RA, Morelli IC: Diet in pregnancy: meddling with the normal or preventing toxemia? Am J Nurs 75:1134−1136, 1975

146. Office on Smoking and Health: Smoking and Health. Rockville, Md., DHEW Publication No. (PHS) 79-50066, 1979

147. Osofsky HJ, Rajan R: The adolescent pregnancy, in Wallace HM, Gold EM, Lis EF (eds): Maternal and Child Health Practices. Problems, Resources and Methods of Delivery. Springfield, Illinois, Charles C Thomas, 1973, pp 884−899

148. Pedersen LM, Tygstrup I, Pedersen J: Congenital malformations in newborn infants of diabetic women. Correlation with maternal diabetic vascular complications. Lancet 1:1124−1126, 1964

149. Perez de Francisco C, Dreyfuss G: Prenatal diagnosis: psychiatric aspects [editorial]. Biol Psychiatry 16:109−111, 1981
150. Phelan JT: Cancer and pregnancy. NY State J Med 68:3011−3017, 1968
151. Pitkin RM, Kaminetzky HA, Newton M, et al: Maternal nutrition: a selective review of clinical topics. Obstet Gynecol 40:773−785, 1972
152. Prasad N, Prasad R, Bushong SC, et al: Ultrasound and mammalian DNA. Lancet 1:1181, 1976
153. Pridham KF, Schutz ME: Preparation of parents for birthing and infant care. J Fam Pract 13:181−188, 1981
154. Primrose T, Higgins A: A study of human antepartum nutrition. J Reprod Med 7:257−264, 1971
155. Pritchard CA, Hufton AP: Low dose obstetric radiography. Radiography 47:85−91, 1981
156. Prout TE: Thyroid disease in pregnancy. Am J Obstet Gynecol 122:669−676, 1975
157. Pugh WE, Fernandez FL: Coitus in late pregnancy. Obstet Gynecol 2:636−642, 1953
158. Pugh WE, Vogt RF, Gibson RA: Primary ovarian pregnancy and the intrauterine device. Obstet Gynecol 42:218−222, 1973
159. Quilligan EJ: Prenatal care, in Romney SL, Gray MJ, Little AB, et al (eds): The Health Care of Women (ed 2). New York, McGraw-Hill Book Co, 1981, pp 579−594
160. Quirk B, Hassanein R: The nurse's role in advising patients on coitus during pregnancy. Nurs Clin North Am 8:501−505, 1973
161. Rich C: A multigravida's work at organization during pregnancy. Matern Child Nurs J 8:195−206, 1979
162. Robinson E: Detection of birth defects by ultrasonography. Birth Defects 17:17−30, 1981
163. Romney SL, Ober WB: The uterus, in Romney SL, Gray MJ, Little AB, et al (eds): The Health Care of Women (ed 2). New York, McGraw-Hill Book Co, 1981, pp 1053−1092
164. Rosenstock IM: What research in motivation suggests for public health. Am J Public Health 50:295−302, 1960
165. Rossi AS: Transition to parenthood. J Marr Fam 30:26−39, 1968
166. Rothman LA, Cohen CJ, Astarloa J: Placental and fetal involvement by maternal malignancy. A report of rectal carcinoma and review of the literature. Am J Obstet Gynecol 116:1023−1034, 1973
167. Rovinsky JJ: Diseases complicating pregnancy, in Romney SL, Gray MJ, Little AB, et al (eds): The Health Care of Women (ed 2). New York, McGraw-Hill Book Co, 1981, pp 697−803
168. Rush D, Stein Z, Susser M: Controlled trial of prenatal nutrition supplementation defended   [letter]. Pediatrics 66:656−658, 1980
169. Sallomi SJ: Rubella in pregnancy. A review of prospective studies from the literature. Obstet Gynecol 27:252−256, 1966
170. Sasmor JL, Grossman E: Childbirth education in 1980. JOGN Nurs 10:155−160, 1981
171. Schifrin BS, Foye G, Amato J, et al: Routine fetal heart rate monitoring in the antepartum period. Obstet Gynecol 54:21−25, 1979

172. Schlesinger ER, Mazundar SM, Logrillo VM: Long-term trends in perinatal death among offspring of mothers with previous child losses. Am J Epidemiol 96:255—262, 1972

173. Smith CA: Effects of maternal undernutrition upon the newborn infant in Holland (1944—1945). J Pediatr 30:229—243, 1947

174. Sokol RJ, Rosen MG, Stojkov J, et al: Clinical application of high-risk scoring on obstetric service. Am J Obstet Gynecol 128:652—661, 1977

175. Standards for Ambulatory Obstetric Care. Chicago, American College of Obstetricians and Gynecologists, 1977

176. Standards for Obstetric, Gynecologic, and Neonatal Nursing. Chicago, Nurses' Association of the American College of Obstetricians and Gynecologists, 1981

177. Standley K, Soule B, Copans SA: Dimensions of prenatal anxiety and their influence on pregnancy outcome. Am J Obstet Gynecol 135:22—26, 1979

178. Stellman JM: Women's Work. Women's Health. New York, Pantheon Books, 1977

179. Streissguth AP: Maternal drinking and the outcome of pregnancy. Am J Orthopsychiatry 47:422—430, 1977

180. Summitt RL: Prenatal genetic diagnosis, in Ryan GM (ed): Ambulatory Care in Obstetrics and Gynecology. New York, Grune & Stratton, 1980, pp 177—203

181. Sweet AY: Classification on the low-birth-weight infant, in Klaus MH, Fanaroff AA (eds): Care of the High-Risk Neonate (ed 2). Philadelphia, WB Saunders Co, 1979, pp 66—93

182. Tartakow IJ: The teratogenicity of maternal rubella. J Pediatr 66:380—391, 1965

183. Task Force Report: Predictors of Hereditary Disease or Congenital Defects. Bethesda, Maryland, National Institute of Child Health and Human Development, 1979

184. Taylor KJW: Ultrasonic damage to spinal cord and the synergistic effect of hypoxia. J Pathol 102:41—47, 1970

185. Teenage pregnancy. Public Health Curr 18(3):1—4, 1978

186. Teenage Pregnancy: The Problem that Hasn't Gone Away. New York, The Alan Guttmacher Institute, 1981

187. Thomson AM: Diet in pregnancy. Brit J Nutr 13:509—524, 1959

188. Timm MM: Prenatal education evaluation. Nurs Res 28:338—342, 1979

189. Tipping VG: The vulnerability of a primipara during the antepartal period. Matern Child Nurs J 10:61—77, 1981

190. Travers CK: Obesity and pregnancy: a review. Obesity/Bariatr Med 5:172—177, 1976

191. Trussell TJ: Economic consequences of teenage childbearing. Fam Plann Perspect 8:184—190, 1976

192. Umphenour JH: Gravidas' responses to realtime ultrasound fetal image. JOGN Nurs 9:77—79, 1980

193. Varney H: Nurse-Midwifery. Boston, Blackwell Scientific Publications, Inc, 1980

194. Vavra HM, Querec LJ: A Study of Infant Mortality from Linked Records: by Age of Mother, Total-Birth Order, and Other Variables, United States, 1960 Live-Birth Cohort. Washington, D.C., Vital and Health Statistics, Series 20, No. 14, 1973

195. Vermeersch J: Maternal nutrition and the outcome of pregnancy, in Worthington-Roberts BS, Vermeersch J, Williams SR (eds): Nutrition in Pregnancy and Lactation (ed 2). St. Louis, CV Mosby Co, 1981, pp 13—36

196. Vermeersch J: Physiological basis of nutritional needs, in Worthington-Roberts BS, Vermeersch J, Williams SR (eds): Nutrition in Pregnancy and Lactation (ed 2). St. Louis, CV Mosby Co, 1981, pp 37—63

197. Vital Statistics of the United States, 1977. Volume I. Natality. Hyattsville, Maryland, DHEW Publication No. (PHS) 81-1113, 1981

198. Vital Statistics of the United States, 1977. Volume II. Mortality, Part A. Hyattsville, Maryland, DHEW Publication No. (PHS) 81-1101, 1980

199. Vital Statistics of the United States, 1977. Volume II. Mortality, Part B. Hyattsville, Maryland, DHEW Publication No. (PHS) 80-1102, 1980

200. Waltzer WC: The urinary tract in pregnancy. J Urol 125:271—276, 1981

201. Wegman ME: Annual summary of vital statistics—1976. Pediatrics 60:797—804, 1977

202. White G: A comparison of home and hospital delivery based on 25 years experience with both. J Reprod Med 19:291—292, 1977

203. Williams SR: Nutritional guidance in prenatal care, in Worthington-Roberts BS, Vermeersch J, Williams SR (eds): Nutrition in Pregnancy and Lactation (ed 2). St. Louis, CV Mosby Co, 1981, pp 64—104

204. Winick M: Fetal malnutrition. Clin Obstet Gynecol 13:526—535, 1970

205. Woods NF, Woods JS: Women and the workplace, in Fogel CI, Woods NF (eds): Health Care of Women. St. Louis, CV Mosby Co, 1981, pp 419—449

206. Worthen N, Bustillo M: Effect of urinary bladder fullness on fundal height measurements. Am J Obstet Gynecol 138:759—762, 1980

207. Worthington-Roberts BS: Nutritional needs of the pregnant adolescent, in Worthington-Roberts BS, Vermeersch J, Williams SR (eds): Nutrition in Pregnancy and Lactation (ed 2). St. Louis, CV Mosby Co, 1981, pp 135—154

208. Zabin LS: The impact of early use of prescription contraceptives on reducing premarital teenage pregnancies. Fam Plann Perspect 13:72—74, 1981

209. Zelnik M, Kantner JF: Sexual and contraceptive experience of young unmarried women in the United States, 1976 and 1971. Fam Plann Perspect 9:55—71, 1977

210. Zelnik M, Kantner JF: Sexual activity, contraceptive use and pregnancy among metropolitan-area teenagers: 1971—1979. Fam Plann Perspect 12:230—231, 233—237, 1980

Teresa Marchese
with
Julia-Harrison Coughlin
Constance J. Adams

4

Childbirth

Each pregnant woman nears the end of her pregnancy and anticipates labor with a mixture of emotions—anticipation, dread, fear or excitement. The birth of her child is an unparallelled event in her life.[121] The nurse-midwife will allow the woman and her family the opportunity to participate in management decisions during the intrapartum period. All health-care procedures during this time should emphasize the woman's control over her care and should increase her sense of mastery.[188]

Normal labor and delivery should be conducted with the minimum of medical intervention and the maximum of patient choice within the framework of safe nurse-midwifery practice. Each family's requests for participation in the birth experience should be respected. Institutional restrictions should not be imposed simply because "it has always been done this way."[8,164,191]

The woman who has received prenatal care from the nurse-midwife will have negotiated through the antepartum period for the kind of birth experience she and her family desire. Nurse-midwives in some settings, however, assume management of the patient in the intrapartum period without the benefit of having known the parturient throughout the prenatal period. It is within the

The author would like to express a special note of appreciation to Sarah Gold, R.N., C.N.M, M.S., for the time and expertise she devoted in review of this chapter.

The sections in this chapter entitled *Analgesia and Anesthesia in Labor* and *Anesthesia for Second-Stage Labor* were contributed by Julia Harrison-Coughlin and Constance J. Adams, respectively.

115

scope of safe nurse-midwifery practice to offer these childbearing women alternatives to routine obstetric practices.

Each labor and delivery should be considered a normal and natural process until proved otherwise. The nurse-midwife continually assesses and updates the data base and evaluates and alters her plan of management for each laboring woman through all the stages of labor and during the early puerperium. One of the purposes of this chapter is to articulate the theoretical bases for nurse-midwifery management decisions; this discussion, however, by no means includes all management areas. It is hoped that nurse-midwives will use this information to allow the pregnant woman and her family greater freedom of personal selection in the childbirth process.

The Place of Birth

The intent of this section is not to rehash an obstetrical controversy over whether birth should take place in the home or hospital, but to review some of the specific literature about the place of delivery. It is known that the demand for and the number of home births are on the rise. Many consumers want to regain control of their birth experiences and to do so have chosen to remain in their homes. Of concern to the medical profession are the increasing number of home births that are unattended or attended by the unqualified.[63] Nurse-midwives dedicated to the concept of family-centered care and self-determination, are attempting to give childbearing families multiple choices of birthing alternatives. Epstein reports on a thriving nurse-midwifery home birth service established in response to overwhelming consumer demand. She and her associates are able to report positive perinatal outcomes.[57,58]

Freestanding alternative birth centers offer another option to families seeking self-determination in their birthings. Lubic and Ernst cite as their first principle of operation: ''A childbearing center is an adaptation of the home, rather than a modification of the hospital.''[116] They have an excellent safety record. Another form of reaching out to childbearing families has been the hospital-based Alternative Birthing Center (ABC). Published reports reveal that the ABC has a high level of family satisfaction and positive outcome statistics.[10,61,95,127] The quality of the ABC seems to vary from hospital to hospital as do the amenities. De Vries studied ABC's in 25 hospitals and found a difference between the ideal and the reality. He feels the popularity of such programs has allowed many hospitals to set up ABC's which really offer no alternatives and do not alter the traditional hospital way of birth in any significant manner.[51]

These alternative situations offer the family a chance to remain together during and after the birth. Family and friends may attend the birth and siblings are welcome. Siblings' attendance at home births is considered to be natural.[7] In hospitals, however, there seems to be some skepticism. As more and more barriers to family-centered care are removed, there is uncertainty in tradition-bound sites. Studies comparing neonates allowed sibling visitation with neonates who have no contact with siblings, show no difference in bacterial colonization.[210] Fears of increasing morbidity rates thus have been allayed. Fears of psychological damage to the children who attend births appear to be unfounded.[7,152] The child who is prepared ahead of time, and supported through the labor and birth has a marvelous, positive experience. Perez was told by a child: "Birth should be a family event. If the children want to be there, they should be. Why separate the family at such an important time?"[152]

The place of birth has been chosen and the family is ready for its new member. The nurse-midwife has many management decisions to make and must continually update the data base of maternal and fetal status. Varney[214] reminds the nurse-midwife that the family must feel welcome in the birthing situation. The nurse-midwife should help "significant others" to support the mother.

MANAGEMENT ISSUES PERTINENT TO THE FIRST STAGE OF LABOR

The Onset of Labor and Admission

As the woman nears the end of her pregnancy, the nurse-midwife is alert for signs and symptoms of the onset of labor. The woman herself may be aware that labor is approaching and often reports one or more prodromal occurrences. Lightening, increased vaginal secretions, discharge of the cervical mucous plug, weight loss, presence of bloody show, persistent backache, false labor pains, gastrointestinal upsets and an increase in physical energy may be noticed.[148,214] The nurse-midwife may observe that the presenting part has settled into the lower uterine segment, engagement has occurred and the cervix has begun to soften and efface.[148] Late pregnancy is often accompanied by discomforts which, though normal, may make the woman quite uncomfortable. The nurse-midwife and the woman must differentiate these discomforts from false and early labor and other complications. Appropriate explanations and support for the woman and her family may help at this time.

When the woman reports the onset of labor, the nurse-midwife must determine that true labor has begun. The critical features of differential diagnosis of true versus false labor are well documented[76,148,160,214] and need not be repeated here. The nurse-midwife needs to be in attendance from the time the woman reports herself to be in labor whether or not actual labor has been documented. It is often difficult to differentiate between false labor and the early latent phase of labor. Institutional policies, personal preference and the reliability of transportation may dictate how management will proceed.[214] False labor is often treated with instructions for relaxation, hydration, and with a sedative for sleep.[135,214] Once active labor is established, the woman is admitted to the birthing center or labor and delivery suite. Nurse-midwives who assist at home births like to be in attendance in the woman's home as soon as possible after labor has begun.[57]

Once the parturient is under her care, the nurse-midwife proceeds with the establishment of a complete data base including history, physical examination and laboratory studies.[214] The results of these will enable the nurse-midwife and the woman to make several decisions which will result in the management plan. Issues surrounding the admission include the routine use of enemas, the perineal shave or "prep" and the routine use of intravenous fluids.

Early Labor

The Enema

A cleansing enema often is ordered early in labor, usually to minimize fecal contamination at the time of delivery. Nurse-midwives generally do not administer an enema routinely; in each case they examine the need, possible harmful side effects, and the woman's own feelings. Many obstetrical and midwifery texts mention the routine administration of enemas.[70,76,135,146,160,173] However, clinicians differ on the efficacy of this procedure to reduce fecal contamination at the time of delivery. In a study by Whitley and Mack, the incidence of fecal contamination in 72 women at delivery was 47 percent. An experimental group with no enema had the highest incidence of fecal contamination (59%). Of the group given enemas, only 5 of 13 (38%) contaminated the delivery field with feces. Although some women who had an enema did contaminate the delivery field with fecal matter this was not termed "gross contamination." The least amount of contamination was from a group who reported diarrhea prior to the onset of labor and who were not given an enema. Whitley and Mack concluded that evacuating the bowel with an enema prior to second-stage labor is still appropriate management. Infection rates were not discussed in this manuscript.[220]

In another, larger study, Romney and associates determined that there was no significant difference in fecal contamination when 149 women were given an enema in early labor and 125 were not. These authors also concluded that the incidence of gross contamination was similar in the two groups and that fecal matter passed following an enema was often liquid and more difficult to control. Seven neonates in each group had infections postnatally. These authors feel that the enema should be reserved for those who have not had a bowel movement in 24 hours and who have stool palpable on examination. In addition, the women who participated in this study thought that they should have a choice.[172] Indeed, more positive results may be obtained from the enema if the woman has participated in the decisionmaking process.[208]

Enemas have often been prescribied for women in order to stimulate contractions.[135,148,214] The enema causes increased intestinal peristalsis which, through a reflex mechanism, stimulates uterine contractions.[22] Opinions of clinicians differ on the benefit of using an enema to stimulate contractions and they usually rely on clinical experience in making this decision. If a decision is made to use an enema, it is now recognized that a small tap water enema is as beneficial as the old-fashioned large, hot, soapsuds enema.

Several other factors also influence the nurse-midwife's decision to administer an enema. A rapidly advancing labor usually contraindicates the use of an enema in order to avoid a precipitous delivery. Many clinicians will avoid enemas when the membranes are ruptured in order to decrease the chance of infection and when the station of the presenting part is high to minimize the possibility of prolapse of the umbilical cord. Enemas are contraindicated when certain complications are present. These can include vaginal bleeding, preeclampsia, malpresentation, premature labor and any other medical condition which would jeopardize the safety of the mother or fetus.[76,148,160,214]

Perineal Preparation

The routine shaving of pubic hair before delivery appears to be a practice which is disappearing. In some settings, however, institutional policies displace the decision from the nurse-midwife and the parturient. Landry and Kilpatrick have undertaken a review of the pertinent literature to determine why this practice persists.[108] Shaving was initiated as part of the move toward asepsis, but as early as 1922 some physicians and nurses questioned its value. Numerous studies have shown no increase in puerperal morbidity among patients who were not shaved prior to delivery.[2,114,171] Landry and Kilpatrick indicate that the reason shaving is still routine in many institutions is that nurses are not aware of research findings that contradict the practice. Landry and Kilpatrick also state that the pubic region may be thought of as "dirty" and shaving provides a more aesthetic perception to some.

The preparation of the perineal area during labor should include a thorough scrubbing with an antiseptic soap.[73,135,160,173] Allowing the woman to take a warm shower following her admission or, for that matter, at any time during labor, is beneficial. Not only will it aid in cleansing, but it also often helps the laboring woman to feel more relaxed. Clipping of longer pubic hairs around the introitus may be desired.[135,214] If an episiotomy is anticipated and the perineal body contains a large amount of hair, the birth attendant may wish to shave only the perineal body. Seropian and Reynolds, however, feel that razor preparation may advance wound infection rather than prevent it.[189] Generally, the perineal body is relatively hair-free and no shaving need be done. It seems clear that whatever the reasons for the persistence of perineal shaving, the normal laboring woman may make the rather simple decision to forego this practice.

Nutrition and Hydration

The management of oral intake during labor varies from allowing the woman to eat if she desires[57,70] to withholding all oral intake during active labor.[76,160,168,173] If no oral intake is allowed, intravenous fluids are used to provide needed nutrients and fluids to the laboring woman. In making the management decision, one must weigh the advantages of adequate nutrition and hydration to the woman against the risks of aspiration. The expressed desires of the parturient must also be considered. Many women do not wish to be limited by the intravenous equipment and will request no intravenous unless there is a definite indication requiring it.

Gastric motility and digestion are inhibited during labor, greatly reducing gastric emptying time.[76,135,160,214] If the woman has eaten prior to the onset of labor or during labor, the food could remain in her stomach for some time. Some clinicians fear that vomiting which may occur in active labor could increase the likelihood of aspiration. Furthermore, if complications arise and a general anesthesia is needed, the woman would be at grave risk for aspiration pneumonia.

Mendelson first described acid aspiration syndrome in 1946.[125] He noted that if the pH of aspirated gastric contents is under 2.5, there is a rise in morbidity and mortality rates. Roberts[168] states that one in four obstetric patients is at risk for aspiration syndrome. He offers that reducing the amount of gastric content to under 25 ml or elevating the pH to over 2.5 can decrease the number of patients at risk. Though Roberts maintains that gastric emptying time is not delayed in the majority of labor patients,[167] he admits that pain, fear, and anxiety may inhibit the process. Roberts states that the single factor influencing gastric emptying is the use of large doses of narcotics. He emphasizes that all patients in labor should be told not to eat or drink anything, and he recommends giving every laboring woman 15 ml of antacid every three hours.[167,168]

Some authors recommend that only solid foods be withheld from the laboring mother and oral fluids be allowed unless general anesthesia is anticipated.[135,148,214] Although highly sweetened juices are not recommended, clear liquids such as weak tea, apple juice, broth or gelatin can be encouraged. Sips of water, ice chips, hard candy, or popsicles often may be all the actively laboring woman requests. Some nurse-midwives will instruct their patients to drink plenty of fluids in early labor. They feel that if a mother starts labor well-hydrated, she will be able to maintain this state throughout labor.

It is appropriate to allow the normal laboring woman who has no complications to labor without an intravenous in place. The nurse-midwife will have guidelines for the initiation of intravenous fluids and these can be shared with the woman so that she will be prepared if the need arises. One of the essentials of excellent first-stage management is a nurse-midwife alert for the signs of maternal dehydration and ketosis. Ordinary signs of dehydration may easily be confused and masked by the physiology of a normal labor. Urinary output is observed for amount, concentration and for ketone bodies. If ketones occur, and metabolic acidosis is suspected, an intravenous of 5 percent glucose in normal saline or lactated ringers may be initiated. Goodwin points out that 1 liter of 5 percent glucose contains 200 calories. In active labor, the mother may require 50 − 100 calories an hour, thus a 10 percent glucose solution may be more appropriate. This solution would provide 15 g of glucose and 60 calories/hour when infused at a rate of 15 ml/hour.[75] Concerned about neonatal iatrognic hyperinsulinism, Rutter and associates advise limiting glucose administration in labor only to the amount which will maintain normal maternal serum glucose levels. These physicians assert that dehydration can be corrected by increasing fluids, and ketosis can be corrected with small amounts of glucose.[179] Nurse-midwives who are managing a lengthy labor may choose to alternate 1 liter of glucose solution with 1 liter of a solution such as lactated ringers.

Despite Roberts' fears that one in four women in labor are at risk for anesthetic morbidity, it is clear that the nurse-midwife who is managing the essentially low risk parturient may offer her patient the choice of intravenous or oral nutrition. It is very unlikely that this patient will be narcotized or have the need for a general anesthetic. The watchful birth attendant may practice within the parameters of safety and still allow oral intake.

Active Labor

Routine Amniotomy

There are a number of management options facing the mother, her family, and the nurse-midwife during active labor. Artificial rupture of the amniotic membranes during labor has become common obstetric practice but it can still be considered optional. When conditions are ideal, amniotomy is effective in initiating labor.[65] It is also widely believed that artificial rupture of the membranes will shorten labor with benefits to both mother and fetus. The routine use of internal electronic fetal monitoring necessitates the performance of amniotomy. The need for internal monitoring of every essentially low-risk fetus is questionable, and nurse-midwives should follow their policy manuals for carefully selecting women who need the monitor. The issue to be considered here is the routine use of amniotomy in labor without medical indication.

Nurse-midwives and their patients often elect to allow a normal course of labor and do not resort to amniotomy. This decision, though safe, often may be contrary to the beliefs of other practitioners and colleagues. A thorough review of the literature concerning amniotomy reveals no absolute response to these critics. However, an excellent review and critique of pertinent research on amniotomy by Lynaugh provides the clinician and patient with reasonable arguments to avoid routine amniotomy.[117]

There is some evidence that amniotomy may shorten labor slight-ly.[109,213,217] Calderyo-Barcia, in a large objective study, found that artificial rupture of the membranes in early labor (4 −5 cms of dilation) significantly shortened the first stage of labor. This difference in the length of the first stage was thought to be caused by the fetal head, acting as a wedge, being a more efficient dilator than the intact membranes.[35] Friedman found no experimental proof to support the widely held clinical notion that amniotomy will stimulate labor progress.[65] With Sachteben,[67] he concluded that amniotomy is "ineffec-tual as a therapeutic procedure in consistently abbreviating any of the phases of labor"[65] Subsequent studies seem to support Friedman's conclusion.[104,157,163] Indeed, Friedman and Poma-Herrera found arrest of labor occurred in certain patients following amniotomy.[65,157]

Results of numerous studies have shown possible adverse effects of amniotomy on the fetus. Though acknowledging the significantly shorter time in labor, Calderyo-Barcia has indicated that the mechanism that may shorten labor carries an increased risk of mechanical trauma to the fetal head.[35] When the membranes have ruptured, the protection of the amniotic fluid afforded the fetal head and umbilical cord is lost.[32,185] This loss of natural protection may cause increased risk to the fetus. A summary of reported hazards to the fetus would include the following:

1. Increase in caput succedaneum.[12,35,186]
2. Disalignment of the fetal cranial bones at birth, with abnormal changes in the fetal EEG.[32,35]
3. Increase in the incidence of Type I decelerations (a pattern associated with fetal head or umbilical cord compression).[32,35,185]
4. Umbilical cord compression.[35,68]
5. Decreased fetal pH.[120]
6. Increase in variable decelerations.[141]
7. Prolapse of the umbilical cord.[214]
8. Increase in neonatal infections if the length of time between rupture of the membranes and delivery is prolonged.[214]

Many of these reported negative results do not appear to have long lasting effects on the neonate,[12,120] though some have been known to continue into the neonatal period for as long as a month.[32]

When the progress of labor is normal and the patient is at low risk, the routine use of amniotomy is unwarranted. Lynaugh points out that no benefit and possible harm may result, thus, its routine use is unjustified.[117] Calderyo-Barcia and Schwarcz state that the normal physiologic process of labor should be allowed to unfold.[32] The membranes naturally stay intact until late labor in most women.[35] Little intervention is needed unless the fetus is in distress or a dysfunctional labor ensues. "When the progress of labor is normal, fetal membranes should not be ruptured artificially—at least not until the first stage is finished and the birth is expected to occur within a few minutes."[184]

Each nurse-midwife has "standing orders" that define when she may perform an amniotomy. These orders usually include such items as: the woman must be in active labor, at least $4-5$ cms dilated, and must have a cephalic, vertex presentation, with the head engaged. The laboring woman and her family are included in the decision as much as possible.

Meconium in the Amniotic Fluid

Once the fetal membranes have ruptured, the nurse-midwife has an opportunity to observe the character of the amniotic fluid. In most instances, the amniotic liquor will be clear or milky and flecked with vernix caseosa. However, in $0.5-30$ percent of labors, the amniotic fluid will be stained with meconium.[125] The nurse-midwife is challenged by the controversy surrounding the significance of meconium-stained amniotic fluid and by the management options available to her.

Meconium passage before or during labor in a cephalic presentation, traditionally was thought to indicate fetal compromise. Clinically, it is obvious, however, that meconium passage may accompany the birth of a perfectly healthy infant and that a compromised fetus may be born attended by clear amniotic fluid. Various mechanisms have been implicated as the causative factors of intrauterine meconium passage. Intrauterine fetal hypoxia induces vasoconstriction, hyperperistalsis of the fetal gut, relaxation of the sphincter ani, and meconium passage. A vagal response due to cord compression also may be responsible for meconium passage. There is most likely no single cause of meconium passage in utero and this leads to a lack of consistency in the reported perinatal morbidity and mortality rates associated with meconium passage. Mandelbaum reported that intrapartum meconium staining, with no other signs of fetal distress yielded a perinatal mortality rate of $1-13.5$ percent.[119] The perinatal mortality rate rises significantly if meconium passage is accompanied by an abnormal fetal heart rate.

In an attempt to define the risks associated with meconium passage, Meis and associates devised a classification of meconium passage according to timing and amount of meconium. In 2933 labors the incidence of meconium passage in cephalic presentations was 22 percent. By grouping amniotic fluid into early-light passage, early-heavy passage and late passage, these researchers determined that the risk to the fetus was associated with the timing of the passage of and with the quantity of meconium. Meconium passage was defined as follows:

Early: Before or during the active phase of labor
Light: Yellow or green, thin
Heavy: Dark green or black, thick
Late: During second stage, when clear fluid had been noted previously

Using these criteria, early-heavy meconium passage was found to be associated with increased risks of perinatal morbidity and mortality including meconium aspiration syndrome. Late meconium passage was found to be associated with meconium aspiration syndrome and lower Apgar scores but no fetal or neonatal deaths. The early-light group had fewer intrapartal problems, no deaths, and higher 1 and 5 minute Apgar scores.[124]

Miller found that 30 percent of his high risk sample experienced meconium passage. The meconium stained fetuses with normal fetal heart rate patterns and normal pH values tolerated labor as well as those with clear fluid.[126] Krebs disagreed, reporting lower Apgar scores, increased perinatal morbidity and mortality, and more abnormal fetal heart rate patterns in meconium stained fetuses than in fetuses with clear fluid. In his sample, heavy meconium did not differ from light meconium in resultant lower Apgar scores or abnormal fetal heart rate patterns.[106]

Because of conflicting reports on the significance of intrapartal meconium passage, nurse-midwifery management of such labors will vary somewhat according to policies, procedures, and the experience and expertise of the clinician. It is recommended that continuous fetal heart rate monitoring be instituted in all cases of meconium in the amniotic fluid.[106,126] Meis[124] states that labors associated with early, light staining of the amniotic fluid can be treated as low risk, though he does not specifically mention the elimination of continuous fetal heart rate monitoring. Fetal scalp blood sampling should be used as a necessary adjunct to the continuous monitoring. Carson has recommended a combined obstetric and pediatric approach to the management of meconium staining. At the birth of the head, a de Lee catheter should be used to suction the nasopharynx. As soon as the birth is complete, the oropharynx should be aspirated carefully with a bulb syringe. If meconium is found, direct visualization of the larynx and tracheal suctioning are essential.[37] Neonates who show signs of asphyxiation are at risk for meconium aspiration syndrome and special care should be taken with resuscitative techniques.[126] Pediatric assistance should be obtained if fetal distress is combined with meconium passage.

Fetal Monitoring

The nurse-midwife managing the essentially low risk mother through labor is continuously watchful for changing maternal and fetal status. Evaluation of the fetal heart rate alerts the nurse-midwife to the condition of her other patient, the unborn. Adaptation of the fetus to the rigors of labor can be inferred from careful evaluation of the fetal heart rate. The fetoscope traditionally was used to auscultate the fetal heart tones. Labor room nurses would listen to the heart tones for 15 seconds, between contractions, and multiply by four in order to establish a rate per minute. It is obvious that use of this method could result in overlooking fetal heart rate changes in the compromised fetus. With technologic advances in medicine it is now possible to continuously evaluate the fetal heart with an electronic monitor. This technology has initiated one of the current controversies in obstetric care. Institutions began reporting dramatically reduced perinatal mortality figures and increased neonatal survival rates following the increased use of electronic fetal monitoring during labor. Many clinicians therefore now advocate electronical monitoring of every laboring woman and fetus. [11,147]

The value of the fetal monitor, when indicated, is not disputed. The debate concerns the relative value of considering every woman and fetus "at risk" and the necessity of using the fetal monitor in all cases. As women and their families have assumed more responsibility for their health care, they have questioned the need for and the desirability of routine electronic monitoring. Laboring families and nurse-midwives who want a family-centered experience find the fetal monitor to be invasive and dehumanizing. Indeed, most of the studies advocating routine fetal monitoring emphasize the perinatal outcome rather than the psychoemotional impact on the childbearing family. Birth has an important psychological as well as physiologic effect which is often overlooked in these studies. Physicians who deny that monitoring can be invasive and depersonalizing seem to have drawn this conclusion from personal observation rather than from studies stressing the psychoemotional aspects of childbirth. [20,21]

The nurse-midwife who chooses to use intrapartum electronic fetal monitoring selectively, functions under established policies and procedures outlining indications for monitoring. The conditions under which the monitor would be applied should be known and understood by the clinician, her medical backup, and most importantly, by the parturient and her family. These participants have the right to know the risks and benefits to them and to their baby and have the right to share in the decision regarding electronic monitoring during labor.

Advocates of routine electronic fetal monitoring. Routine electronic fetal monitoring is credited with the reduction of perinatal mortality and morbidity by many clinicians. Quilligan and Paul[162] examined the results of fetal monitoring in their institution and noted a reduction in perinatal mortality. The rates decreased from 49/1000 births to 23/1000 births over a 4 year period. In a retrospective study spanning 3 years (1970−1972), Paul and Hon reviewed over 27,000 deliveries at Los Angeles County Hospital/University of Southern California. They found a reduction in intrapartum and perinatal mortality of monitored patients over unmonitored patients. [151] Other retrospective studies have demonstrated that monitored patients have improved perinatal outcomes. [192,207] Many of these early studies have been criticized for faulty research design, and retrospective analysis limits interpretation of data. The parturients selected for monitoring often differed in significant ways[16] from the unmonitored patients. Study samples were not randomized and did not allow for such differences among patients as use of analgesia, anesthesia, or oxytocin. [28]

Hughey and associates report a decline in perinatal mortality from 19.9/1000 in 1968 −1969 to 14.9/1000 in 1974 −1975. During this period, obstetrical practice in their institution allowed for an increase in the use of fetal monitors from 0−85 percent. However, these investigators are careful to note that other advances in perinatal care were concurrent. They conclude that electronic fetal monitoring has a beneficial effect though perinatal survival in this group was influenced by multiple factors.[87]

Mueller-Heubach and colleagues examined both perinatal outcome and obstetric practice in their retrospective study of fetal monitoring. They reported that intrapartum stillbirth and severe neonatal asphyxia were lower in their study population in 1977 than in 1970. Severe asphyxia was defined as the need for positive-pressure ventilation with oxygen at delivery. None of the patients had been monitored in 1970 while 72.7 percent were monitored in 1977. In their analysis of the data, the authors controlled for changes in obstetric practice and patient population including all cases of breech presentation, prolonged labor, traumatic delivery, congenital malformation, and Rh disease. They concluded that electronic fetal monitoring significantly decreased the intrapartum stillbirth rate and the incidence of severe birth asphyxia. The neonatal death rate remained the same.[132]

Another recently published retrospective study compared elective and nonelective fetal heart rate monitoring. The nonelective group included those women who had indications for monitoring according to guidelines published by the American College of Obstetricians and Gynecologists.[5] Those who did not were assigned to the elective group. The first 30 minutes of tracings after admission to the hospital and the last 30 minutes of tracings before delivery were analyzed. Krebs and associates reported that the nonelective or risk group demonstrated three times the perinatal mortality of the elective group. They also reported a significantly higher number of low 5 minute Apgar scores in the nonelective (risk) group. Using a previously devised fetal heart rate score based on monitor tracings, these researchers found that poor fetal prognosis correlated with the height of the fetal heart rate score. They concluded that (1) fetal heart rate patterns known to indicate hypoxia occur more frequently in the risk than in the nonrisk group, and (2) low-risk fetuses are at the same risk of cord incidents as high risk fetuses. In the low-risk group 72 percent of low 5 minute Apgar scores occurred in conjunction with variable decelerations which are known to indicate cord compression. These authors have presented a strong argument for the routine monitoring of every patient in labor.[105]

In an attempt to elucidate the fetal monitoring controversy, Parer combined results from ten fetal monitoring studies. Sufficient data were obtained to show a statistically significant decrease in intrapartum stillbirths when fetuses were monitored. The combined results showed that intrapartum stillbirth rates dropped from 2.4−0.5/1000 in association with electronic fetal monitoring. The neonatal death rate decreased from 8.1−3.6/1000. Parer obtained a large amount of data, but he combined data from a variety of studies each of which had methodologic defects. The studies differed in population selection and in

obstetric management; randomization of subjects was not used. Parer nevertheless concluded that intrapartum stillbirths and neonatal deaths are significantly
reduced in association with monitoring. He was careful to acknowledge that
this strong association does not imply cause-and-effect, while stating that even
low-risk patients would benefit from routine electronic fetal monitoring.[150]

Baumgarten[12] pleaded for the electronic monitoring of all laboring wom-
en, and has claimed a reduction of perinatal mortality of 30 percent in his
department in the first 2 years after fetal monitoring was introduced. His
support of routine electronic fetal monitoring, as that of many clinicians, has
evolved from the unpredictable occurrence of fetal distress in some cases.

As impressive as these studies are, the nurse-midwife and pregnant
woman who wish some choice in the matter of electronic fetal monitoring will
find support in the literature for selective fetal monitoring.

Advocates of selective fetal monitoring.   Opponents of routine fetal
monitoring often have cited the rising cesarean section rate which seems to
have accompanied the increased use of fetal monitoring in labor. Banta and
Thacker pointed out that in 1956 the cesarean section rate in the United States
was 4.5 percent of all deliveries and by 1976 it was 12.1 percent of all
deliveries.[9] Many physicians have noted an increase in cesarean sections which
occurred concurrently with a rise in the use of the electronic fetal monitor.[87,90,207] Others, however, have reported no such increase. In evaluating the
effect of electronic fetal monitoring on the rate of cesarean sections, care must
be exercised. It is difficult to attribute the rising rate to a single factor. The use
of cesarean section for cephalopelvic disproportion, dystocia and breech presentation has also increased. The reported use of cesarean section for fetal
distress alone is 15 − 20 percent.[9] Parer indicated that part of the cause of the
expanding cesarean section rate may be due to misuse of the monitor and
misinterpretation of the fetal heart rate pattern.[150] Haverkamp determined that
mothers who were electronically monitored were at risk for cesarean section.
An increased diagnosis of fetal distress and failure to progress in labor were
found in monitored patients over patients whose fetal heart rates were determined by auscultation.[82]

The research of Haverkamp and co-workers is widely quoted by advocates
of less intervention in the birth process. In two controlled studies, these
investigators demonstrated no difference in immediate fetal outcomes in an
electronically monitored group and an auscultated group.[81,82] In their 1976
study, high risk women were randomly assigned to one of two groups.
Evaluation of the monitored group was based on electronic fetal monitoring,
while in the other group fetal heart rate was determined by a nurse who
auscultated according to a stringent protocol. These women also had electronic
monitors, but management decisions supposedly were based on data from
auscultation only.[81] In a more recent investigation, Haverkamp and coworkers
allowed for a third group which had electronic fetal monitoring plus an option

for fetal scalp blood sampling as needed.[82] The researchers concluded that electronic fetal monitoring alone or with fetal scalp blood sampling did not improve perinatal outcome over auscultation alone. "It would seem very unlikely that a low risk term patient experiencing a normal labor would benefit from monitoring if she is properly auscultated."[82]

Neutra and colleagues evaluated over 15,000 live births, and, as a result of their findings, questioned the value of routine electronic fetal monitoring for the low risk patient.[140]

Goodlin and Haesslein attempted to define fetal distress. They compared prepartum fetal monitoring (fetal activity and other diagnostic tests) with intrapartum monitoring. They concluded that the prepartum monitoring appeared to be more effective than the intrapartum monitoring in avoiding perinatal deaths; the normal, term fetus tolerated labor well; and that accidents, such as cord prolapse or placental abruption, were diagnosed by good nursing care and observation, not continuous fetal heart rate monitoring.[74]

Banta and Thacker's highly critical and much criticized study of electronic fetal monitoring has added fuel to the debate.[9] These authors intensively reviewed the available literature on monitoring and concluded that the procedure has become a routine without proper consideration for the risks to mother and fetus and to the cost effectiveness of continuously monitoring every laboring woman. This report touched off a storm of controversy. Perhaps it will encourage more controlled studies of the effects of fetal monitoring.

There are certain risks reportedly associated with fetal monitoring that the nurse-midwife needs to disclose to the laboring woman and her family so they can make an informed decision and give informed consent for the procedure. Fetal risks include neonatal infection, scalp abscess, rare hemorrhage, and the previously mentioned loss of protection of the amniotic fluid when the internal electrode is used. The long range effects of ultrasound, used in the external monitor, have yet to be documented. Monitored mothers are at an increased risk for postpartum infection, especially if they undergo cesarean section.[71] Other side effects are uterine perforation, placental perforation or abruption, and cord prolapse.[13,214]

Psychological aspects of fetal monitoring. In nearly all of the previously mentioned studies, the psychoemotional component of electronic fetal monitoring is barely mentioned. Haverkamp[81] pointed out that the careful attention given to the auscultated patients in his study possibly could have benefited the fetus. A reassuring atmosphere may have contributed to the excellent fetal outcomes in this group.

Does electronic fetal monitoring dehumanize the birth experience, and what are the responses of laboring women to this technology? Starkman conducted interviews of postpartum women who had been monitored and found a variety of responses.[197,198] Some of the women viewed the monitor as reassuring—confirming the viability of the fetus. Other women said the monitor was a help in passing the time and in allowing optimal interactions with their partners. The monitor gave information about the beginnings and peakings of contractions and allowed the couples to work together. This working together and knowing when the contractions were starting gave the women an increased sense of mastery over their labors. Other positive responses from these women indicated the monitor helped them by giving the staff information they could not give or did not feel able to give.

Some of the interviewed women had negative feelings about the monitor. There were reports of a feeling of competitiveness with the monitor—the staff seemed to give more attention to the machine than to the woman. In some instances the monitor contributed to the laboring woman's discomfort. Application of the internal monitor was considered by many to have been painful and the belts associated with external monitoring often caused the women distress. Restriction of movement was also considered a problem by some of the women. Other negative remarks about the monitor included annoyance caused by the noise of the machine and a few women found that the presence of the monitor increased their anxiety.

Starkman determined that women who had a previous pregnancy loss had highly positive feelings for the monitor while women who expressed the most dissatisfaction had prior uncomplicated labors and healthy neonates. She concludes that personality characteristics as well as the outcome of prior pregnancies affect the way women view the monitor.[198]

Starkman and Youngs[199] have examined the psychological and physiologic implications of fetal monitoring and have clearly stated their suggestions concerning the routine use of this technology, as follows:

1. Not all women need to be monitored. The fetal monitor should be used when necessary to augment normal labor management.
2. The monitor should not replace an attentive staff.
3. All partners involved in the birth process should have anticipatory guidance regarding possible use of the monitor and equipment involved. Ideally, this should occur both prenatally and on admission in labor.
4. The implementation of electronic monitoring methods that allow ambulation, such as telemetry,[177] should be encouraged.
5. If a monitor is necessary, careful attention to the maintenance of privacy is very important.
6. The staff should have a healthy respect for the anxiety-producing potential of the monitor and be prepared to deal with it.[199]

Several studies have shown that prenatal teaching about the monitor reduces anxiety and negative feelings toward the monitor.[53,115] It behooves all clinicians involved in prenatal care to brief their patients on the monitor, even if its use is not anticipated.

For nurse-midwives and their patients who do not choose to use continuous electronic fetal monitoring, continual attention must be given to fetal status. The time-honored method of auscultating and counting the fetal heart tones for 15 seconds, then multiplying by four, is no longer recognized as adequate monitoring. For nurse-midwives who will use auscultation, Varney has described a method of obtaining reliable fetal heart information. She recommends beginning auscultation between contractions. The fetal heart rate should be counted for 10 seconds, multiplied by 6, then a rest for 5 seconds, then counted again for 10 seconds and multiplied by 6. This should continue through a contraction and to a point midway before the next contraction. The uterus should be palpated simultaneously to determine the relationship between fetal heart rate and uterine activity.[214] A fetoscope can be used but the use of a small portable doppler instrument will allow the nurse-midwife to evaluate the fetus with little disturbance to the mother. Parer,[150] though vehemently supporting routine electronic monitoring, offers a suggestion for intermittent electronic monitoring or fetal heart rate sampling. Critics may find his request of a 5 minute tracing every 30 minutes to be as invasive as continuous electronic monitoring. However, this does offer the nurse-midwife working in a tertiary or large medical center an option that may meet her needs, those of her patient, and institutional demands as well. It is important for the nurse-midwife to stay abreast of this controversy surrounding intrapartum care and to be aware of options she might offer. In this way she can provide optimal and satisfying service to her patient.

Psychoemotional Support in the First Stage of Labor

"The pregnant patient has the right to be accompanied during the stress of labor and birth by someone she cares for, and to whom she looks for emotional comfort and encouragement."[79] The nurse-midwife has elected to participate in a profession dedicated to family-centered care—this is stated in the philosophy of her professional organization.[4] Some nurse-midwives, however, must practice in institutions in which family-centered care is not a priority. In some hospitals, especially in large, city institutions, lack of personnel is often cited as the reason for failing to offer family-centered care. Another objection is that the patient's support person often is unprepared and might "faint" or "interfere." For whatever reasons, the pregnant woman's significant other is not allowed to participate in the labor and birth despite studies incontrovertibly showing the value of this involvement to participants. The consumer movement, which has done so much to reform the birthings of the middle class, has not yet reached the poor residents of inner cities. The nurse-midwives, lacking administrative, medical and staff nurse support, must, quite literally, fight city hall. It is hoped this section will assist nurse-midwives in compiling more data essential to generating needed reforms.

The nurse-midwife's initial contact with the family occasionally may be at admission to the labor and delivery area. In some larger institutions the nurse-midwife shares the work load with the medical staff and will assume management of a woman who was not a nurse-midwifery patient prenatally. In these situations frequently neither the woman nor her family is prepared for labor and birth. The nurse-midwife working with unprepared patients may find the following discussion helpful in providing support to her patients during labor.

The nature of support.   Adequate support of the woman in labor does much to increase her command over the situation and give her a satisfying birth experience. Increasing her sense of control is likely to decrease her anxiety. Varney states that, "Effective supportive care is worth 100 to 200 milligrams of Demerol, two to three hours of labor duration, and uncountable psychological benefits."[214]

Support is an elusive term and is a concept difficult to define. Anderson attempted to give support an operational definition. She discovered that support means many things to many people—help or encouragement, guidance, strength, reassurance, understanding, praise, or relief from discomfort, mental pain, and fear. She reviews many nurses' thoughts on support and concludes, "The goal of support ... is to enhance the patient's participation in the labor process and to foster activity which enables the participants to maintain control."[6] She affirms that the psychological, emotional, and physical facets of support cannot be separated.[6] This seems to strengthen Lesser and Keane's ideas. In their classic work they recognized five areas of support for the laboring woman:

1. Sustaining the woman with human presence.
2. Relieving the pain.
3. Delivering physical care.
4. Reassuring the couple of a positive outcome.
5. Accepting the couple's behaviors and attitudes.[112]

Although there may be many definitions of the term "support," one certainty emerges—support cannot be routinized. Every labor is different and every laboring family has different needs to be met. In this discussion of support it will be helpful to consider support to include the care of a nurturing nurse-midwife or other birth attendant, the presence of at least one significant other, provision of physical care, and attention to the informational needs of the laboring woman and her family.

Physiologic and psychological benefits of support.   Shainess states that almost all labors are accompanied by some degree of fear and anxiety,[190] and nurse-midwives know this from clinical experience. The behavioral manifestations of anxiety are familiar to those who attend women in labor. Not as evident, however, are the physiologic changes anxiety can produce that can be detrimental to both mother and fetus.

Newton and associates manipulated the environment of pregnant mice and found that the onset of labor was delayed or the interval to the next pup's birth was lengthened when laboring mice were disturbed after the birth of the first pup. A more troubling result of this study was that 54 percent more pups died when the mother received environmental stress than when she was left in familiar surroundings.[138] Though extrapolation from mice to humans might be considered questionable, one can only wonder what the birth atmosphere would be like if laboring humans were as obvious in their reactions to environmental stress as these other mammals.

When pregnant rhesus monkeys were exposed to stress, Morishma noted a significant elevation in maternal arterial blood pressure and heart rate. Accompanying these changes were caridac arrhythmias and increased uterine activity. Fetal deterioration in the form of bradycardia and lower oxygenation was associated with maternal agitation. Morishama attributed this to an increase in uterine activity and resultant reduction in uteroplacental circulation. He infers from his findings that a stress, which causes excitability in the mother, can damage the unborn fetus. The situation was reversed by removing the stressful stimulus. Projecting the same results to human mothers should be done with care. Considering the typical American delivery room, however, it is stunning to discover the nature of the environmental stress given the monkeys—they were subjected to a bright light shining in their eyes.[130]

It is known that catecholamine secretion increases in response to anxiety. Rosenfeld demonstrated that reproductive tissues are more sensitive to epinephrine than other tissues in the body.[176] Findings from a number of studies have suggested that this response to the increase in catecholamines can decrease the blood supply to the fetus and inhibit uterine contractions.[26,45,226] Norepinephrine produces increased uterine contractility while epinephrine elicits the opposite effect.[111] Lederman and associates assayed catecholamine levels during labor in 32 primigravidae who had also been measured for anxiety. They found, as expected, that there was a significant correlation between epinephrine and anxiety levels. In their sample an increase in plasma epinephrine was related to a decrease in uterine activity and a lengthening of labor. Their findings confirmed an interrelationship among the catecholamine epinephrine, anxiety in the mother, and progression of labor.[111]

Suspecting that women who scored high on a measure of anxiety would be likely to develop uterine dysfunction or fetal hypoxia, Crawford designed a study to test this hypothesis. Women in late pregnancy were asked to complete a questionnaire designed to determine if they had experienced symptoms of muscle tension. Behavioral manifestations of anxiety during labor were recorded by nurses. Finally, physiologic data that would indicate anxiety, such as systolic blood pressure and pulse, were obtained from the delivery summary sheet. From these observations Crawford determined that women who reported more than average muscle tension in pregnancy and exhibited more than average behavioral and physiologic symptoms of anxiety at the beginning of labor, developed uterine dysfunction and uterine hypoxia. Seventy-two percent of the primiparae who scored high on measures of anxiety developed physiologic disturbances of labor. When scores of anxiety in this group of women were above the median, Apgar scores of the neonate were lower than when anxiety scores were below the median. The author contends that this information lends support to a vasoconstrictive effect of anxiety which reduces oxygen to the fetus. These findings suggest that the nurse-midwife who is alert for muscle tension, behavioral clues, and physiologic signs of anxiety can provide support in labor which will result in more efficient labors and better fetal outcomes.[45]

Does human contact affect the mother's perception of pain during labor? Is she more in control when another is with her? Is interaction with another important for the mother in labor? Support implies that someone is with her, whether it is husband, partner, a family member, a significant other or the birth attendant. In an often-cited 1976 study on continuous electronic fetal monitoring, women who had only auscultation experienced the bonus of extensive physical contact with a nurse. These nurses provided individualized care while the monitored group did not receive this attention. The study's authors consider that this extra human contact could have had a significant effect on the fetus. In the auscultation group of women, there were significantly fewer mothers who had cesarean sections and postpartum infections and there were less ominous fetal heart rate patterns in early labor than in the group of women that received electronic monitoring.[81]

Perception of pain and sense of control in childbirth are affected not only by the moral support of a significant other, but also by practical help. If the support person is not only with the woman but also offers help with breathing, massage, and other comfort measures, then her control is increased. The helping hand of the support person is often the only cause of a difference in the woman's perception of pain.[19]

The conscientious nurse-midwife will realize that a possible source of environmental stress for the parturient could be the manner in which the staff interacts with her. Danzinger[49] observed interactions between laboring women and staff. She found a possible source of conflict when the staff attempted to control the experience and expected certain behaviors to be exhibited. Certainly all nurse-midwives have had the experience of having a staff member place a value judgment on the laboring mother's behavior or on her requests for variation in care. Danzinger's valuable study cautions caregivers to individualize the care of the family in labor. Pressure to behave in a certain manner can only increase anxiety.

Meeting the informational needs of the laboring woman and her family requires the nurse-midwife to educate, to some extent. The nurse-midwife shares information as labor progresses, but also is aware of the value of education throughout pregnancy. Prenatal education for childbirth has greatly increased the support to laboring women and their families. Dick-Read was the originator of the concept of the fear-tension pain cycle.[52] He felt that education and some preparation for labor would ease the cycle. He also believed that support and reassurance during labor was vitally important. There are a number of methods of childbirth education and it is beyond the scope of this chapter to discuss these methods in detail here, but all are directed toward helping the childbearing woman and her family have a positive birth experience. Though most of the education takes place antenatally, the benefits are reaped in the intrapartal period. This author suggests that the nurse-midwife supporting the unprepared family may use the techniques of the various education methods and see some of the same positive results.

Several studies have examined the outcomes of labors of prepared gravidas. A specific method of prepared childbirth was examined by Hughey. Five hundred Lamaze-prepared couples were compared to 500 unprepared couples to determine the obstetric effects of such preparation. The parturients who were Lamaze prepared had fewer cesarean sections, less fetal distress and febrile morbidity, as well as fewer perineal lacerations. Apgar scores were higher in the Lamaze group, though this difference was not significant. In this sample the Lamaze-prepared group had a more positive obstetric performance than the unprepared group.[88]

A second study, by Scott and Rose, that matched prepared and unprepared patients resulted in findings somewhat different from Hughey's. Scott and Rose, however, examined different variables. There was no difference between the prepared and unprepared groups on fetal distress, Apgar scores, length of labor, or maternal complications. The chief dissimilarity in the groups involved the use of medication. The prepared mothers received narcotics less frequently, had less conduction anesthesia, and had more spontaneous vaginal deliveries.[187] Since many of the risks of narcotics and forcep deliveries are known, one can reason that the prepared women had better outcomes.

Prepared primiparae requested significantly less medication and were in better control than their unprepared counterparts in a small sample studied by Rutter et al. Labors were shorter in the prepared group, but the difference was not significant. The researchers discerned that the husbands of the prepared women contributed to a very positive birth experience.[89]

Moore provides a historical review of the prepared childbirth movement and uses this background to emphasize the mutuality of a couple who work together in birth. She reasons that a couple's relationship would be strengthened by sharing the birthing experience.[129] Peterson and Mehl believe that the parents' activities and experience during labor and birth affect their relationship and their interaction with the neonate; a negative birth experience may cause many later problems in family interaction, but with a positive birth experience there will more likely be a positive maternal self-image. This, in turn, will initiate a mutual positive regard among all members of the family.[153]

There can be no doubt that support to the woman in labor is of great importance. Support encompasses the physical, emotional, and psychological realms of the woman's being. It has immediate ramifications for the intrapartal period, and probably long-term meaning for the childbearing woman and her family. It is the essence of nurse-midwifery intrapartal care.

Providing support to the childbearing woman and her family. The woman who has attended childbirth classes and has received individual anticipatory guidance during pregnancy is usually the best prepared for the event. The woman who begins labor without the advantage of childbirth education may be apprehensive as she proceeds through admission. Her anxiety level—with associated psychological and physiologic disadvantages—may be increased by unfamiliar and embarrassing procedures, recalling exaggerated tales of childbirth horrors, or by separation from her family. Assisting the unprepared woman and her family to have a positive intrapartum experience is therefore challenging for the nurse-midwife.

In a study directed particularly to childbirth educators, Stevens[200] reviews the psychologic aspects of pain management. He identifies five psychological strategies that have been found to reduce the perception of pain in the laboratory. These seem to encompass the teachings of most childbirth education classes and many of these strategies can be used to help the unprepared woman if the nurse-midwife encounters her in the early stages of labor.

Systematic relaxation is a technique used to promote muscular relaxation. The mother tightens a muscle group and maintains the contraction. Then the muscle group is relaxed. The nurse-midwife encourages the woman (and her partner) to notice and concentrate on the feelings of both tension and relaxation. Then another muscle group is contracted and relaxed. While the muscle group is in contraction, the nurse-midwife helps the woman recognize the feeling of relaxation in all of the other muscle groups. Touch is an important tool here for giving support; gentle pressure on tense muscles will clue the mother to relax them. This absence of tension diminishes the perception of pain and the anxiety which may accompany it.

Cognitive control is another strategy to control pain perception; the laboring woman is encouraged to occupy her mind with something other than pain. The woman uses dissociation to focus on a nonpainful stimuli such as the contraction of the uterus rather than the labor pain. Cognitive control includes two other techniques—distraction and attention focusing. A stimulus such as noise, music, or voice may be used to distract the laboring woman. In Starkman's study of electronic fetal monitoring, she noted that some women found the clicking and noise of the monitor to be a distractor.[199] Attention focusing directs the mother's attention to another process; being absorbed in various breathing rhythms and massage procedures can alter her perception of pain.

The nurse-midwife can describe for the woman the experiences of progression through labor. This anticipatory guidance—the strategy of cognitive rehearsal—will allow the woman to ''rehearse'' her fears and will reduce her anxiety. Stevens points out that the parturient benefits from having objective and subjective knowledge and both are needed to reduce anxiety and pain. Objective information includes statements about labor progress and exactly what procedures will be used and reassurance that the labor is normal.

Subjective information is more experiential and, to be effective, the mother needs to be told how procedures will affect her and what she will feel.

The fourth strategy has been mentioned indirectly in the earlier discussion of the nature and value of support in labor. A subject in a psychological experiment will perform any task more successfully when he or she has received special attention or a greater amount of attention than the other subjects (the Hawthorne effect).[86] Strategies to reduce the perception of pain in a laboring mother are therefore more effective when the woman has a support person with her. The data supporting the Hawthorne effect would suggest that the woman should be attended throughout her labor.[200]

Systematic desensitization is a combination of all of the previously mentioned techniques. Mothers who have completed childbirth education classes often have been taught all of the strategies. The woman who is unprepared probably will not reach the stage of systematic desensitization.

These strategies are incorporated into a number of specific steps which may be taken to assist the woman in labor. Kitzinger has written an excellent article for the birth attendant of the unprepared mother that reinforces a belief of many nurse-midwives; the unprepared woman can be given a "quick" course in childbirth education that can help her cope with her labor.[97] The earlier the nurse-midwife encounters the woman in labor, the more effective the measures will be. Kitzinger emphasizes the value of touch and a firm, confident tone of voice.[97]

Finally, the nurse-midwife who gives support during labor is referred to several common-sense approaches by Varney.[214] She points out that it is vitally important to individualize support if it is to be successful. But perhaps her most important piece of advice is to the nurse-midwife who may feel like a failure. "Be realistic in your expectations of what you can accomplish with your support and comfort measures."[214]

The nurse-midwife who practices support as described above and allows birthing family members the freedom to behave as they desire will have contributed as much as possible to a gratifying birth experience and deserves a measure of self-satisfaction.

Analgesia and Anesthesia in Labor

One of the continuing controversies in obstetrics revolves around the intrapartum use of analgesia and anesthesia. In the early eighteenth century, the newly developed use of inhalation anesthesia at birth was questioned by the clergy who advised that the Lord's will dictated that, "In sorrow thou shalt bring forth children."[72] Women continued to seek relief, however, and by the twentieth century it was common for mothers to sleep through their deliveries.

Various developments in the twentieth century changed the attitudes of the professionals and the public toward usage of obstetric analgesia and anesthesia. As physicians became more sophisticated in their understanding of maternal—

fetal physiology, they sought methods which would not compromise the fetus while making the mother comfortable. More and more women, influenced by the teachings of Grantly Dick-Read and and Ferdinand Lamaze, chose to deliver without any medication. These women wanted to experience the birth process fully, to be "awake and aware," and to be active participants in their infants' births. Klaus and Kennell described the influence of early maternal— infant contact, "bonding," on subsequent maternal nurturing behaviors and infant development. Since drugs given to the mother during labor could alter the infant's or mother's responsiveness in the first hours of life,[100] many well-read mothers began refusing medication. These women wished to facilitate optimal bonding with their infants.

These and other developments generated the lively interest in obstetrical analgesia and anesthesia that exists today. There is a great deal of research in this area by a wide range of interest groups including obstetricians, anesthesiologists, pediatricians, neonatologists, perinatologists, nurses, childbirth educators, and parents. The nurse-midwife must evaluate the research critically. Since she manages labor and birth, she must remain current in her understanding of obstetric analgesia and anesthesia. In many nurse-midwifery practices, it is she who will decide, in conjunction with her patient, whether or not, when, and with what to medicate. Depending on her practice, she will have a variety of methods from which to choose. Some techniques are administered by her or another nurse. Others require the expertise of an anesthesiologist. Whether or not she is responsible for the medication decision, the nurse-midwife must always assume the responsibility of informing the woman of the available choices and of the risks and benefits of each.

Drugs Effective in Reducing Maternal Pain and/or Anxiety

The methods most often used are narcotic analgesia, local anesthesia, regional anesthetic blocks with pudendal, paracervical, epidural, and spinal, and inhalation analgesia and anesthesia. Sedative hypnotics and ataractics also play a role. There is no method affecting only the mother's perception of pain.

There is evidence that if medication is administered too early or in too large a dose it may inhibit the progress of labor.[3,65] If labor has been dysfunctional, however, judicious use of medication may actually potentiate progress.[3,193]

The nurse-midwife must consider potential effects of medication on the fetus and neonate. Some studies suggest that the effect of medication on an infant lingers well into the first year of life.[15,174] The immediate effects may be respiratory depression or hypothermia.[182] Long-term effects may be evidenced by subtle changes in neurologic behaviors.[25] Whether or not these changes are a result of direct drug effect or of indirect effect on maternal infant bonding is not yet known.

The nurse-midwife should be aware that not every fetus will respond similarly to the same drug. Pre-term infants have less mature kidneys and livers than term infants, and they will take longer, therefore, to metabolize drugs and will experience the effects longer than term infants.[182] A fetus who is acidotic will actually receive a larger percentage of the total maternal dose than a more stable fetus would due to alterations in placental transfer.[182]

When faced with the possible deleterious effects of drugs on the newborn, many nurse-midwives become reluctant to medicate under any circumstances. Another element of maternal response to labor complicates the issue, however. The release of maternal catecholamines in labor can also affect the infant adversely and slow the progression of labor. The work of Myers and Myers suggests that in some women with acute anxiety, medication may actually benefit the fetus and the labor progress.[134]

Further research is also required in the possible effects of the mother's attitudes towards pregnancy, childbearing, and family on her expectations of pain relief. These attitudes may be confounding variables in all research concerning the effect of maternal medication on neonatal outcome. Does the mother with unresolved feelings towards parenting require more medication as Yang et al. suggest?[222] Does only the medication alter newborn response?

Recent research into brain biochemistry has revealed that the body produces opiate-like substances called endorphins that raise pain threshold. Csantos et al. demonstrated that pregnant women have significantly higher levels of endorphins than nonpregnant controls.[48] In addition, the levels increase throughout labor, returning to nonpregnant levels at one day postpartum. It would be interesting to measure endorphins in laboring women to determine whether higher individual levels correlate with decreased perception of pain. Oyama et al. recently reported that they had good success decreasing pain perception by the intrathecal injection of synthetic endorphins into laboring women. The researchers were pleased with the results, stating that excellent pain relief was achieved with no untoward effects on the fetus or the labor. Since the medication must be introduced into the spinal fluid, however, side effects secondary to spinal fluid leakage may result.[149]

Perhaps when endorphins are better understood, the drugs we use now will no longer be necessary. In the meantime the nurse-midwife must consider the appropriateness of their use in each birthing experience.

Sedative Hypnotics

Sedative hypnotics allay anxiety and decrease excitability. In higher doses these drugs induce a hypnotic state similar to natural sleep. Those most commonly used in labor are the barbituates secobarbitol (Seconal) and pentobarbitol (Nembutal). The nurse-midwife should note that these drugs are not analgesics and that if given to a woman whose anxiety is a response to pain, they may merely decrease her ability to cope with that pain.[23] In such a case, a narcotic analgesic would be more appropriate.

The barbituate may be more useful for the parturient in early labor if she is frightened but not experiencing a great deal of pain. Using pregnant monkeys, Myers and Myers[133] demonstrated that high levels of catecholamines can adversely affect fetal status. When a barbituate is administered, maternal catecholamine production is decreased, uterine perfusion is increased, and fetal status is improved. The authors suggest that barbituates used in human labor would have the same beneficial effects. Other researchers, however, caution that if the drug is given once labor is well established it may affect the neonate adversely.

The placental transfer of barbituates is rapid. If the infant is born within 6–12 hours after maternal administration he may suffer significant respiratory depression.[193] Narcotic antagonists are not effective in reversing neonatal respiratory depression caused by barbituates. Other reported neonatal effects include neonatal hypotension, hypotonia, low Apgar scores, poor sucking, and decreased infant responsiveness.[44,59] Perhaps, because of the fetal effects, barbituates are used less frequently than the ataractics.

Ataractics

Ataractics are commonly used in obstetrics to allay anxiety and to decrease the dose of narcotic required to affect pain perception. Some of the ataractics have antiemetic properties which are useful if nausea occurs secondary to labor itself or secondary to concomitant narcotic use. The ataractics include the phenothiazines and some tranquilizers. Among the phenothiazines used in labor are chlorpromazine (Thorazine), prochlorpromazine (Compazine), promazine (Sparine), propiomazine (Largon), and promethazine (Phenergan). Hydroxyzine (Vistaril), diazepam (Valium) and meprobamate (Equinil) are all tranquilizers with ataractic properties. Some of the more commonly used tranquilizers will be discussed briefly.

Often a woman becomes quite anxious in early labor and reacts strongly to her relatively mild contractions. Medicating her with an ataractic such as intramuscular hydroxyzine and providing emotional support might calm her enough to allow her to cope beautifully with the rest of her labor.

If maternal tension and anxiety are slowing the progress of labor, administration of hydroxyzine theoretically will facilitate labor progress. There are no studies, however, which indicate that the drug has any effect on labor.[65] Some maternal side effects include drowsiness, dry mouth and dizziness.[9,59] Petrie et al. have shown that hydroxyzine is associated with a change in fetal heart rate variability.[154] What long term neonatal effects, if any, this may have is not yet known. Apgar scores are not affected when hydroxyzine is given in conjunction with a narcotic although the mother receives greater relief.[193]

Another frequently used ataractic with properties similar to hydroxyzine is promethazine. Unlike hydroxyzine, it can be given intravenously but this must be done with caution since it can significantly damage subcutaneous tissue. When used alone, promethazine decreases uterine contractility.[155] When used in conjunction with a narcotic, however, labor progression may be enhanced.[43,165] Perhaps this is due to decreased activity of the maternal sympathetic nervous system. Like hydroxyzine, promethazine reaches fetal blood quickly. Petrie noted an effect on fetal heart rate variability and findings of an earlier study documented decreased muscle tone in the infant at birth.[122] Most authors agree that at obstetrical doses there are no known sustained neonatal effects.[3,154,122,193] Like hydroxyzine, promethazine has effective antiemetic properties in addition to tranquilizing and narcotic potentiating effects.

Diazepam is a potent tranquilizer and narcotic potentiator. Its uses in labor include early labor sedation, narcotic potentiation in later labor, and as an adjunct to operative anesthesia and anticonvulsant therapy in preeclampsia. Since it does not alter maternal hemodynamics, it is a drug of choice in women with known cardiac disease.[3]

Whether or not it directly affects uterine contractility is debated, but Friedman reports that diazepam does not affect the course of labor except in those instances in which administration of the tranquilizer decreases the dose of narcotic analgesic used. In a woman whose high level of anxiety is thwarting the progress of labor, diazepam may block catecholamine release and thereby permit labor to progress.

The controversy concerning diazepam's use in healthy women with normal labors centers around reported fetal effects. The drug easily enters the fetal circulation and is found to be more highly bound to fetal serum protein than to maternal albumin.[44] When the mother has received relatively high doses, as in preeclampsia, diazepam has been found in the blood of neonates as old as 8 days.[46] The most commonly reported side effects in the newborn are hypothermia and hypotonia.[3,46,62] The hypotonia may be the cause of the poor sucking that has also been reported. These responses are dose related and most authors agree that in small doses (2.5—10.0 mg) diazepam is a useful drug in obstetric management.[3,193]

One potentially complicating factor in diazepam use is the ability of its buffer, sodium benzoate, to displace bilirubin from its albumin binding site. This conceivably could lead to a higher incidence of hyperbilirubinemia in infants whose mothers received diazepam, but in animal studies no increase has been reported.[136]

Narcotic Analgesics

Currently, narcotic analgesics are the drugs the nurse-midwife is most likely to use when her patient requires pain relief. They are potent analgesics acting directly on pain receptors in the brain. They are also easily administered and do not require the skills of an anesthesiologist. If used judiciously and with proper monitoring of the mother and the fetus they can provide pain relief with relatively minor side effects. In addition to raising the pain theshold, these narcotic analgesics also promote physical and mental relaxation and increase rest between contractions.

The narcotics also have respiratory depressant effects. These are usually counteracted in the mother by the stimulus of her contractions. If a large dose is given, however, so that either the contractions decrease significantly or the mother no longer feels them, her respirations may be sufficiently depressed to cause relative hypoxia and hypercarbia. This is most likely to occur if the mother receives an epidural shortly after a large intramuscular injection of a narcotic. She no longer feels any pain and, therefore, there is no counteraction to the narcotic-induced respiratory depression.[3]

The nurse-midwife should be aware that narcotics cause vasodilation and peripheral pooling with resultant orthostatic hypotension. The patient therefore should be encouraged to stay in bed on her left side to promote adequate uterine perfusion and to prevent dizziness after a narcotic injection. The hypotensive effect is potentiated by the concomitant use of a phenothiazine.[3]

Effects on labor are dependent on time of administration and dose. If given before labor is well established, narcotics can inhibit or arrest the progress of labor.[66] Although some authors report that once labor is well established, the analgesics do not inhibit progress,[44,193] others state that they can lengthen first-stage labor and interfere with maternal pushing efforts in the second stage.[3] This discrepancy may be dose related. In smaller doses the analgesic may counteract anxiety reactions and facilitate labor progress. In larger doses the efficiency of the contractions is affected and the mother may become too sleepy to cooperate.

Narcotics are given with the intent of affecting contractions in the "test of true labor,"[66] which might proceed as follows:

A parturient at term presents with a history of regular, frequent, and intense contractions. The cervix is not significantly dilated and perhaps is only minimally effaced. The fetus is stable. Several hours later labor has not progressed despite contractions confirmed by palpation or by an electronic monitor. The nurse-midwife may then decide to rest the woman and the uterus. A narcotic, sometimes with a sedative hypnotic, is given. If the woman awakens later not having contractions, the previous contractions are referred to as "false labor." If, however, the contractions resume and the cervix begins to dilate, it is assumed that the earlier contractions were dysfunctional.

In such cases of dysfunctional latent labor, sedation will facilitate the development of an effective labor pattern.

Practitioners' greatest concern about the obstetric use of narcotic analgesics is the direct and indirect effects of these drugs on perinatal status. Narcotic analgesics readily cross the placenta to the fetus who is actually more sensitive to them than the mother.[3] The blood brain barrier of the perinate is more permeable than that of the adult. His liver is less mature, therefore, metabolism is slower. Renal excretion of the drugs is also slower. Intrapartum hypoxia and birth asphyxia potentiate placental transfer and the depressant effects. These effects are dose related. The small doses that are currently used in obstetric practice result in few severely depressed neonates.

Petrie and Crawford[154] report that when the mother receives a narcotic there is a decrease in fetal heart variability. If the dose is too great, the infant's respiratory efforts will be depressed at birth. Interference with thermoregulation is evidenced by hypothermia.[3] In addition to direct central nervous system effects, narcotics also depress the infant by indirectly causing maternal hypotension. If the mother suffers hypotension, uterine perfusion is decreased and the infant can become hypoxic. In such instances the effects of the drug are enhanced.[3]

Findings from recent studies indicate that narcotics have more subtle and perhaps more disturbing effects on the newborn than previously thought. Changes in newborn neurobehavior which may affect parent—infant bonding have been identified. Decreased motor activity[56] and increased quiet sleep in the neonatal period may result in decreased infant—parent interaction. Brower et al.[30] report that when the mother receives analgesics the infant is less likely to respond to auditory stimuli. How these changes in neurobehavior affect maternal—infant bonding and subsequent infant development is currently a matter of speculation.

Of the narcotics, morphine is one of the longer acting drugs. It is therefore the drug of choice when a test of labor is required. Unlike meperidine, it does not increase myocardial work and is useful in the management of parturients with cardiac disease. While some authors suggest that morphine is responsible for greater neonatal depression than meperidine,[215] others discount this theory stating that the effects are similar in equipotent analgesic doses.[23] Neonatal depression is greatest in the infant born 1—4 hours after maternal sedation.[59] Naloxone is an effective antagonist.

Meperidine currently is the favored narcotic in obstetrics. It has shorter onset and duration of action than morphine. Recent research on the effects of narcotics on labor and on neonatal behavior has been centered on meperidine. Effects on the newborn are most apparent if given to the mother 2—3 hours before birth, but even if 6 hours elapse before birth, the infant will demonstrate side effects. One theory for this infant susceptibility is the toxicity of the metabolites of meperidine.[107,131] Another theory stems from the mechanisms of fetal/neonatal brain uptake of the drug.[131] Whether the persistence of the drug in the perinate is unique to meperidine or a characteristic of all the narcotics is not well defined. There are few, if any, recently published studies in which the neonatal effects of the various narcotic analgesics have been compared. Some question persists about whether or not the effects of meperidine metabolites are easily counteracted by naloxone.[203]

Other narcotics used in obstetrics include alphaprodine (Nisentil), pentazocine (Talwin), fentanyl (Sublimase), and butorphanol (Stadol).

Local Anesthesia

Local anesthetic drugs reversibly terminate nerve conduction, thereby interfering with the perception of painful stimuli. In obstetrics they are administered by numerous routes including local infiltration of the perineum for episiotomy or laceration repair; infiltration of the pudendal nerves for relief of second stage discomfort; paracervically to alleviate pain of first stage labor dilatation; into the epidural space for first and second stage discomfort and vaginal or operative birth; and in the intrathecal space for vaginal or operative birth. All nurse-midwives should be skilled in local and pudendal use. Some nurse-midwives also will choose to become proficient in paracervical block administration. Although nurse-midwives do not actually perform the epidural or spinal, they may make the decision along with the patient, to request the use of one of these methods. Nurse-midwives must be well versed in the effects of paracervical blocks in order to adequately inform patients and to postadministratively monitor patients.

Local anesthetics consist of two classes of drugs distinguished from one another by either an amide or ester linkage. Those with ester linkage (procaine, tetracine, chloroprocaine, piperocaine, and propoxycaine) are rapidly hydrolyzed by maternal plasma cholinesterases. They are shorter acting and are considered less toxic to the fetus than the amides.[181] The amides (bupivacaine, mepivicaine and lidocaine) are longer acting and affect the fetus more readily than other local anesthetics. The individual drugs differ from one another on the basis of onset of action, scope of action, duration of action, and toxicity, among other factors. One amide, bupivicaine, is strongly bound to maternal plasma and is therefore less likely to cross the placenta than the others. Choice of drug and dose administered are dependent on method of administration employed.

Inherent in the use of local anesthetics, regardless of the mode of administration, is the risk of toxicity. This can occur if a large dose is inadvertently injected into maternal vasculature or if a large dose accumulates after repeated injections. Signs of maternal toxicity include generalized twitching, convulsions, respiratory distress and loss of consciousness.[181] Signs of fetal toxicity can occur at lower levels than those tolerated by an adult. These, too, may be a result of accumulation or of rapid placental transfer of one maternal dose as sometimes seen after a paracervical block. Rarely, the local anesthetic is injected directly into the fetus during the administration of a caudal block.[193] Fetal local anesthetic toxicity is evidenced by tachycardia, bradycardia, acidosis, apnea, convulsions, and death.[181] Any nurse-midwife using these drugs should be prepared to sustain the patient should toxicity occur.

Paracervical Block

A paracervical block is the injection of a local anesthetic into the fornices lateral to the cervix. It affects sensation from the upper vagina, cervix, and uterus,[43] and is best employed in active labor before 8 cm dilatation. A paracervical block can be an effective means of obliterating the pain of first stage labor.[3] It does not, however, affect the discomfort of vaginal and perineal distention during second-stage labor.

Among the advantages of a paracervical block are the ease of administration and the quick onset of effect. Unlike the epidural and spinal routes, the paracervical mode of local anesthetic administration does not cause sympathetic nervous system blockade and therefore is not associated with maternal hypotension.[3] Since a local anesthetic is used, however, safeguards must be taken against maternal toxicity. The mother should receive fluids intravenously, oxygen should be available, and a means of resuscitation should be at hand.

Studies on the labor effects of paracervical blocks give contradictory evidence.[43,66] It has been reported that they enhance labor progress, deter it, and leave it unaffected. In instances of labor dysfunction caused by a uterine constriction ring or spasm in the lower uterine segment, a paracervical block may be helpful.[43]

The major concern about paracervical blocks is their fetal effect. In a number of cases, the fetal heart rate will decrease significantly within 2–10 minutes after administration and the effect may last up to twenty minutes.[43,181,193] Greiss has shown that one cause is a dose-related decrease in uterine blood flow leading to fetal acidosis and bradycardia.[77] With an increase in fetal acidosis, more of the drug is transferred across the placenta facilitating the direct depressant effect of the drug. Rarely, this bradycardia leads to fetal death.[44,193] When there has been previous evidence of fetal distress, all sources agree that the paracervical block should not be employed. Some authors suggest that, because of the fetal effects, the paracervical block is "doomed to eclipse."[44]

Epidural Analgesia and Anesthesia

The epidural route of local anesthetic administration currently is popular in obstetrics. The anesthetic is injected through a lumbar vertebral interspace into the spinal canal but not through the dura and, thus, not into the spinal fluid. Depending on dose, placement, and choice of medication, the epidural route provides the parturient with complete pain relief in the first and second stages of labor and in operative birth. The technique most often employed currently is the continuous epidural. Using a large bore needle as a guide, a catheter is placed in the epidural space. The catheter is secured and the mother's comfort can be maintained with repeated local anesthetic doses. The nurse-midwife should refer to an anesthesiology text to familiarize herself with the techniques so that she might assist both the mother and the anesthesiologist during the procedure.

The epidural has numerous advantages in obstetrics. Unlike the narcotics, which cause some central nervous system depression, local anesthetics given per epidural cause no maternal depression.[3,43,193] Effective epidural analgesia minimizes maternal stress responses. Less hyperventilation and lactic acid accumulation is seen in mothers receiving epidural than in those receiving systemic narcotic analgesia.[91] Women receiving epidural pain relief do not evidence the rise in corticosteroids seen in women who receive narcotics or who take no medication. While its effect on normal labor is in dispute,[29,43] many authors suggest that it is useful in facilitating progress thwarted by abnormal or incoordinate uterine activity.[29,43] If given for a cesarean birth—instead of a general anesthetic—the mother is awake at birth and, therefore, immediate maternal–infant interaction is promoted. Results of several studies indicate that local anesthetics given epidurally readily cross the placenta and may have adverse fetal effects.[206] In Standley's research, lidocaine, tetracaine, mepivicaine, and bupivicaine were the drugs given.[196] Infants of mothers recieving these drugs were more irritable and less mature in motor activity than controls. No distinction was made between the drugs. Rosenblatt et al. studied infants whose mothers received epidural bupivicaine. They found dose-related poor motor organization, poor self-quieting skills,[174] and decreases in visual skills and alertness. Despite these findings, many authors suggest that in the absence of maternal hypotension and large anesthetic doses, there are few adverse fetal effects from epidural bupivicaine.[29,38,43]

Although the epidural has been called the "cadillac of obstetrical anesthesia," the method does have significant side effects and potentially life-threatening complications. The most common side effect is maternal hypotension due to vasodilation in the lower extremities.[3] This decrease in blood pressure can usually be controlled by intravenous hydration, left uterine displacement, avoidance of a high vertebral block, and the judicious use of a vasoconstrictor such as ephedrine if the blood pressure falls significantly.[193] In those instances in which hypotension is severe or prolonged, however, not only is the mother's life in danger, but the fetus suffers acidosis and bradycardia secondary to decreased uterine perfusion.[38,193] Rare but serious complications include dural puncture with resultant spinal headache; inadvertent injection of the epidural dose into the spinal fluid, which may lead to total spinal anesthesia, respiratory arrest, and loss of consciousness;[3,161,193] and injection into the vascular bed, which can result in maternal convulsions and high fetal drug levels.[29] Although these complications are rare, the epidural should not be presented glibly to the patient, nor should it be administered without appropriate personnel and equipment available for resuscitation.

Another disturbing consequence of epidural anesthesia is its association with an increased incidence of forceps deliveries.[43,202] When the motor neurons of the pelvic musculature are affected by the anesthetic, the muscles do not provide enough resistance to facilitate fetal flexion and internal rotation.[43] Local anesthetics that cause relatively little motor blockade, but adequate analgesia, minimize the problem.[29] If a motor blockade has occurred, Friedman recommends waiting for the effect to wane so that the mother can deliver spontaneously.[66] In deciding whether or not to recommend epidural analgesia, the nurse-midwife must consider maternal status, maternal perception of pain, labor progress, fetal status, and the availability of skilled personnel and resuscitation equipment. Epidural analgesia must not be considered a routine procedure, only a useful tool for labor and pain management in individual situations.

Caudal Anesthesia

Caudal anesthesia is the placement of local anesthetic through the sacro-coccygeal ligament into the lowest point of the epidural space—the caudal canal.[193] Although similar to lumbar epidural anesthesia, caudal anesthesia is less popular because larger doses of medication are needed to effect pain relief in first-stage labor; there is a higher incidence of pelvic floor relaxation, which is associated with more forceps deliveries; and it is technically a more difficult procedure. The anesthetic rarely is injected directly into the fetus.[193]

Spinal Anesthesia

Spinal anesthesia is the injection of local anesthetic through the dura into the subarachnoid space. It is recommended for use in second-stage labor for cesarean birth only. The advantages of spinal anesthesia are that it requires less medication to effect pain relief than the epidural and less of that medication reaches the fetus.[23] Continuous lumbar epidural can be used earlier in labor.

MANAGEMENT ISSUES PERTINENT TO THE SECOND STAGE OF LABOR

When labor has progressed normally, the woman and her family are physically and psychologically ready for the birth. The nurse-midwife, having watchfully assisted the family through the first stage, is ready to attend the birth. This is the climax of the pregnancy and the labor. Many families have planned and negotiated during the pregnancy for the birth experience they desire. Others have not had this opportunity. The nurse-midwife will adhere as closely as possible to the family's requests while maintaining the highest standards of maternal and perinatal safety. Families often request the presence of siblings or grandparents at the birth. They may insist that early family—infant interaction be allowed to unfold without interruption. They may request adherence to the principles of Leboyer and severance of the umbilical cord only after it ceases to pulsate. The mother or father may desire to deliver their own child. They may request that the birth attendant not do an episiotomy unless absolutely necessary. The woman may elect a position other than on her back for delivery. All of these choices enter into the nurse-midwifery management of second-stage labor.

Maternal Expulsive Efforts of Second-Stage Labor

Once the second stage of labor has begun, the descent of the fetal presenting part is accomplished by uterine contractions and maternal endeavor. Traditionally, as soon as the cervix was completely dilated, the woman was coached to strenuously bear down. It is still taught in obstetrical textbooks that, once the second stage is reached, the woman should take deep breaths and "with her breath held ... exert downward pressure exactly as though she were straining at stool."[160] This method of conducting the second stage of labor is now known to be neither the safest nor necessarily the most efficient.

Once the presenting part reaches the pelvic floor as a result of uterine contractions, a spontaneous urge to bear down usually is felt by the mother. The mother will bear down for several seconds, breathe, and then bear down once again. If left to her own devices, rarely will she hold the expulsive effort for very long. When spontaneous bearing down efforts are allowed, the average number per contraction has been reported to be 4.29.[34] Skeptics of the physiologic soundness of aggressive pushing propose that nature has provided the mother with the forces necessary for fetal expulsion. Not every contraction of the second stage may result in a spontaneous maternal expulsive effort. Kitzinger[98] fosters maternal attention or "listening" to the contraction with pushing only if and when the contraction demands it.

Strenuous and sustained expulsive efforts may result in harm to the fetus. Prolonged bearing down, defined as longer than 6−7 seconds, with closure of the glottis, produces an increase in intrathoracic pressure. The elevated intrathoracic pressure causes a drop in maternal cardiac output and arterial pressure with a resultant decrease in placental perfusion and oxygenation to the fetus. Fetal acidosis may be the ultimate outcome.[33] A transient fetal heart rate dip is often associated with maternal expulsive efforts.[126] Abdominal aortic compression occurs with maternal bearing down even if the maternal position is such that the uterus is displaced.[11] Fetal outcome can be meliorated if the bearing down efforts last about 4−5 seconds and if the mother is directed not to close her glottis.[33]

If maternal and fetal status continue to be normal, the nurse-midwife and the mother may conduct second-stage labor as naturally as they wish. The uterine contractions will bring the presenting part low enough to initiate spontaneous pushing efforts. These spontaneous pushing efforts should be allowed to continue until crowning when the nurse-midwife and mother will control the birth of the baby. The concept of having the mother keep the glottis open as recommended by Caldeyro-Barcia coincides with opinions of some authors who feel that the mother should have an image of "openness" during second stage. Those authors believe that relaxing the mouth and throat will help the mother to relax the perineal floor and effect a smoother delivery.[70,98]

Occasionally a spontaneous urge to bear down does not occur. Assisting the mother into a position, such as squatting or kneeling, which will allow some gravitational force, often will help to bring the presenting part down to the pelvic floor and the urge to push will soon be apparent. Sometimes it is appropriate to use coached bearing down. If this is the case, the woman should be taught to bear down, with her glottis open, for 5−6 seconds at a time. Helping her to relax her arms rather than pulling back on hand grips may increase the efficiency of the pushing effort. There is no place for the protracted, intense bearing down that has been so much in style.

Anesthesia for Second-Stage Labor

The use of local anesthetic agents to induce perineal numbness is indicated when the need for an episiotomy seems likely. Since there is some evidence indicating that the use of local anesthetics may be associated with an increased incidence of perineal lacerations,[54] the question of whether or not they should be administered primarily to assist an uncomfortable mother with a more controlled delivery remains unanswered.

Depending upon the circumstances surrounding the childbirth event, either a pudendal block or local infiltration of an anesthetic agent into the perineum may be appropriate. Both procedures for administration of an anesthetic carry very little risk of potential harm to the mother or baby as long as appropriate medications are used in judicious amounts. Care must be taken to be certain that no medication is injected intravenously. Only rarely do women have toxic reactions to these anesthetic agents.[173]

Pudendal block. A pudendal block consists of transvaginal injection of a local anesthetic agent bilaterally at sites immediately posterior to the tip of each ischial spine.[173] This allows for an anesthetized pudendal nerve which results in numbness of the perineum and vulva, including the clitoris, labia majora, labia minora, perineal body, and rectal area.[214] There is no effect on the uterus or uterine contractions. The bearing-down reflex, however, is likely to be lessened and may be lost completely.

Local infiltration. Local infiltration of an anesthetic agent into the midline or mediolateral area of the perineum before delivery is appropriate when the second-stage has progressed so rapidly that there is no time to do a pudendal block or when the decision to perform an episiotomy cannot be made until just before the delivery. It is also indicated when administration of a pudendal block has been unsuccessful or when the mother has requested that a pudendal block not be used.[214]

Episiotomy

Incising the perineal body has become routine practice in American obstetrics. This procedure, designed to prevent severe perineal tears during childbirth, has grown to be deemed necessary in almost all deliveries. Pritchard and MacDonald cite episiotomy as the most common operation in obstetrics.[160] The reported incidence of episiotomy in hospitals is 70–95 percent.[201] This rate is much less in alternative settings, however. Mehl reports a 9.8 percent episiotomy rate in home birth,[123] Gaskin reports a 22 percent rate,[70] and Barton and colleagues[10] report an episiotomy rate of 33.7 percent in their Alternative Birthing Center. As women have questioned more and more of the matters associated with their health care, it is natural that episiotomy would be scrutinized. In 1977 Cogan and Edmunds reviewed the existing literature regarding episiotomy and asked for a more conservative approach to episiotomy than was in practice.[40]

Episiotomy is presented as necessary to avoid perineal lacerations, to protect the fetal head from intracranial injury, to shorten the second stage of labor, and to avoid permanent relaxation of the pelvic floor.[160] In responding to the critics of routine episiotomy, one author says that it is obvious that since the advent of hospital deliveries with the use of episiotomies, "There has been an appreciable decrease in the number of women subsequently hospitalized for treatment of symptomatic cystocele, rectocele, uterine prolapse, and stress incontinence."[160] This exclamation is, of course, totally unsupported by any longitudinal comparison studies of perineal muscle integrity following deliveries with or without episiotomy.

Since the future condition of the pelvic floor is cited as a reason for episiotomy, Schrag has reviewed the literature on the subject. She found that there are many factors that affect the pelvic floor only one of which is childbirth. She describes three categories of factors:

1. *Conditions inherent in the woman's situation:* heredity, development, ethnic considerations, fetal size and presentation, pelvic-type labor pattern, and maternal age and parity.
2. *Factors the woman can influence:* good nutrition, muscle tone of the pelvic floor, ability to relax, and perhaps prenatal perineal massage.
3. *Variables the nurse-midwife can control:* prompt treatment of any vaginitis, selection of an optimal delivery situation, and the skill with which second stage is conducted.[183]

It is no doubt true that the perineal musculature is stretched and injured somewhat in every delivery. Levitt found a moderate negative correlation between the number of vaginal births and intravaginal, contracted pressure as measured with a perionometer. He does not specify whether episiotomies were performed on the women in the sample.[113] Since it is true that other muscle stretching and damage can be repaired with exercise it would seem that this would also be true of the perineal area. Kegel avers that these muscles can recuperate and a number of authors give specific instructions for pre- and postnatal exercises.[93,128,142]

Kitzinger elucidates an important element relative to episiotomy that is often overlooked. Episiotomy is a genital injury and must be considered within the context of the psychosexual and emotional adjustment of the woman and her partner. If an episiotomy is needed the woman may construe this as some sort of genital injury and may suffer afterward.[96] If a woman wishes to attempt delivery with an intact perineum, it is therefore necessary for the nurse-midwife to be supportive but also to be careful in her prenatal discussion. The parturient should know the conditions under which an episiotomy would be needed and should be prepared to accept the possibility.

Crediting episiotomy with reducing the incidence of perineal lacerations has been questioned by some authors. Cogan and Edmunds report that the incidence of perineal lacerations prior to the institution of episiotomy as a routine was from 20–30 percent in nulliparae and 5–10 percent in multiparae.[40] Mehl reports a 15.9 percent laceration rate among women experiencing home birth. Coupled with the episiotomy rate (9.8%) in this group of women, one can see that about 74 percent of the women were able to deliver with intact perineums. Of the parturients in this sample 57.7 percent were primigravidas.[123] Gaskin reports that 25 percent of the women in her sample had tears which means that 53 percent were able to deliver over an intact perineum.[70] Barton reports that 20.5 percent of women had repairable lacerations without episiotomy and the intact perineum rate was 37.3 percent in his sample.[10] There is a very real risk of a parturient sustaining a laceration in addition to the episiotomy. Reported rates of the incidence of laceration with episiotomy have been from 9.5 percent to about 13 percent.[18,80] Although the figures vary in each situation, it is clear that an episiotomy does not guarantee that no perineal laceration will occur.

Episiotomy has been advocated to shorten second-stage labor and to avoid injury to the fetal head. The fetal head is described as a "battering ram" against perineal obstruction in one of the premier obstetrical textbooks.[160] The necessity of protecting a pre-term infants's head or the fetus who is overly stressed by labor is not disputed. The healthy, term fetus will tolerate the second stage nicely. The correct management of the expulsive efforts of second stage will minimize deleterious effects to the fetal head.

Many clinicians believe that allowing the woman to follow her natural instincts in pushing, rather than coaching her to push with all her might, will aid in reducing the need for episiotomy and the danger of perineal laceration. It also may be advantageous for the fetus.[34] Some fear that this type of gentle pushing may protract the second stage with dangers to the mother and fetus. Beynon allowed 100 primigravidas to push as they were inclined and compared them with 100 mothers who were coached to push in the conventional way. Eighty-three of the women in the experimental group experienced spontaneous vaginal deliveries with just two having a second stage longer than the recommended 2 hours. Episiotomy was needed in less than half of these women as compared with 63 percent of the controls. The average length of the second stage of labor for these primigravidas was 1 hour and 3 minutes.[17] Cohen has responded to critics of slow descent by studying 4403 nulliparas. He analyzed the perinatal mortality rate, the neonatal death rate, 1 and 5 minute Apgar scores, and maternal fever and postpartum hemorrhage. He found no increase in perinatal mortality with a progressive lengthening of the second stage of labor and concluded that terminating the second stage of labor simply because the parturient has been in the second stage for longer than 2 hours is unjustified. He does recommend the use of the fetal monitor, scalp blood sampling, and careful observation and recording of descent.[41]

It is clear that, despite the fact that many clinicians have strong feelings about episiotomy, the literature does not abound with carefully controlled studies documenting its necessity or its worthlessness. If a woman requests the birth attendant to deliver her over an intact perineum, they may work together toward this goal throughout the pregnancy.

Preparation and management of an intact perineum. When the mother decides she would like to avoid an episiotomy, she and her health care practitioner may find suggestions in a wide variety of publications supporting her goal. The steps both mother and clinician can take have been detailed by several authors and are summarized in the following discussion.

Optimal nutritional status of the mother should be maintained, including prevention of anemia and attention to adequate protein and Vitamin C intake. This will ensure good perineal tissue condition.[183,201]

Vaginitis, which may cause poor tissue turgor and lead to laceration, should be promptly diagnosed and treated.[183,201]

Perineal massage may be used prenatally. It is thought that this will stretch the perineal muscles. It will also help the woman to identify which muscles will need to be relaxed during the second stage.[183]

Kegel's exercises, practiced prenatally, may aid in strengthening perineal tissue and teaching pelvic floor relaxation.[183]

Prenatal childbirth education will enable the woman to help conduct the second stage to allow for maximum control of delivery of the fetal head. If the parturient is carefully taught proper pushing techniques and has practiced them, she will be able to effect slow delivery.[128]

Control of the expulsive forces of the second stage using gentle pushing will also help to maintain an intact perineum.[96,128] Several authors recommend delivery of the head by the mother pushing between contractions.[133,214] At least one author, however, states that this can lead to cardinal ligament damage and future uterine prolapse.[121] Others mention that better control of the delivery of the fetal head can be maintained if the parturient blows out or "breathes the baby out" during contractions rather than pushing during contractions.[135]

A delivery position allowing the most efficient use of natural forces and a minimum of trauma to the perineum should be selected. Some clinicians suggest that the dorsal recumbent or side-lying positions cause less perineal tearing than the lithotomy; this is not well documented, however.[201]

Massage of the perineum during second stage in order to stretch, soften and relax the perineal tissues can be helpful.[105,108,183,201] Substances used include vegetable oil, baby oil, Vitamin E, green soap, and KY jelly. The use of hot compresses during second-stage labor also has been reported to soften the tissues and increase the circulation.[58] Some birth attendants find the compress aids in reducing the burning sensation accompanying late second-stage labor, thus giving the woman more control over her expulsive efforts. If massage is done in the second stage it must be done firmly but gently to avoid injury to the perineum.[14]

Careful delivery of the fetal head and body is essential to maintaining the perineum. It is clear that the skill of the nurse-midwife is important in preventing perineal tears.[92,183,201] Myles defines the principles of management of the delivery, "The smallest diameter of the head and shoulders should be allowed to deliver and the birth of the head should be permitted to take place slowly.''[135] Flexion needs to be maintained until the parietal bosses are born.[135,214] Some nurse-midwives declare that judicious application of a modified Ritgen's maneuver will allow for greater control of delivery of the fetal head. Others maintain that this intervention is not necessary. Another method of preventing tears at the time of birth of the fetal head is described by Varney.[214] This so-called ''guarding [of] the perineum,'' a method of perineal support, is advocated by some practitioners and not by others.

Perineal anesthesia may be used. In some studies the use of a local anesthesia has been found to be associated with perineal lacerations.[54] It is thus advised that local anesthesia not be given unless episiotomy is inevitable. Some nurse-midwives will use pudendal anesthesia to help in maintaining an intact perineum. They feel that this will assist the unprepared mother in a more controlled delivery when the fetal head is causing distention and burning. Other clinicians dispute this saying the anesthesia will increase the risk of lacerations. It is clearly a matter for further study.

The nurse-midwife, concerned about allowing the woman to make choices about her birthing, will cooperate with the mother who requests delivery over an intact perineum. As an expert clinician, however, the nurse-midwife is aware of the value of the episiotomy as an obstetric procedure when necessary. It is the responsibility of the nurse-midwife to share with the woman and her partner the circumstances dictating the need for episiotomy. A fully informed mother will be less likely to give a connotation of failure to the necessity for episiotomy. She will know that the procedure was used to provide the safest birth for her and her infant.

Midline versus mediolateral episiotomy. When it becomes clear that an episiotomy is necessary, the nurse-midwife must decide whether a midline or mediolateral incision should be made. Part of the decision rests on the reasons why an episiotomy is needed. The median, or midline, episiotomy is preferred by many clinicians because of the ease in repairing. It is less painful for the mother, there is less bleeding, healing is superior, and there is less dyspareunia.[18,148] If extension into the rectal sphincter and rectum are to be avoided, a mediolateral episiotomy would be preferred.[135] A mediolateral is advised when the patient has a short perineum, the infant is large, there is persistent occiput posterior, and in midforceps operations and breech births, and for the management of shoulder dystocia.[148,214] Some authors and clinicians, however, feel that a mediolateral episiotomy is not justified even when extension into the rectum is probable.

Nel affirms that a midline incision is the most efficient way to enlarge the orifice—the same way the orifice enlarges naturally.[137] Gaskin reminds us that even a very small cut of 1/8″ in the midline enlarges the opening 1/4″.[70] Kaltreider points out that the midline episiotomy enlarges the anterior-posterior diameter of the orifice—the best diameter, since the head delivers in this diameter.[92]

Kaltreider's 1948 study gives us some insight into the controversy of median versus mediolateral episiotomy. He examined the sequelae of over 15,000 midline episiotomies and found the incidence of rectal extension to be 0.6 percent and the incidence of third degree lacerations to be about 5 percent. Other researchers have found larger percentages.[18,81] Kaltreider and Dixon summarize the causes of third and fourth degree lacerations to be forceps deliveries, inexperience of the operator (the more skilled, the fewer extensions), occiput posterior positions, and prolonged labors. Breech birth and large infants, which are often cited as reasons for mediolateral episiotomy, were not proven to be related to extension in this study. In examining the sequelae of the rectal extensions, these authors concluded that later gynecologic repairs were done less frequently in women who had midline episiotomies than in those who had mediolateral episiotomies. They also include an interesting anecdotal note from two gynecologists who feel that the midline episiotomy affords better postpartum perineal support and diaphragm fitting.[92]

Harris reports a 13 percent rate of laceration following midline episiotomy, with a 4.6 percent chance of rectal extension.[80] He found only 7 infections reported in 7477 midline episiotomies and only one of these occurred with a perineal laceration. He acknowledges a high patient acceptance rate of the midline episiotomy based on complaints of discomfort and ease of ambulation postpartally. A significant finding of this study was that the incidence of laceration was five times higher among primigravidas after midline episiotomy than among primigravidas without episiotomy. As the degree of experience of the operator increased the incidence of third- and fourth-degree lacerations decreased. Given the low rate of infection and other effects, however, he concludes, "Fears regarding midline episiotomy are more theoretical than real, and its advantages far outweigh the disadvantages of the mediolateral episiotomy."[80]

Beynon cites a 3 percent risk of third degree extension with a midline episiotomy and less than 1 percent with a mediolateral. She maintains that a fear of extension into the rectum does not justify the use of the mediolateral episiotomy. The advantages of the midline episiotomy to the patient far outweigh its disadvantages.[18]

A randomized, prospective study was conducted by Coats and associates in 1980.[39] They examined 407 primigravidas, half had mediolateral episiotomies and half had midline episiotomies. The patients' estimates of pain were not significantly different in either group. Anal sphincter injury occurred more commonly with the midline but no fistulae developed. In postpartum examinations, scarring was less noticeable in the midline episiotomy and these women reported resumption of intercourse earlier than the mediolateral episiotomy group. There were not significant differences in dyspareunia or achievement of orgasm in the two groups. These researchers experienced an unexpected difficulty in conducting their research. The staff at the institution were extremely reluctant to use the midline episiotomy, even for the purpose of a controlled study.

If the obstetrical staff does not acknowledge the advantages of midline episiotomy over mediolateral episiotomy, the nurse-midwife who is pressured to avoid third and fourth degree lacerations may find herself using the mediolateral episiotomy more frequently. Nurse-midwives in large, teaching institutions often remark that more mediolateral episiotomies are cut because of the rather large numbers of inexperienced clinicians.

Timing of Cord Clamping

With the successful completion of the second stage, the immediate care of the neonate becomes a priority of the birth attendant. When the head has delivered, it is gently wiped dry and secretions from the mouth and nares are either wiped away or suctioned gently with a soft syringe. The body of the infant is born slowly and then held safely by the nurse-midwife or placed immediately on the mother's abdomen.[214] One of the management issues confronting the practitioner is the optimal time for clamping the umbilical cord. There is no unanimous resolution of the controversy over early versus delayed cord clamping. The umbilical blood flow continues after birth and it is certain that a transfusion of blood from placenta to fetus does take place, though reported amounts vary.[225] The controversy revolves around the possible benefits and risks to the neonate of either allowing or disallowing this placental transfusion. Advocates of a family-centered approach to birth are in favor of not clamping and cutting the cord until pulsations have ceased and many expectant parents will request this variation in care. The nurse-midwife must acquaint these parents with the known risks and benefits and with situations under which the cord will be cut immediately. As with all management decisions, the ultimate goal is a safe and satisfying birth experience for the woman and her family. When delayed cord clamping is practiced, the amount of placental transfusion varies. Blood quantities of 30ml−80ml and even as high as 100ml of blood in a full term infant, have been reported.[204,211] Taylor cites an average transfusion of 73ml for a full term fetus following a delay of 3 minutes between birth and cord clamping.[204] Yao and Lind[225] have reported that placental transfusion is 75 percent complete at the end of one minute following birth, and complete at three minutes.

Uterine contractions, gravity, and maternal blood pressure influence the amount and duration of placental transfusion.[145,204] To confirm their belief that uterine contractions of the third stage contribute to the placental transfer, Yao and colleagues administered methylergonovine maleate to mothers immediately after birth and observed that the time of complete transfusion was shortened from 3 minutes to 1 minute.[223] Gravity is also known to influence the placental transfusion. If the infant is held 40 cm below the level of the placenta, complete placental transfusion is accomplished in about 30 seconds, rather than 3 minutes. When the neonate is held 50−60 cm above the placenta for three minutes, there is no advantage of placental transfusion.[225] In most normal vaginal deliveries, the newly delivered infant is held at the level of the introitus and placental transfusion is most likely accomplished by uterine contractions. An infant held 10 cm above or below the introitus will not experience the gravitational effect of the transfusion. The data from Yao et al. indicate that a neonate held at intermediate levels between the introitus and 60 cm above will experience some impediment to transfusion directly related to the height at which he is maintained. This is significant information for the nurse-midwife who places the infant on the mother's abdomen or chest immediately following birth. The baby is often not many centimeters above the placenta, but the cord is curved up and around the pudenda, and may be quite taut. There are at present no published studies indicating the amount of placental transfusion or the effects of neonatal and cord position when the mother receives the infant directly onto her chest or abdomen. Ogata's research implies a relationship between maternal blood pressure and placental transfusion. Low maternal blood pressure will decrease the amount of placental transfer.[145]

Benefits of Placental Transfusion

Potential benefits of placental transfusion are derived from the supplementary blood the neonate receives if cord clamping is delayed. Klebe studied residual placental blood volume and declared early cord clamping unphysiologic because about 30ml of the infant's own blood are left in the placenta.[103] This amount has the potential of adding about 50 mg of iron to the neonate's stores.[160] The hematocrit of infants allowed placental transfusion has been measured to be about 60 mg% at 72 hours of life compared with 44 mg% in an early-clamped group.[211] Leboyer advocates late cord clamping because he believes that the cord blood provides auxiliary oxygen to the transitional neonate in the first 4 or 5 minutes after birth.[110] Because of the increased hematocrit and oxygen, there is a potential benefit to the anemic neonate or to infants who have been subjected to intrauterine hemorrhage.[42]

The neonatal respiratory system is also affected by placental transfusion, although researchers report both positive and negative effects. There are conflicting reports on whether late cord clamping causes fetal respiratory problems.[73,211,225] Emmanouildes and Moss indicate that umbilical cord clamping prior to lung expansion may be associated with respiratory distress.[55] Oliver and Oliver found a smoother initiation of respiration with less gasping in Leboyer (late-clamped) infants when they were compared with early-clamped infants.[147]

Thermoregulation of the infant may be positively affected by late cord clamping.[75] Gimbel mentions an advantage of late clamping not discussed in other literature. The late clamping prevents stagnation of blood in the cord thereby reducing the chance of neonatal oomphalitis.[73]

There are possible maternal advantages of placental transfusion. Botha's observation of Bantu women giving birth led him to believe that their customs decreased postpartum hemorrhage and retained placentae. After a Bantu baby is born, the mother remains squatting until the placenta delivers by gravity. Only then does she attend to the cord. The newborn receives an estimated 89ml of blood, but Botha has stated that the chief advantage is to the mother. Since the cord is not clamped, placental volume is decreased and the placenta detaches and is propelled rapidly into the lower uterine segment and vagina with only a small blood loss to the mother.[24] The implications of this information for nurse-midwifery management of third-stage labor will be discussed later in this chapter.

Risks of Placental Transfusion

As in all aspects of nurse-midwifery management, the clinician must consider both the risks and benefits of any procedure. There are some worrisome reports of potential problems following placental transfusion. Late-clamped infants reportedly spend a larger amount of time in quiet sleep while early-clamped babies spend longer periods in the quiet awake state. Since this state is the most favorable one for mother—infant interaction, the delayed clamping may affect bonding.[225]

A significant correlation has been found between neonatal hyperbilirubinemia and late cord clamping.[225] The increased red cell mass causes an increase in bilirubin turnover and breakdown of red cells.[211] Renal flow is increased in the late-clamped neonate and there is evidence that the placental transfusion and hypervolemia may inundate the neonatal circulatory system.[225] Late clamping results in increased respirations and pulmonary arterial pressure and decreases lung compliance.[73] The onset of respirations may be delayed by late cord clamping, though this conclusion is controversial,[211,225] and expiratory grunting has been noted in late-clamped infants.[225]

Because of conflicting ideas about whether the benefits outweigh the risks, the optimal time for cord clamping is an open question. This question may not be crucial in the healthy, full-term neonate. Yao and Lind feel strongly that the late-clamped infant has increased effort in transition from intrauterine life and state categorically that even in the normal spontaneous vaginal delivery, the cord should be cut within 30 seconds after birth.[225] Others feel that the transition is made easier by the placental transfusion and think it would do no harm if the infant is not stressed by other factors.[42,110,147] If the infant is anemic or in shock from fetoplacental hemorrhage, he may benefit from the transfusion of blood.[225]

The normal full-term infant can be held at the level of the introitus or placed on the mother's abdomen and allowed placental transfusion, if desired. The cord usually stops pulsating within 3—5 minutes after birth and then can be severed. Assiduous attention must be given to maintaining a thermal environment conducive to healthy neonatal transition. Chilling of the infant should be avoided. It is not recommended that the cord be stripped. Late cord clamping is contraindicated in fetal asphyxia, prematurity, polycythemia, intrauterine growth retardation, and infants born of diabetic mothers or mothers sensitized to Rh antibodies. Some practitioners avoid late cord clamping in all Rh negative mothers. In all instances, the priority of the nurse-midwife remains delivery of a healthy infant. The management plan regarding cord clamping may need to be altered at the last minute if neonatal condition so warrants. Clearing the air passages, maintaining respiration, or attention to thermoregulation may supercede parental desire for late cord clamping.

Immediate Care of the Newborn

Allowing early parent—infant contact immediately after birth is a goal of all clinicians concerned with family-centered care. Expectant parents, aware of the importance of this early contact, are seeking birth alternatives allowing early and extended encounters with their newborns. For the family experiencing birth at home or in an alternative birthing center, immediate contact with the newborn is expected and automatic, and sometimes occurs before the birth is complete.[101] The majority of births in the United States occur in hospitals, most of which have long standing care practices precluding early and extended parent—infant interactions. Unfortunately, many nurse-midwives know first hand the complaint of Klaus and Kennell, "There are still large hospitals that have never provided for early and extended contact, and the mothers who miss out are often those at the limits of adaptibility and who may benefit the most— the poor, the single, the unsupported, the teenage mothers."[101]

Accompanying the desire to provide parents with early newborn contact is the very real need for the nurse-midwife to attend to the immediate condition of the neonate. It is necessary to maintain an environment minimizing cold stress to the infant, yet maximizing newborn—parent interaction. Neonatal thermoregulation is of prime importance in the immediate postbirth minutes. The neonatal core temperature can drop by $2°-3°$ C at delivery and the resultant stress on the newborn may lead to metabolic acidosis, respiratory problems and other difficulties in transition to extrauterine life.[99] The desire to provide the thermal environment necessary for optimal transition is not in conflict with the parents' need to interact with their newborn. The nurse-midwife can modify traditional hospital practices during the intrapartal period to satisfy these concurrent needs. The following discussion will examine the importance of the parent—infant bond and the principles of neonatal thermoregulation. The author will suggest some nurse-midwifery intrapartal provisions for both requirements. Perhaps these suggestions will enable the practitioner in more traditional settings to alter services provided.

Bonding

A sensitive period uniquely affecting maternal attachment is known to exist shortly after the birth of a newborn animal. The importance of early animal mother—infant interaction also has been demonstrated. Studies have shown that early mother—infant separation in animals may result in deviant mothering behavior,[83] and even death of the offspring.[175] Weinenger reported that early handling (holding and stroking) caused the albino rat pup to increase in weight gain, skeletal length and ambulatory activity.[216] Rat and mice pups depend on maternal tactual stimulation in order to excrete and experience normal development.[205] McKinney discovered that the removal of Collie puppies from the mother immediately after birth seriously impeded the mother's recovery from the whelping process. He suggested that similar results may occur in the human mother.[118] Klaus and Kennell suggest that a sensitive period, similar to the one in animals, may exist in the human adult parent.[101]

Observers have noted that the maternal exploration of the neonate is orderly and progressive. It proceeds from a fingertip touch and moves from the baby's smaller peripheral areas to the chest and abdomen, where the mother will use the palm of her hand.[178] The sequence of behaviors is predictable, though variations may occur in the rapidity with which the mother proceeds.[36] The open eyes of the infant seem to be important to the mother for interaction. Mothers seek out the stimulus—rich eyes of their neonates and the newborns frequently fixate on their mother's eyes. The *en face* position is attained to allow for optimal eye to eye contact.[169] Mothers speak to their newborns in a high pitched voice, while they speak to health care personnel in a normal tone of voice. The infant is most responsive to this high pitched voice.[101]

Fathers given their naked newborns within 15 minutes of birth also respond in an orderly and progressive way. Paternal behaviors include hovering, fingertip stroking, palming, eye-to-eye contact and use of the *en face* position.[170] These behaviors are notably similar to maternal interactive behaviors.[101] Interestingly, unrelated males (medical students) also respond to the newborn in a way quite similar to the mother and father.[101] Perhaps these activities are part of a "claiming" behavior on the part of the human adult.

The opportunity to interact immediately after birth has positive effects, which are immediately apparent and long lasting, for both the neonate and the parents. Many research findings have demonstrated that mothers allowed early, extended contact with their newborns exhibit more maternal attachment and affectionate behaviors than mothers whose infants are removed immediately after birth.[50,94,101,102,166] Breastfeeding is likely to continue longer[195] and there are fewer reported incidences of child abuse, neglect, and failure to thrive if mothers are given an opportunity for early and extended interaction with their babies.[143] There are a few early studies indicating that positive effects extend over time when fathers are allowed extra interaction with their newborns.[98]

The reactions of the mother and father to their newborn encompass complex behaviors learned over many years. The influences on parental behavior are numerous and varied. The practitioner can alter some of these influences and others are stable but must be considered in the nurse-midwifery management of the early postnatal period. Unalterable influences include the caregiving the new parents received from their own mothers and fathers, heredity, cultural background, interfamily relationships, the outcome and conduct of previous pregnancies, and the progress of the present pregnancy.[101] Infant weight, sex, and birth order also have been shown to affect mother−infant interaction.[31]

Certain events affecting early parent−infant interaction can be influenced by the practitioner and the parents. Klaus and Kennell cite the behaviors of health care personnel, institutional rules, provision of supportive care during labor, and separation of parent and infant after birth as factors that can influence parental behavior. Parents should be allowed to plan for and have control over their birth experience as much as possible. Behavioral variations should be expected and accepted in a nonjudgmental way by health care personnel. Most mothers who receive considerate, concerned care and remain relaxed during labor will show positive behaviors toward their babies.[139]

Drugs administered to the mother during labor and birth can interfere with positive interactions between parent and infant.[25] Depressed neonates and sleepy mothers cannot participate in the reciprocal behaviors necessary for early interaction. Repair of an episiotomy usually takes place in the immediate postdelivery period. The discomfort caused by episiotomy or laceration repair can greatly distract the mother and hamper her immediate involvement with the newborn. Klaus recommends delaying the interaction until the repair is complete.[101] Practitioners who are convinced that the need for early interaction supercedes the necessity for immediate repair, will delay suturing until after the first parent−newborn interaction period. Early interaction should not coincide with uncomfortable procedures and the mother should not be given her newborn to hold as a distractor from pain.

Parents and newborns must be given the opportunity to exchange behaviors and pave the way for later interaction. The nurse-midwife is able to provide the family with the atmosphere necessary for this early care. Individual responses to labor are varied and individualization of care to the childbearing family should be a priority. To reduce anxiety, supportive labor care should be continuous, attentive, and particular to each family's needs. If possible the same room should be used for laboring and delivery to alleviate upheaval at the time of birth.[101]

The health care practitioner assisting the birth should be observant for maternal cues of readiness to accept the newborn. A mother who has experienced a long and exhausting second stage may appreciate the chance for a rest period before receiving her infant. Other mothers reach for their babies before the birth is complete and are eager and ready to begin immediate contact and interaction.

Because eye contact is an important component in initiating parent−infant bonding, prophylactic antigonorrheal eye medications should be delayed until after the interaction period is complete. The neonate is usually alert and quiet in the first 30−60 minutes following birth. Eyes are open, responses are alert, and caretaking behaviors are elicited from the parents. The new family needs privacy and a quiet time together as soon as possible after birth in order to integrate the new member and unify. Siblings and other close family members may benefit from participation in this special time.

The very young mother who has delivered without the benefit of her family's presence also needs time alone with her infant. The mother not engaging spontaneously in acceptable interactive behaviors may need some help. The nurse-midwife who hands her the baby can assist by pointing to the open eyes, sucking behaviors, clenched fists or other normal features of the neonate. Some practitioners actually help the mother to begin stroking activities. The importance of vocal stimulation of the infant can be emphasized and supported. The initial newborn examination can be done while the mother holds the baby with the practitioner identifying distinctive aspects of newborn appearance and behavior. If maternal or paternal behavior is considered to be maladaptive, appropriate support can be offered and referrals made to assist the new family.

All early parent−infant contact is predicated on the excellent condition of mother and baby. If maternal or infant condition enforces delay of early interaction, the nurse-midwife should be supportive of the family. Parents aware of the importance of early contact may fear they will be unsuccessful as parents if circumstances prevent it and may need reassurance. Other opportunities for neonate−parent interaction should be sought, and flexible institutional regulations should allow as much contact as possible. It is obvious that, though the immediate 30−60 minutes postnatally are a rich possibility for family integration, other occasions exist for enhancing the future health of the family.

Thermoregulation

One of the aims of family-centered intrapartal care is to return the healthy infant to the mother as soon as possible after birth. When the birth occurs at home or in a homelike setting, the baby usually is lifted directly onto the mother's abdomen as soon as the body is born. In more traditional settings, concern about neonatal hypothermia usually takes precedence over family−newborn interactions. The newborn is hustled off to a warming crib and the interaction of the new family is delayed. As more families request immediate contact with their newborns, health care practitioners are becoming aware that early bonding and neonatal thermoregulation are not mutually exclusive goals.

The rectal temperature of the newborn at delivery is 37.6°−37.8° C and this temperature can fall 2°−3° C rapidly after birth.[221] Slight cooling of the skin receptors may be a part of the impetus for the neonate's first breath and also probably helps to stimulate initial thyroid function.[99] Severe and sudden cold stress to the newborn, however, results in an increased metabolic rate with consequences including increased glucose and oxygen consumption, and metabolic and/or respiratory acidosis. Hypoglycemia and an increased incidence of kernicterus also have been reported to be results of sudden cold stress. Severe neonatal hypothermia also may affect clotting factors and cause bleeding disorders either directly or from asphyxia.[221]

The human neonate is described by Klaus as a homeotherm—an animal possessing the physiologic mechanisms needed to maintain body temperature at a constant level despite changes in the environment. A newborn will involve itself in increased muscle activity and shivering in order to compensate for heat loss. When the newborn flexes its body, the total amount of body surface exposed to the air is reduced, thereby promoting heat retention. The primary mode of neonatal heat production is nonshivering thermogenesis.[99] Neonatal temperature rises are generated through increased metabolic activity and oxygen consumption and an increase in the circulation through brown fat deposits. The four major mechanisms of newborn heat loss to the environment are conduction, evaporation, convection, and radiation, and each of these can be affected by physical properties in the birth room. Ambient room temperature and humidity are important considerations in neonatal thermoregulation. It is possible to assure thermal balance in the newborn if the ambient room temperature is 1.5° C less than the newborn's skin temperature.[167] An environment that maintains neonatal skin temperature at 36.2°−37° C is referred to as the neutral thermal environment. In such an environment, the newborn's metabolic rate is normal, oxygen consumption is minimal, and the body temperature is normal.[221] The nurse-midwife should endeavor to provide an acceptable or neutral thermal environment for all neonates, regardless of the place of birth.

Because neonatal temperature stabilization is so important, it is common practice in delivery rooms to have the newborn placed in a radiant heater immediately after birth. The radiant heater warms the peripheral blood and, since the blood is then circulated to the deeper tissues, the warmer provides an excellent way to prevent neonatal heat loss. Compensation must be made for insensible water loss which is increased with the use of the radiant heater.[219] The simplest, cheapest, and most convenient way of conserving neonatal thermal energy seems to have been overlooked for many years. A newborn infant, dried and wrapped, can be given to the mother to be held without experiencing problems with temperature stabilization.[27,85,156,212] Gardner, Gulezian, and Van Art have demonstrated in separate studies that skin-to-skin contact with the mother will provide the neonate with an acceptable thermal environment.[69,78,212]

Färdig used a three group study to compare the effects of mother−infant skin contact with the effects of radiant heat. The treatment groups consisted of newborns who had no skin-to-skin contact, but were placed under a radiant heater; newborns who received routine care under a radiant heater and then had skin-to-skin contact with their mothers; and a group who had immediate skin-to-skin contact with their mothers. The protocol required that each baby be dried thoroughly. This investigator was able to conclude that rapid drying of the neonate and skin-to-skin contact with the mother under a warm blanket provided a neutral thermal environment while, in her study, the radiant heated crib did not. The warmest neonates in this study were those that had the earliest and longest skin contact with their mothers. [60]

At the time of delivery, the nurse-midwife must take steps to prevent neonatal heat loss from the four major mechanisms. Conduction involves the direct transfer of heat from a warmer surface to a cooler surface. This can occur, for example, if the newborn is placed on a cold table, sheet or blanket. Protecting the newborn from cooler surfaces by placing a warm blanket between the surface and the infant will prevent conductive heat loss. Placing the naked newborn on the mother's chest or abdomen will also minimize conductive heat loss. Heat loss through evaporation occurs when heat is dissipated as the amniotic moisture from the infant's skin dries. Evaporation heat loss also occurs with respirations. Careful drying of the neonate will reduce heat loss from this mode and babies dried well have higher temperatures than those dried carelessly. [60] Both Gulezian and Färdig point out that birth attendants varied greatly in method and completeness of drying the infant. [60,78] Nurse-midwives assisting at births must be attentive to this feature of care. The fetal head can be dried before delivery of the body is accomplished if there is time, and the newborn should be carefully dried by the birth attendant or helper even before the cord is severed. Careful drying should not include removal of vernix caseosa as this seems to provide the newborn with some thermal protection. [158] Convective heat loss involves loss of heat from the infant's body to the air. Drafts or air currents, swinging doors, the flow of cold oxygen over the newborn's face, even hustling personnel may increase air flow over the newborn, potentially causing heat loss. Covering the neonate with a warm blanket reduces exposure to convective currents. Oxygen, if needed, should be warmed and it would be helpful if birth rooms could be kept quiet and free from hurry to reduce the flow of air currents. Newborns may also transfer body heat through radiation to cooler objects, such as a stethoscope, that are in direct contact with their bodies. The infant should be kept away from cold windows and walls. Skin-to-skin contact with the mother will reduce heat loss to surfaces and provide a source of radiant heat from the mother. [60,78,221]

Parents who desire immediate and continuous skin-to-skin contact with their newborns can be supported in this desire by the nurse-midwife. A newborn placed near the mother's nipple may lick or suckle, initiating oxytocin release from the maternal pituitary which will cause uterine contractions and diminish postpartum bleeding. [180] A mutually beneficial interdependence may occur in these early moments, physiologically sound for mother and baby. The normal term newborn and his or her parents must be permitted to take full advantage of these benefits.

MANAGEMENT ISSUES PERTINENT TO THIRD-STAGE LABOR

Following the birth of the infant, the nurse-midwife is responsible for the safe conduct of the third stage of labor and the immediate postpartum period. The management issues during this stage of labor concern the technique employed in placental delivery, the routine use of oxytocins in the third stage and immediate postpartum period, and the estimation of maternal blood loss.

Diligence is necessary in the third stage in order to prevent devastating maternal complications. Third stage hemorrhage and uterine inversion, though they may occur without apparent cause, are generally the result of mismanagement of the third stage of labor.[76,160,214] Hemorrhage in the immediate postpartum period is usually caused by uterine atony.[214] Myles indicates that a woman in optimal physical condition as a result of excellent prenatal care and nutrition is least likely to suffer complications of the third stage.[135] The nurse-midwife who has been managing the woman's pregnancy from early in the first trimester therefore is in a position to minimize the complications of the third stage. The nurse-midwife will also be familiar with any risk factors that potentially could cause problems in this period. These include such factors as history of a previous postpartum hemorrhage, precipitous birth, dysfunctional labor, uterine overdistention, and grand multiparity.[214] Prevention of problems of the third stage of labor can begin long before the actual birth.

Placental separation usually takes place spontaneously as the fetus is born or shortly thereafter. It is brought about by a diminution in the size of the uterus and by the force of strong uterine contractions. The nurse-midwife awaits the classic clinical signs of placental separation.[148] Greenhill indicates that these signs may not be temporarily associated with placental separation, but may occur several minutes after actual separation has occurred.[76] Since separation occurs spontaneously there are no real management decisions necessary. The foremost duty of the birth attendant at this time is one of vigilant anticipation.[160,214] Most sources agree that the nurse-midwife may await spontaneous expulsion of the placenta. As long as there is no active or unusual bleeding, no aggressive management steps are necessary.[76,160,214] Although sound management of the third stage of labor is based on patience while waiting, occasionally there is reference to a more active management of the third stage. For example, Romney alleges that if the third stage of labor is allowed to progress spontaneously, complications are more likely to occur.[173] Active management of third stage includes routine manual removal of the placenta,[74] use of the Crede procedure forcing the expulsion of the placenta,[76] use of umbilical cord traction, and the administration of a uterotonic agent with the birth of the anterior shoulder.[24,135,194] Most of these procedures have been criticized for creating more problems than they cure. In a normal birth the nurse-midwife most likely will employ a method of controlled cord traction while "guarding" the fundus of the uterus, a modified Brandt-Andrews maneuver.[214] It is generally acknowledged that spontaneous expulsion of the placenta is difficult if the woman is in a recumbent or lithotomy position. The placenta is much more readily expelled with the mother in the squatting position. Many birth attendants will have the mother assume this position for third stage. Cord traction is not usually necessary in this case.[70,135,214] Botha has reported that the placenta will deliver spontaneously by gravity without maternal effort in a woman who is in the squatting position.[24]

Some practitioners believe that draining the placenta before delivery will hasten the third stage with an attendant reduction in the amount of maternal blood loss.[24,214] Botha studied this problem and found that the duration of the third stage and measured blood loss were less following placenta drainage than when the cord was left clamped. He has claimed that if the cord is left unclamped, spontaneous expulsion of the placenta should occur within 3 minutes.[24] When the nurse-midwife utilizes this process, the amount of blood drained from the placenta should not be included in the estimated blood loss. Oxytocic drugs often are used routinely as part of third stage management in order to reduce bleeding.[194] Some authors recommend administration before the second stage is complete,[24,135] while others caution that this could cause the placenta to become trapped within the uterus, with subsequent difficulty in delivery.[76] The routine use of an oxytocic following delivery of the placenta is practiced in many institutions in an effort to reduce postpartum hemorrhage. Friedman found that approximately 22 percent of women not receiving a uterotonic agent following placental delivery will develop subsequent atonia and hemorrhage.[64]

Nurse-midwives working within large medical centers are often expected to use an oxytocic routinely; many birth attendants, however, do not use oxytocics as a matter of routine. These practitioners find that following a normal, spontaneous delivery, there is minimal bleeding and there is no call for routinized drug use.[47,84,173] Prevention of hemorrhage can be accomplished by allowing a slow delivery of the body of the infant.[47,135] Several authors mention breast stimulation, which causes reflex secretion of oxytocin and consequent uterine contractions, as an effective method of reducing the chance of a portpartum hemorrhage.[47,70,101,180] By careful attention to third-stage management, the nurse-midwife can reserve the use of oxytocics following delivery of the placenta for those who are at risk for postpartum hemorrhage.

When the nurse-midwife considers it necessary to administer an oxytocic agent, she should be aware of the different actions and side effects of such drugs, as well as the usual routine of administration. These drugs must be used judiciously. Hendricks and Bonner reported instances of severe maternal hypotension following direct intravenous injection of oxytocin.[84] There is also a known antidiuretic effect of oxytocin, and when the infusion is administered at a high rate of speed, water intoxication may result.[160,218] The recommended method of oxytocin use is in a slow, dilute intravenous infusion.[84] Ergonovine and methylergonovine may exert a pressor effect, and a severe hypertensive reaction may result in some women, especially in those known to be hypertensive.[84] A mother occasionally will express a preference regarding the use or nonuse of an oxytocic drug at her birth. As always, the nurse-midwife allows maternal determination within the parameters of safety.

Estimating the amount of blood lost by the mother following parturition is another step in management of the labor and birth process. Obstetric hemorrhage is defined as the loss of 500 ml or more of blood as a result of all stages of labor. The nurse-midwife is presented with a dilemma as there are several published reports indicating that the amount of blood loss at a normal spontaneous delivery is greater than 500 ml. Pritchard measured blood loss and found the average amount lost at delivery to be 505 ml.[159] Uleland observed a mean decline in blood volume at one hour postpartum of 610 ml.[209] Notably, the postpartum hematocrits of women in these studies did not decrease appreciably. Haswell, using an under-buttock drape designed for this purpose, measured blood loss in 156 women who experienced normal spontaneous vaginal deliveries. He found the average blood loss to be 237.6 ml. In this study the least-experienced practitioners had the highest incidence of postpartum hemorrhage and the most blood loss. Odell and Seski reported that the mean amount of blood loss from episiotomy alone equals 253 ml.[144]

The purpose of estimating blood loss is to ensure the mother of maximum health during the postpartum period. The woman who has lost a large amount of blood at delivery will tend to have a longer convalescence and is at risk for postpartum complications. Because the definition of obstetric hemorrhage is narrow, the birth attendant may tend to underestimate blood loss following a normal delivery. Uleland found that most woman compensated well for blood lost during a normal vaginal delivery, probably due to the hypervolemic state of pregnancy. He recommended that postpartum hemorrhage be redefined to signify loss of blood from a vaginal delivery which results in a decreased hematocrit at 24 hours postpartum.[209]

In the interest of the mother's safety, the nurse-midwife should be conscientious in her estimation of blood loss. New practitioners will find it helpful to measure blood in graduated containers in order to become accustomed to amounts of blood lost at delivery.

The first hour following the delivery of the placenta is an important one for the nurse-midwife and the family. Because particular attention must be given to the mother, the neonate and the new family, this hour is sometimes referred to as the Fourth Stage of Labor. The nurse-midwife is attentive to the physical condition of both the mother and the infant and to the developing psychosocial relationships within the new family group. Often during this first hour, the birth attendant is still involved with procedures surrounding the birth. As soon as the stability of the mother and baby are secured, the new family should be allowed private time together.

REFERENCES

1. Adamsons K: The role of thermal factors in fetal and neonatal life. Pediatr Clin North Am 13:599−619, 1966
2. Adeleye JA: Perineovulvovaginal preparation in labor. Int Surg 62:106−107, 1977
3. Albright GA: Anesthesia in Obstetrics. Menlo Park, Addison-Wesley, 1978
4. American College of Nurse-Midwives: Philosophy. Adopted, 1972, Washington, D.C.
5. American College of Obstetricians and Gynecologists Technical Bulletin: Intrapartum fetal monitoring. ACOG 44, Chicago, 1977
6. Anderson C: Operational definition of support. JOGN Nurs 5:17−18, 1976
7. Anderson SV: Siblings at birth: A survey and study. Birth Fam J 6:80−87, 1979
8. Arms S: Immaculate Deception: A New Look At Women and Childbirth in America. Boston, Houghton-Miflin, 1975
9. Banta HD, Thacker SB: Assessing the costs and benefits of electronic fetal monitoring. Obstet Gynecol Surv 34:8−10, 1979
10. Barton J, Rovner S, Puls K, et al: Alternative birthing center: Experience in a teaching hospital. Am J Obstet Gynecol 137:377−382, 1980
11. Bassell GM: Maternal bearing down another fetal risk. Obstet Gynecol 56:39−41, 1980
12. Baumgarten K: Advantages and disadvantages of low amniotomy. J Perinat Med 4:3−11, 1976
13. Baumgarten K: The benefits and hazards of fetal monitoring under competent and objective aspects. J Perinat Med 9(Suppl 1):62, 1981
14. Bekhit SM: The use of episiotomy. Nursing Times 72:1231−1233, 1976
15. Belsey EM, Rosenblatt DB, Lieberman BA, et al.: The influence of maternal analgesia on neonatal behavior: I. Pethidine. Br J Obstet Gynaecol 88:398−406, 1981
16. Berger GS, Maynard L: Intrapartum fetal heart-rate monitoring and perinatal mortality. Perinat/Neonat Sept:22−25, 1978
17. Beynon C: The normal second stage of labor: A plea for reform in its conduct. J Obstet Gynaecol Br Commonw 6(164):815−820, 1957
18. Beynon C: Midline episiotomy as a routine procedure. Obstet Gynecol Surv 29:614−617, 1974
19. Block CR, Block R: The effect of support of the husband and obstetrician on pain perception and control in childbirth. Birth Fam J 2:43−50, 1975
20. Bloom SL: Differential effects of fetal monitoring (Discussion). Am J Obstet Gynecol 134:411, 1979
21. Boehm FH: Differential effects of fetal monitoring (Discussion). Am J Obstet Gynecol 134:411, 1979
22. Bonica JJ: Principles and Practice of Obstetric Analgesia and Anesthesia. Philadelphia, FA Davis, 1969
23. Bonica JJ: Obstetric Analgesia and Anesthesia (ed 2). Amsterdam, World Federation of Societies of Anaesthesiologists, 1980
24. Botha, MC: The management of the umbilical cord in labor. SAJ of Obstet Gynecol 24:30−33, 1968

25. Brazelton TB: Psychophysiologic reaction in the neonate. II. Effects of maternal medication on the neonate and his behavior. J Pediatr 58:513−518, 1961
26. Breggin PR: The psychophysiology of anxiety. J Nerv Ment Dis 139:558−568, 1964
27. Britton G: Early mother−infant contact and infant temperature stabilization. JOGN Nurs 9:84−86, 1979
28. Brody H, Thompson JR: The maxim strategy in modern obstetrics. J of Fam Practice 12:997−986, 1981
29. Bromage PR: Epidural Anesthesia. Philadelphia, WB Saunders, 1978
30. Brower KR, Crowell DH, Cashman TM: Neonatal electroencephalographic patterns as effected by maternal drugs administered during labor and delivery. Anes Analg 57:303−307, 1978
31. Brown J, Bekeman R, Snyder P, et al: Interactions of black inner-city mothers with their newborn infants. Child Dev 46:677−686, 1975
32. Caldeyro-Barcia R: Some consequences of obstetric interference. Birth Fam J 2:1−5, 1975
33. Caldeyro-Barcia R: The influence of maternal bearing down efforts during second stage on fetal well-being. Birth Fam J 16:19−23, 1979
34. Caldeyro-Barcia R, Guissi G, Storch E, et al: The bearing down efforts and their effects on fetal heart rate, oxygenation and acid-base balance. J Perinat Med 9(Supple I):63−67, 1981
35. Caldeyro-Barcia R, Schwarcz R, Belzian JM, et al: Adverse perinatal effects of early amniotomy during labor, in Gluck L (ed): Modern Perinatal Medicine. Chicago, Year Book Medical Publishers, 1974, pp 431−449
36. Cannon RB: The development of maternal touch during early mother−infant interaction. JOGN Nurs 28−33, 1977
37. Carson BS, Losey RW, Simmons MA: Combined obstetric and pediatric approach to prevent meconium aspiration syndrome. Am J Obstet Gynecol 126:712−715, 1976
38. Clark RB: Conduction anesthesia. Clin Obstet Gynecol 24:601−617, 1981
39. Coats PM, Chan KK, Wilkins M, et al: A comparison between midline and mediolateral episiotomies. Br J Obstet Gynaecol 87:408−412, 1980
40. Cogan R, Edmunds EP: The unkindest cut? Contemporary OB/Gyn 9:55−59, 1977
41. Cohen WR: Influence of the duration of second stage labor on perinatal outcome and puerperal morbidity. Obstet Gynecol 49:266−269, 1977
42. Colozzi AE: Clamping of the umbilical cord. N Engl J Med 250:629−632, 1965
43. Cosmi EV: Obstetric Anesthesia and Perinatology. New York, Appleton-Century-Crofts, 1981
44. Crawford J: Principles and Practice of Obstetric Anesthesia (ed 4). Oxford, Blackwell Scientific Publications, 1978
45. Crawford MI: Physiological and behavioral cues to disturbances in childbirth. Bull Sloan Hospital Women XIV:132−142, 1968
46. Cree JE, Meyer J, Hailey DM: Diazepam in labor: Its metabolism and effect on the clinical condition and thermogenesis of the newborn. Br Med J 4:251−256, 1973
47. Crisp WE: Postpartum oxytocics. Obstet Gynecol 7:470−471, 1956

48. Csantos K, Rust M, Holt V, et al: B endorphin levels in pregnant women. Life Sci 25:835−844, 1979

49. Danzinger SK: Treatment of women in childbirth: Implications for family beginnings. Am J Pub Health 69:895−901, 1979

50. de Chateau P: The influence of early contact on maternal and infant behavior in primiparae. Birth Fam J 34:149−155, 1976

51. De Vries RG: Evaluating the role of the hospital alternative birth center. Paper given at Second Conference on Technological Approaches to Obstetrics: Benefits and Risks. San Francisco, 1981

52. Dick-Read, Grantley: The Birth of a Baby. New York, Vanguard. 1950.

53. Dulock HL, Herron M: Women's response to fetal monitoring. JOGN Nurs 53:68−70, 1976

54. Dunne K: Characteristics associated with perineal condition in an alternative birthing center. Unpublished Master's Thesis, University of Illinois at the Medical Center, 1981

55. Emmanouilides GC, Moss AJ: Respiratory distress in the newborn: Effect of cord clamping before and after onset of respirations. Biol Neonate 18:363−368, 1971

56. Ende RN, Swedborg J, Suzuki B: Human wakefulness and biological rhythms after birth. Arch Gen Psychiatry 32:780−784, 1975

57. Epstein JL: Setting up a viable home birth service run by CNM's, backed by doctors and hospitals, in Stewart D and Stewart L (eds): 21st Century Obstetrics Now! Chapel Hill, NAPSAC, 1977, pp 327−358

58. Epstein JL, McCartney M, Brew J, et al: A safe home birth program that works, in Stewart D and Stewart L (eds): Safe Alternatives in Childbirth. Chapel Hill, NAPSAC, 1976, pp 101−125

59. Ericson AJ: Medications Used During Labor and Birth. Milwaukee, International Childbirth Education Association, 1978

60. Färdig JA: A comparison of skin-to-skin contact and radiant heaters in promoting neonatal thermoregulation. J Nurs Midwif 25:19−28, 1980

61. Faxel AM: The birthing room concept at Phoenix Memorial Hospital Part I: Development and eighteen months statics. JOGN Nurs 9:151−155, 1980

62. Flowers CE, Rudolph AJ, Desmond MM: Diazepam as an adjunct in obstetric anesthesia. Obstet Gynecol 36:68−81, 1969

63. Freeman RK (moderator): Symposium: Where will your patient deliver—at home? in a hospital? in an alternative birth center? Contemporary OB/Gyn 12:104−130, 1978

64. Friedman EA: Clinical evaluation of postpartum oxytocics. Am J Obstet Gynecol 73:1306−1311, 1957

65. Friedman EA: Labor: Clinical Evaluation and Management (ed 2). New York, Appleton-Century-Crofts, 1978

66. Friedman EA: Correspondence. Br J Obstet Gynaecol 88:464, 1981

67. Friedman EA, Sachtleben MR: Amniotomy and the course of labor. Obstet Gynecol 22:755−770, 1963

68. Gabbe SG, Ettinger BB, Freeman RK, et al: Umbilical cord compression associated with amniotomy: Laboratory observations. Am J Obstet Gynecol 126:353−355, 1976

69. Gardner S: The mother as incubator—after delivery. JOGN Nurs 8:174−176, 1979

70. Gaskin IM: Spiritual Midwifery. Summertown, The Book Publishing Co, 1978
71. Gassner CB, Ledger WJ: The relationship of hospital acquired maternal infection to invasive intrapartum monitoring techniques. Obstet Gynecol Survey 32:282−283, 1977
72. Genesis Chapter 3 Verse 16: The Jerusalem Bible. New York, Doubleday, 1968
73. Gimbel J, Nocon JJ: The physiological basis for the Leboyer approach to childbirth. JOGN Nurs 6:11−15, 1977
74. Goodlin RC, Haesslein HC: When is it fetal distress? Am J Obstet Gynecol 128:441−447, 1978
75. Goodwin JW, Godden JO, Chanel GW: Perinatal Medicine: The Basic Science Underlying Clinical Practice. Baltimore, Williams and Williams, 1976
76. Greenhill JP, Friedman EA: Biological Principles and Modern Practice of Obstetrics. Philadelphia, Saunders, 1974
77. Greiss FC, Gobble FL: Effect of sympathetic nerve stimulation on the uterine vascular bed. Am J Obstet Gynecol 97:962−967, 1967
78. Gulezian GZ: Effect of skin-to-skin contact on transitional newborn infants' temperature. Unpublished Master's Thesis, University of Illinois at the Medical Center, 1980
79. Haire D: The Pregnant Patient's Bill of Rights. New York, Committee on Patient's Rights, 1977
80. Harris RE: An evaluation of the median episiotomy. Am J Obstet Gynecol 106:660−665, 1970
81. Haverkamp AD, Thompson HE, McFee JG, et al: The evaluation of continuous fetal heart rate monitoring in high-risk pregnancy. Am J Obstet Gynecol 125:310−320, 1976
82. Haverkamp AD, Orleans M, Langendoerfer S, et al: A controlled trial of the differential effects of intrapartum fetal monitoring. Am J Obstet Gynecol 134:399−412, 1979
83. Hersher L, Richmond J, Moore A: Modifiability of the critical period for the development of maternal behavior in sheep and goats. Behavior 20:311−320, 1963
84. Hendricks CH, Brenner WE: Cardiovascular effects of oxytocic drugs used postpartum. Am J Obstet Gynecol 108:751−760, 1970
85. Hill ST, Shronk LK: The effect of early parent−infant contact on newborn body temperature. JOGN Nurs 8:287−290, 1979
86. Homans G: Group factors in worker productivity. In Proshansky H and Seidenberg S (eds): Basic Studies in Social Psychology. New York, Holt, Rinehart and Winston, 1965.592−604.
87. Hughey MJ, LaPata RE, McElin TW, et al: The effect of fetal monitoring on the incidence of cesarean section. Obstet Gynecol 49:513−518, 1979
88. Hughey MJ, McElin TW, Young T: Maternal and fetal outcomes of Lamaze-prepared patients. Obstet Gynecol 51:643−647, 1978
89. Huttel FA, Mitchell I, Fisher WM, et al: A quantitative evaluation of psychoprophylaxis in childbirth. J Psychosom Res 16:81−92, 1972
90. Johnstone FD, Campbell DM, Hughes GJ: Has continuous fetal monitoring made any impact on fetal outcome? Lancet:1298, 1978
91. Jouppila K, Hollmein A: The effect of segmental epidural analgesia on maternal and foetal acid−base balance, lactate, serum potassium and creatine phosphokinase during labour. Acta Anaesth Scan 20:259−268, 1976

92. Kaltreider DF, Dixon DM: A study of 710 complete lacerations following a central episiotomy. South Med J 41:814−820, 1948

93. Kegel A: Progressive resistance exercises in the functional restoration of the perineal muscles. Am J Obstet Gynecol 56:238−248, 1948

94. Kennell J, Jerauld R, Wolfe H, et al: Maternal behavior one year after early and postpartum contact. Dev Med and Child Neurol 16:172−179, 1974

95. Kieffer MJ: The birthing room concept at Phoenix Memorial Hospital Part II: Consumer satisfaction during one year. JOGN Nurs 9:155−159, 1980

96. Kitzinger S: Emotional aspects of episiotomy and postnatal sexual adjustment, in Kitzinger S (ed): Episiotomy-Physical and Emotional Aspects. London, National Childbirth Trust, 1972, pp 18-24

97. Kitzinger S: Challenges in antenatal education Part 2: Giving support in labour. Nursing Mirror 7:20−22, 1977

98. Kitzinger S: Challenges in antenatal education Part 3: A fresh look at second stage. Nursing Mirror 7:17−20, 1977

99. Klaus MH, Fanaroff AA: Care of the High Risk Neonate. Philadelphia, Saunders, 1973

100. Klaus MH, Kennell JH: Maternal−Infant Bonding. St. Louis, Mosby, 1976

101. Klaus MH, Kennell JH: Parent−Infant Bonding (ed 2). St. Louis, Mosby, 1982

102. Klaus MH, Kennell J, Plumb N, et al: Human maternal behavior at the first contact with her young. Pediatrics 46:187−192, 1970

103. Klebe JG, Ingomer CJ: The fetoplacental circulation during parturition: Evidence from residual placenta blood volume. Pediatrics 54:213−216, 1974

104. Krapahl A, Myers G, Calderyo-Barcia R: Uterine contractions in spontaneous labor. Am J Obstet Gynecol 106:378−387, 1970

105. Krebs HB, Petres RE, Dunn LJ, et al: Intrapartum fetal heart rate monitoring. IV: Observations on elective and nonelective fetal heart rate monitoring. Am J Obstet Gynecol 138:213−219, 1980

106. Krebs HB, Petres RE, Dunn LJ, et al: Intrapartum fetal heart rate monitoring. III: Association of meconium with abnormal fetal heart. Am J Obstet Gynecol 137:936−943, 1980

107. Kuhnert BR, Kuhnert PM, Ann-Sheng LT, et al: Meperidine and normeperidine levels following meperidine administration during labor. II: Fetus and neonate. Am J Obstet Gynecol 133:909−913, 1979

108. Landry KE, Kilpatrick, DM: Why shave a mother before she gives birth? Maternal Child Nursing 2:189−190, 1977

109. Laros RK, Work BA, Wetting WC: Amniotomy during the active phase of labor. Obstet Gynecol 39:702−704, 1972

110. Leboyer F: Birth Without Violence. New York, Knopf, 1976

111. Lederman RP, Lederman E, Work BA, et al: The relationship of maternal anxiety, plasma catecholamines, and plasma cortisol to progress in labor. Am J Obstet Gynecol 132:495−500, 1978

112. Lesser MS, Keane VR: Nurse−Patient Relationships in a Hospital Service. St. Louis, Mosby, 1956

113. Levitt EE, Konovsky M, Freese MP, Thompson JF: Intravaginal pressure assessed by the Kegel perinometer. Arch Sex Behav 8:425−430, 1979

114. Long AE: Unshaved perineum at parturition. Am J Obstet Gynecol 99:333−336, 1967

115. Long VE: Orientation of high risk pregnant women to antepartal fetal monitoring. Unpublished Master's Thesis, University of Illinois at the Medical Center, 1978

116. Lubic RW, Ernst EK: The childbearing center: An alternative to conventional care. Nursing Outlook 26:754—760, 1978

117. Lynaugh KH: The effects of early elective amniotomy on the length of labor and the condition of the fetus. Nurse-Midwif 25:3—9, 1980

118. McKinney BM: The effects upon the mother of removal of the infant immediately after birth. Child-Family Digest 10:63—65, 1954

119. Mandelbaum B: Gestational meconium in the high-risk pregnancy. Obstet Gynecol 42:87—92, 1973

120. Martell M, Belizan JM, Nieto F, et al: Blood acid—base balance at birth in neonates from labors with early and late rupture of the membranes. J Pediatr 89:963—967, 1976

121. Martin L: Health Care of Women. Philadelphia, Lippincott, 1978

122. Marx GF, Bassell GM: Obstetric Analgesia and Anesthesia. Amsterdam, Excerpta Medica, 1980

123. Mehl L: Scientific research on childbirth alternatives: What it can tell us about hospital practice, in Stewart L and Stewart D (eds): 21st Century Obstetrics now! Chapel Hill, NAPSAC, 1977, pp 171—208

124. Meis PJ, Hall M, Marshall JR, et al: Meconium passage: A new classification for risk assessment during labor. Am J Obstet Gynecol 131:509—513, 1978

125. Mendelson CL: Aspiration of stomach contents into the lungs during obstetric anesthesia. Am J Obstet Gynecol 52:191—205, 1946

126. Miller FC: Meconium staining of the amniotic fluid. Clin Obstet Gynecol 6:359—365, 1979

127. Moloni JA: The birthing room: Some insights into parents' experience. Maternal Child Nursing 5:314—319, 1980

128. Montgomery E: Teaching patients about the pelvic floor, in Kitzinger S (ed): Episiotomy-Physical and Emotional Aspects. London, National Childbirth Trust, 1972, pp 5-8

129. Moore DS: Prepared childbirth: The pregnant couple and their marriage. J Nurs Midwif 22:18—26, 1977

130. Morishma HO, Pederson H, Finster: The influence of maternal psychological stress on the fetus. Am J Obstet Gynecol 131:286—291, 1978

131. Morrison JC, Wiser WL, Rosser Sl, et al: Metabolites of meperidine related to fetal depression. Am J Obstet Gynecol 115:1132—1137, 1973

132. Mueller-Huebach E, MacDonald HM, Joret D, et al: Effects of electronic fetal heart rate monitoring on perinatal outcome and obstetric practice. Am J Obstet Gynecol 137:758—763, 1980

133. Myers RE: Maternal psychological stress and fetal asphyxia: A study in the monkey. Am J Obstet Gynecol 122:47—59, 1975.

134. Myers RE, Myers SE: Use of sedative, analgesic and anesthetic drugs during labor and delivery: Bane or boon? Am J Obstet Gynecol 133:83—104, 1979

135. Myles M: Textbook for Midwives (ed 8). London, Churchill-Livingston, 1975

136. Nathanson G, Cohen MI, McNamara T: The effect of nabenzoate on serum bilirubin in the gonn rat. J Pediatr 86:799—803, 1975

137. Nel JJ: Episiotomy, in Kitzinger S (ed): Episiotomy-Physical and Emotional Aspects. London, National Childbirth Trust, 1972, pp 12-17

138. Newton N: The effect of fear and disturbance on labor, in Stewart L and Stewart D (eds): 21st Century Obstetrics Now! Chapel Hill, NAPSAC, 1977, pp 61–72

139. Newton N, Newton M: Mothers reactions to their newborn babies. JAMA 181:206–210, 1962

140. Neutra RR, Fienberg SE, Greenland S: Effect of fetal monitoring on the incidence of neonatal death rates: N Engl J Med 299:324–326, 1978

141. Nishijima M, Majima T, Amano K, et al: Comparison of fetal heart-rate patterns and acid–base balance between early and late rupture of the membranes. J Perinat Med 9(Suppl 1):1–171, 1981

142. Noble E: Essential Exercises for the Childbearing Year. Boston, Houghton Mifflin, 1976

143. O'Connor S, Vielze PM, Sherrod KB, et al: Reduced incidence of parenting inadequacy following rooming-in. Pediatrics 66:176–182, 1980

144. Odell LD, Seski A: Episiotomy blood loss. Am J Obstet Gynecol 54:51–56, 1947

145. Ogata ES, Kitterman JA, Kleinberg F, et al: The effect of time of cord clamping and maternal blood pressure on placental transfusion with cesarean section. Am J Obstet Gynecol 128:197–200, 1977

146. Olds SB, London ML, Ladewig PA, et al: Obstetric Nursing. Menlo Park, Addison Wesley, 1980

147. Oliver CM, Oliver GM: Gentle birth: Its safety and its effects on neonatal behavior. JOGN Nurs 7:35–40, 1978

148. Oxorn H: Oxorn-Foote Human Labor and Birth. New York, Appleton-Century-Crofts, 1980

149. Oyama T, Metsuki A, Taneichi T, et al: B-endorphin in obstetric analgesia. Am J Obstet Gynecol 137:613–616, 1980

150. Parer JT: FHR monitoring: Answering the critics. Contemporary OB/Gyn 17:163–174, 1981

151. Paul RH, Hon EH: Clinical fetal monitoring versus effect on fetal outcome. Am J Obstet Gynecol 118:529–533, 1974

152. Perez P: Nuturing children who attend the birth of a sibling. Maternal Child Nursing 4:215–217, 1979

153. Peterson GH, Mehl LE: Comparative strategies of psychological outcome of various childbirth alternatives, in Stewart L and Stewart D (eds): 21st Century Obstetrics Now! Chapel Hill, NAPSAC, 1977, pp 209–238

154. Petrie RH, Sze-Ya Y, Yugi M, et al: The effect of drugs on fetal heart rate variability. Am J Obstet Gynecol 130:294–299, 1978

155. Petrie RH, Wo R, Miller FC, et al: The effect of drugs on uterine activity. Obstet Gynecol 43:431–436, 1976

156. Phillips CR: Neonatal heat loss in heated cribs vs. mothers' arms. Nursing Digest Jan:49–50, 1976

157. Poma-Herrerra P, Webster A, Kuth L: The effect of amniotomy on progress in the first stage of labor: A retrospective study. Chicago Med School Q 29:184–189, 1970

158. Porth CM, Keylor LE: Temperature regulation in the newborn. Am J Nurs 78:1691–1696, 1978

159. Pritchard JA, Baldwin RM, Dickey JC, et al: Blood volume changes in pregnancy and the puerperium.II: Red blood cell loss and changes in apparent blood

volume during and following vaginal delivery, cesarean section, and cesarean section plus total hysterectomy. Am J Obstet Gynecol 84:1271–1282, 1962

160. Pritchard JA, MacDonald PC: Williams Obstetrics (ed 16). New York, Appleton-Century-Crofts, 1980, pp 405–434
161. Pritchard JA, Macdonald PC: Williams Obstetrics (ed 15). New York, Appleton-Century-Crofts, 1976, p 369
162. Quilligan EJ, Paul RH: Fetal monitoring: Is it worth it? Obstet Gynecol 45:96–100, 1975
163. Retnam SS, Tow SH: Amniotomy in labour. Singapore Med J 10:50–53, 1969
164. Rich A: Of Woman Born: Motherhood as Experience and Institution. New York, Norton, 1976
165. Riffel HD, Nochinson DJ, Paul RH, et al: Effects of meperidine and promethazine during labor. Obstet Gynecol 42:738–744, 1973
166. Ringler NM, Kendall JH, Jarvello R, et al: Mother-to-child speech at two years: Effects of early postnatal contact. J Pediatr 86:141–144, 1975
167. Roberts RB: Aspiration and its prevention in obstetric patients. Int Anesthesiol Clin 15:49–70, 1977
168. Roberts RB, Shirley MA: The obstetrician's role in reducing the risk of pneumonitis. Am J Obstet Gynecol 124:611, 1976
169. Robson K: The role of eye-to-eye contact in maternal infant attachment. J Child Psychol 8:13–15, 1967
170. Rodholm M, Larsson K: Father–infant interaction at the first contact after delivery. Early Hum Dev 3:21–27, 1979
171. Romney ML: Predelivery shaving: An unjustifiable assault? Br J Obstet Gynaecol 1:33–35, 1980
172. Romney ML: Is your enema really necessary? Br Med J (Clin Res) 282:1269–1271, 1981
173. Romney SL, Gray MJ, Little AB, et al: Gynecology and Obstetrics. The Health Care of Women (ed 2). New York, McGraw Hill, 1981
174. Rosenblatt DB, Belsey EM, Lieberman BA, et al: The influence of maternal analgesia on neonatal behavior. II: Epidural bupivacaine. Br J Obstet Gynaecol 88:407–413, 1981
175. Rosenblatt JS, Lehrman D: Effects of separation on maternal behavior in rats, in Rheingold HR (ed): Maternal Behavior in Mammals. New York, Wiley, 1963
176. Rosenfield CR, Barton MD, Meschia G: Effects of epinephrine on distribution of blood flow in the pregnant ewe. Am J Obstet Gynecol 124:156–163, 1975
177. Roux JF, Neuman MR: Electronic fetal monitoring by telemetry. Contemporary OB/Gyn 16:67–72, 1980
178. Rubin R: Maternal touch. Nurs Outlook 11:828–831, 1963
179. Rutter N, Spencer A, Mann N, et al: Glucose during labor. Lancet 2(8186):155, 1980
180. Sala NL, Luther EC, Arballo JC, et al: Oxytocin reproducing reflex milk ejection in lactating women. J Appl Physiol 36:154–158, 1974
181. Salts L, Oh M, Walson PD: Local anesthetic agents—pharmacological basis for use in obstetrics: A review. Anesth Analg 55:829–838
182. Scanlon JW: Anesthetic management of the high risk pregnancy: Consequences for the newborn. Clin Obstet Gynecol 24:671–681, 1981

183. Schrag K: Maintenance of pelvic floor integrity during childbirth. Nurse-Midwif 24:26–31, 1979

184. Schwarcz R: Amniotomy. ICEA Review 3, Summer, 1979

185. Schwarcz R, Althabe O, Belizky R, et al: Fetal heart rate patterns in labours with intact and ruptured membranes. J Perinatal Med 1:153–167, 1973

186. Schwarcz R, Diaz A, Belizian J, et al: Influence of amniotomy and maternal position on labor, in Proceedings of the VII World Congress of Gynecology and Obstetrics. Mexico, 1976, pp 377–391

187. Scott JR, Rose NB: Effect of psychoprophylaxis (Lamaze preparation) on labor and delivery in primiparae. N Engl J Med 294:1205–1207, 1976

188. Seiden AM: The maternal sense of mastery in primary care obstetrics. Primary Care 3:717–726, 1976

189. Seropian R, Reynolds BM: Wound infections after preoperative depilatory versus razor preparation. Am J Surg 121:251–254, 1971

190. Shainess N: The psychologic experience of labor. New York State J of Med 15:2923–2932, 1963

191. Shaw NS: Forced Labor: Maternity Care in the United States. New York, Pergamon Press, 1974

192. Shenker L, Post RC, Seiler JS: Routine electronic monitoring of the fetal heart rate and uterine activity during labor. Obstet Gynecol 46:185–189, 1975

193. Shnider SM, Levinson G: Anesthesia for Obstetrics. Baltimore, Williams, 1979

194. Sorbe B: Active pharmacological management of the third stage of labor: A comparison of oxytocin and ergotomine. Obstet Gynecol 52:694–697, 1978

195. Sosa R, Klaus MH, Kennell JH, et al: The effect of early mother–infant contact on breastfeeding, infection and growth, in Breastfeeding and the Mother. Ciba Foundation Symposium 45:Amsterdam, Elsevier, 1976, pp 179–193

196. Standley K, Klein RP, Soule AB: Local-regional anesthesia during childbirth and newborn behavior. Science 180:634–635, 1974

197. Starkman MN: Psychological responses to the use of the fetal monitor during labor. Psychosom Med 38:269–277, 1976

198. Starkman MN: Fetal monitoring: Psychological consequences and management recommendations. Obstet Gynecol 50:500–540, 1977

199. Starkman MN, Youngs DD: Reactions to electronic fetal monitoring, in Youngs DD, Ehrhardt AA (eds): Psychosomatic Obstetrics and Gynecology. New York, Appleton-Century-Crofts, 1980

200. Stevens RJ: Psychological strategies for management of pain in prepared childbirth. I: A review of the research. Birth Fam J 3:157–164, 1976

201. Stiles D: Techniques for reducing the need for episiotomy. Issues in Health Care of Women 2:105–111, 1980

202. Studd JW, Crawford JS, Duignan NM, et al: The effect of lumbar epidural analgesia on the rate of cervical dilation and the outcome of labour of spontaneous onset. Br J Obstet Gynaecol 87:1015–1021, 1980

203. Szeto HH, Clapp JF, Abrams R, et al: Brain uptake of meperidine in the fetal lamb. Am J Obstet Gynecol 138:528–532, 1980

204. Taylor PM, Bright NH, Birchard EL: Effect of early versus delayed clamping of the umbilical cord on the clinical condition of the newborn infant. Am J Obstet Gynecol 86:893–898, 1963

205. Thompson WR: Early development: Its importance for later behavior, in Hoch PH, Zubin (eds): Psychopathology of Childhood. New York, Grune & Stratton, 1955, pp 120–139

206. Tronick E, Wise S, Als H, et al: Regional obstetric anesthesia and newborn behavior: Effect over the first ten days of life. Pediatr 58:94–100, 1976

207. Tutera G, Newman RL: Fetal monitoring: Its effect on the perinatal mortality and cesarean-section rates and its complications. Am J Obstet Gynecol 122:750–754, 1975

208. Tryon PA: The effect of patient participation in decision making on the outcome of a nursing procedure. ANA Clinical Sessions Monograph 19:14–18, 1962

209. Ueland K: Maternal cardiovascular dynamics: VII. Intrapartum blood volume changes. Am J Obstet Gynecol 126:671–677, 1976

210. Unphenaur JH: Bacterial colonization in neonates with sibling visitation. JOGN Nurs 9:73–75, 1980

211. Usher R, Shepard M, Lind J: The blood volume of the newborn infant and placental transfusion. Acta Pediatr 52:497–519, 1963

212. Van Art L: A descriptive study of thermal regulation in newborn infants held skin-to-skin by their mothers shortly after birth. Unpublished Master's Thesis, University of Illinois at the Medical Center, Chicago, 1977

213. Van Praegh I, Hendricks C: The effect of amniotomy during labor in multiparas. Obstet Gynecol 24:258–265, 1964

214. Varney H: Nurse-Midwifery. Boston, Blackwell, 1980

215. Way NL, Costley EC, Way EL: Respiratory sensitivity of the newborn infant to meperidine and morphine. Clin Pharmacol Ther 6:454–461, 1965

216. Weininger O: The effects of early experience on behavior and growth characteristics. J of Comp Psychol 49:1–9, 1956

217. Wetrich D: Effect of amniotomy upon labor. Obstet Gynecol 35:800–806, 1970

218. Whalley PJ, Pritchard JA: Oxytocin and water intoxication. JAMA 186:601–603, 1963

219. Whiteside D: Proper use of radiant warmers, Am J Nurs 78:1694–1696, 1978

220. Whitley N, Mack E: Are enemas justified for women in labor? Am J Nurs 80:1339, 1980

221. Williams JK, Lancaster J: Thermoregulation of the newborn. Maternal Child Nursing 1:355–360, 1976

222. Yang RK, Zweig AR, Douthitt TC, et al: Successive relationships between maternal attitudes during pregnancy, analgesic medication during labor and delivery and newborn behavior. J Dev Psychol 126, 1976

223. Yao AC, Hervensalo M, Lind J: Placental transfusion rate and uterine contraction. Lancet 1:380–383, 1968

224. Yao AC, Lind J, Vuorenkoski V: Expiratory grunting in the late clamped normal neonate. Pediatrics 48:865–876, 1971

225. Yao AC, Lind J: Placental transfusion Am J Dis Child 127:128–141, 1974

226. Zuspan FP, Ciblis LA, Pose SV: Myometrial and cardiovascular responses to alterations in plasma epinephrine and norepinephrine. Am J Obstet Gynecol 84:841–851, 1962

Diane B. Boyer

5
Early Parenthood

The postpartum period, or puerperium, has been the most neglected aspect of modern maternity care. Although its length, usually considered to be the 8 weeks following parturition, makes up 15 percent of the total maternity cycle, less than 5 percent of the space in current obstetric textbooks is devoted to it.[3]

The existing literature deals primarily with the physical and pathologic aspects of the puerperium, although these may not be the most important factors for new parents. Many mothers are as concerned about coping with the stress of parenthood and changes in family relationships as in their own physiologic changes. This critical period in the maternity experience, called by some "the fourth trimester," deserves more attention by health-care professionals. Successful integration of the infant into the family unit is the vital culminating event in the process of childbearing.

Pregnancy and the intrapartum period are times of relative dependence for a woman. During the postpartum period she must return to a more independent state while meeting the needs of a totally dependent new being. Gruis has identified four tasks of all women in the puerperium:[24]

1. physical restoration;
2. learning to care for and meet the needs of a dependent infant;
3. establishing a relationship with that infant;
4. altering life-style and relationships to accommodate a new family member.

It is the responsiblity and joy of the nurse-midwife to foster the mother's process of moving from dependence to independence and to assist her in accomplishing these tasks.

177

This chapter is not intended to be a complete review of the postpartum period. Several excellent treatments of postpartum assessment, teaching needs, and basic management already exist.[45,68] Rather, it will review several aspects of physical restoration and emotional adjustment and examine issues important in making nurse-midwifery management decisions. For convenience, physical and emotional aspects will be separated, although these factors in an individual mother are often not so easily divided.

The following definitions applying to the puerperium will be used:[45]

1. immediate puerperium—the first 24 hours after delivery
2. early puerperium—days 2−7
3. remote puerperium—from day 8 through completion of involution, about 8 weeks

NURSE-MIDWIFERY MANAGEMENT OF PHYSICAL ASPECTS OF THE PUERPERIUM

Uterus

During pregnancy, largely under the influence of estrogen, the myometrial cells undergo marked hypertrophy and some hyperplasia, and the weight of the uterus is increased by twentyfold at term. In the puerperium there is a rapid decrease in tissue mass, so that by 7 days after delivery, uterine weight is half that at term. This rapid reduction is accomplished by lysosomal hydrolytic enzymes catalyzing the degradation of extra-cellular collagen and ground substance and by intracellular autodigestion of cellular organelles and actomyosin. Macrophages also migrate into the myometrium and endometrium. As a result of these processes, myometrial cells rapidly decrease in size, and degenerating decidua is sloughed as part of the lochia, leading to involution.[1,41,45]

Normally there is complete restoration of the proliferative endometrium by 16 days postpartum, except for the placental site, which takes about 6 weeks to regenerate. Cells in the deeper layer of the decidua are not shed with the placenta or lochia, and take an active part in the regeneration of the endometrium.[56]

Involutional processes in the uterus result in a progressive decrease in the height of the fundus, which the nurse-midwife will note during her postpartum evaluation of the mother. The mother should be taught how to palpate for and evaluate this decrease. Most midwifery and obstetric texts have diagrams indicating the average height of the fundus on various days in the puerperium.[45,68] Immediately after the delivery of the placenta, the fundus is usually found several centimeters below the umbilicus, but it rises up to the level of the umbilicus within a few hours. By the fifth day postpartum, the fundus is usually found halfway between the umbilicus and the symphysis pubis, and by the tenth day is just palpable above the symphysis.

The importance of an empty bladder to correctly assess fundal height cannot be overstressed. Even a partially-full bladder can result in an increase of several centimeters in fundal height. Although the woman may have voided recently and may feel no urge, the extreme diuresis found in the puerperium coupled with the decreased sensation of the pressure of bladder contents that most women experience may result in sufficient amounts of urine in the bladder to distort the results of the exam. If there is any question the woman should be asked to void again and the fundus palpated immediately thereafter.

Another important factor to remember is that the fundal height given in texts as being appropriate to a particular day postpartum is an average, and there may be considerable individual variation. Differences in parity and size of the baby may lead to variations from the norm. More important than absolute size is a progressive decrease in height at successive daily examinations. The most accurate way to evaluate this is to have the same practitioner perform all of the examinations and carefully record her findings as centimeters below the umbilicus for at least 3 days after delivery.

Subinvolution is the result of interference with the normal processes of decreasing myometrial size and sloughing of degenerating decidua and clots. This is most commonly caused by retained placental fragments, or membranes, or by infection. As a consequence of any of these factors, fundal height will not decrease as expected.

What is appropriate nurse-midwifery management if the fundus is found, even immediately after voiding, to be the same height on two successive postpartum days in the early puerperium? Preferences may vary among nurse-midwives, but if there are no signs of infection—such as fever, foul-smelling lochia, or uterine tenderness—the condition can be safely managed without medication. The mother should be taught to massage the uterus every 2 or 3 hours, void frequently, increase ambulation, and sleep prone with a pillow under her lower abdomen. In most cases this treatment will result in a decrease in fundal height by the next day. If there is no improvement after 2 days, an ergot preparation may be given (Ergotrate [ergonovine maleate] or Methergine [methylergonovine maleate] 0.2 mg p.o. q 4 hours X 6 doses). Since the medication will probably cause painful cramping, a pain medication should be given with each dose. The blood pressure should be taken prior to giving each dose, and the medication held if the pressure is >140/90. Since infection is one of the causes of subinvolution, the mother must continue to be screened for signs of such an infection. Subinvolution, even in the absence of infection, may result in a low-grade fever (>100.4°F or 38°C), but in these cases the pulse rate generally is normal.

Some practitioners routinely give a series of an ergot medication to all mothers in the early puerperium. This use is questionable, since ergot may interfere with lactation by inhibiting prolactin release and may cause temporary hypertension in susceptible individuals.[45] Breastfeeding ad lib from birth is a more physiologic and safer way to promote involution.

Adequate involution may proceed in the early puerperium while the mother is under observation by the nurse-midwife in the hospital or at home, but may later decrease or stop at a time when she is not in direct contact with any health-care personnel. For this reason, and to promote a sense of involvement and control in the mother regarding the changes in her body, she should be taught to palpate for and to evaluate the height of the fundus daily for the first 10−14 days postpartum. If the fundus is still palpable above the symphysis at 2 weeks, she should notify her nurse-midwife.

By 6 weeks postpartum, the uterus should be nearly involuted to a nonpregnant, although not prepregnant, size. The normal nulliparous uterus ranges in size from 5.5−8 cm long, 3.5−4 cm wide and 2−2.5 cm thick, while the multiparous uterus is larger than this by 1−4 cm in length, 1.5−2.5 cm in width and 0.5−1.5 cm in thickness.[68] The cervix may still be somewhat edematous at 6 weeks. The os will be transverse, and the external os may be gaping. The reddish, granular-appearing columnar epithelium of the endocervix may be visible, since retraction of this epithelium occurs to a variable degree in postpartum women.[41]

Lochia

Lochia is the vaginal discharge following delivery. For 2 or 3 days this is composed mainly of bits of decidua and blood and is known as *lochia rubra*. After this time the bleeding decreases and the discharge becomes paler and is known as *lochia serosa*. By about day seven, the flow is composed mainly of serum and leukocytes and is known as *lochia alba*. By 3 weeks, the amount of lochia is greatly diminished, although some may persist up to 6 weeks.[41] *Lochia rubra* may contain an occasional small clot, but the presence of many or large clots is abnormal and may be due to abnormal involution.[53] Mothers should be instructed to save large clots for inspection by the nurse-midwife or nurse to detect pieces of placental tissue.

Arterioles supplying the former placental site in the uterus constrict after delivery of the placenta, become fibrinized, and later hyalinized. New vessels of smaller diameter develop to supply the involuting uterus.[41] Failure of the uterine musculature to constrict in the immediate and early puerperium before vessels are permanently occluded, may result in hemorrhage, which is traditionally considered to be blood loss exceeding 500 ml. Since results of studies have indicated that 500 ml is an average blood loss at delivery, some authors think a loss in excess of 1000 ml would be a more realistic criterion for hemorrhage.[53] Underestimation of blood loss at delivery is very common.

Frequent evaluation of the amount of bleeding and consistency of the uterine fundus during the postpartum period are essential. These assessments should be made every 15 minutes during the first hour, every 30 minutes during the next 3 hours, every hour during the next 4 hours, then every 4 hours for the remainder of the first 24 hours. Daily evaluation by the nurse-midwife is essential for the first 2 or 3 days, either in the hospital or at home. The mother should be taught to evaluate the uterus for atony, what to expect as a normal amount of bleeding, and to report any deviations to her caregiver promptly.

The nurse-midwife should be especially alert for uterine atony and hemorrhage in women who have had a multiple gestation, a large baby, hydramnios, high parity, rapid delivery, or prolonged labor. A prophylactic oxytocic drug may be administered in these cases.

Hemorrhage resulting from uterine atony usually is treated with expression of any clots from the uterus, followed by fundal massage, and infusion of an oxytocic drug (i.e., 20 units Pitocin in 5% dextrose and water to run at 20–50 milliunits/minute), and ergonovine [Erogtrate] or methylergonovine [Methergine] 0.2 mg 1M.) If these measures are not effective, bimanual compression of the uterus between one hand placed in the vagina and the other on the abdomen or massage of the lower uterine segment with a hand placed in the vagina often are useful. Over-massage of the uterus should be avoided because it may lead to relaxation of the uterine muscles. Packing of the uterus is less effective than compression.[53] Continued bleeding calls for reevaluation of the vagina and cervix for lacerations and manual exploration of the uterus for retained placental fragments. Vital signs should be monitored carefully, assessment should be made for shock, and blood should be crossmatched for possible transfusion. The physician should be consulted if fundal massage does not control bleeding. Hypogastric artery ligation or hysterectomy are drastic measures to control life-threatening hemorrhage.

Although chance of hemorrhage is greatly reduced after 24 hours, a late postpartum hemorrhage may occur up to several weeks after delivery. This is due to subinvolution of the placental site or to retained placental fragments.[53] The mother should be instructed to report to her nurse-midwife any increase in bleeding after the lochia has become pale and scant. A return of the menses is not likely before 6 or 8 weeks postpartum, and bleeding in the late puerperium needs to be evaluated.

Interpretation of Vital Signs

Blood Pressure

Blood pressure should be monitored carefully in the new mother, even if it has been normal during the antepartum and intrapartum periods. Readings every 15 minutes during the first hour after delivery, every hour for the next 3 hours, then every 8 hours for the remainder of the first 24 hours are recommended. Daily assessment should continue for 3 or 4 days. Abnormal readings will require more frequent monitoring and physician consultation. If available, the prepregnant or first trimester blood pressure should be used as a baseline for evaluating changes.

Low blood pressure (<90/60) in the puerperium commonly may be caused by hemorrhage with subsequent shock or may result from anesthetic and analgesic drugs. Careful evaluation for occult hemorrhage needs to be made in such cases, checking for a uterus filling with blood or for a hematoma. Unless there has been an actual overdose or an allergic reaction, drug effects generally do not require treatment.

Hypertension in the postpartum period may result from excessive use of oxytocic or vasopressor drugs.[45] Obviously the best cure is prevention in such cases. Overdoses must be treated promptly with a vasodilator drug (chlorpromazine, 5–15 mg slowly IV).[45]

Elevated blood pressure during the puerperium can also be a sign of impending eclampsia, even in women whose antepartum and intrapartum courses have been normal. Although some authors state that true eclampsia occurs within 48 hours of delivery, others disagree. Sibai and colleagues report six cases of eclampsia occurring three or more days past delivery from a series of 3699 deliveries.[60] Four of the six had no prenatal complications, normal blood pressures during the intrapartum period and for the first 24 hours postpartum, and negative intrapartum urinary protein. Although the incidence of postpartum eclampsia is low, the possiblity must be considered when assessing postpartum women.

Pulse

During the puerperium the pulse rate may be elevated for a number of reasons. Shock, anemia, infection, pain, and anxiety will need to be considered in such cases. Some women will have a low pulse (50–60/minute) in the early puerperium, and this is not abnormal.

Temperature

Increases in temperature above the norm of 37°C (98.6°F) are very common in the puerperium. Determining the significance of such increases is one of the more challenging tasks for the nurse-midwife. Studies have shown that over one-third of mothers in this period have at least one temperature elevation above 38°C (100.4°F), with no ensuing morbidity if this was a single, isolated rise.[18] Low-grade temperature elevations in the puerperium have been attributed to dehydration, breast engorgement, infusion of fetal protein, and blockage of lochial flow, among other things.[18]

Nurse-Midwifery Management of Puerperal Infections

Infection is, of course, one cause to consider when evaluating a temperature increase. The standard definition of puerperal morbidity is a temperature of >38°C occurring on any two of the first ten days postpartum, exclusive of the first 24 hours, with the temperature being taken at least four times daily using an appropriate technique. This definition may not apply to many documented cases of infection today, when early use of antibiotics is common. Various authors have developed different definitions of puerperal morbidity, which often complicates comparison of studies.[16,45]

One large study involving 10,181 deliveries found a puerperal infection rate of 5.9 percent. Other investigators have found rates from 1.0−7.2 percent.[16] Not all investigators, however, used the same definition of morbidity.

Although the rates are not high, infection is one of the most common causes of maternal mortality, along with hemorrhage and hypertension.[50] Death from infection is most common among women undergoing cesarean section. While the maternal death rate in the United States in 1975 was 12.8/100,000 live births,[50] the death rate from infection in a study of 120,684 women in 1974 who underwent cesarean section was 80/100,000 operations.[16] Novy states that the death rate in cesarean section is 26 times that of vaginal delivery, although it is not clear whether this is from all causes, or infection alone.[45] In 162,656 deliveries occurring in Rhode Island between 1965 and 1975, the death rate from sepsis was 81 times greater in those undergoing cesarean section than in those having vaginal deliveries.[17] These statistics serve to emphasize the importance of good prenatal care and meticulous management of the intrapartum period to avoid, as much as is possible, the need for cesarean section.

Endometritis

Most authors consider infection of the genital tract to be most common infection in the puerperium.[45,50] These infections generally are termed *endometritis*, although Pritchard and MacDonald prefer the term *metritis*, since the myometrium underlying the infected decidua is often involved.[50]

Besides cesarean section, other predisposing factors related to endometritis are low socioeconomic status, prolonged rupture of membranes, intrauterine manipulations for delivery of the baby or placenta, traumatic delivery, prolonged labor, and breaks in aseptic technique during labor and delivery.[22] Numerous vaginal examinations in labor have been associated with higher puerperal infection rates, but since more examinations generally are found with greater duration of labor, cause-and-effect relationships are not clear.[16] Anemia and poor nutrition during the antepartum period have long been suggested as predisposing factors, but proof is lacking.[50,52] Sexual intercourse close to term has been proposed, but not clearly demonstrated, to be a factor. Studies investigating internal fetal monitoring as a causative factor in endometritis are difficult to interpret because monitored and nonmonitored groups are often not comparable. Internal monitoring is often used for women whose labor is abnormal in some way, and prospective, randomized studies have not been done. In women having vaginal deliveries, however, it appears that internal fetal monitoring does not greatly increase the risk of puerperal infection.[22] Episiotomy and lacerations occurring during delivery provide a portal of entry for pathogenic organisms. Although hemorrhage has been suggested as a predisposing factor, a clear relationship has not been demonstrated. Hematomas provide a good culture medium and thus increase the chance of sepsis.[50]

Numerous organisms have been linked with puerperal infection. Most common are those that normally inhabit the bowel, vagina, and cervix. Aerobic and anaerobic organisms have both been demonstrated, and many infections are polymicrobial. Eschenbach and Wager have done a thorough review of the organisms implicated in puerperal infection.[16] The infection may be contained within the uterus, or may be disseminated as pelvic cellulitis or peritonitis, or may be associated with pelvic thrombophlebitis.[50]

One symptom of endometritis is fever, which often begins on the second or third postpartum day, commonly to $38.8-39.4°C$ ($102-103°F$).[45] The fever remains elevated, although with diurnal fluctuations. Infection may exist in the absence of fever, however, and not all women who show an elevated temperature are infected. Other signs and symptoms are malaise, uterine tenderness, and tachycardia. Many women in the early puerperium have mild tenderness of the uterus on firm palpation, but this decreases rapidly as involution proceeds. In cases of endometritis, the tenderness usually is more pronounced and may increase with time. The lochia may be profuse and have a foul odor or, as in the case with Group A beta-hemolytic *Streptococcus* infection, be scant and odor-free.[45] More serious infections may be accompanied by systemic manifestations such as repeated chills and hypotension. The white blood cell count is often elevated to $15,000-30,000/mm^3$, but since leukocytosis is normal in the early puerperium, this value is difficult to interpret.

Medical treatment of endometritis consists of intravenous antibiotic therapy, usually with a combination of drugs effective against a broad range of aerobic and anaerobic organisms, such as penicillin and tetracycline or penicillin and an aminoglycoside.[16] Other measures are hydration, maintenance of electrolyte balance, and bed rest in semi-Fowler's position to promote uterine drainage.[45]

Preventive measures for endometritis include optimum nutrition during pregnancy, education of mothers to report rupture of membranes promptly, good aseptic technique during vaginal examinations, minimal number of vaginal examinations in labor, maintenance of aseptic technique during delivery, and good perineal hygiene and uterine drainage in the early puerperium.

Urinary tract infection

The urinary tract is another common site of infection in the postpartum period—the most common according to some investigators.[19,63] Antepartum urinary tract infection (UTI), trauma during delivery, catheterization in the intrapartum period, and a tendency toward urinary retention in the immediate puerperium are predisposing factors. In a prospective study of 3554 women in Finland, the incidence of bacteriuria in those delivering vaginally without catheterization was 4.0 percent, in those with a single catheterization was 8.7 percent and after two catheterizations was 42.9 percent.[51] Patients having a urinary tract infection diagnosed and treated during pregnancy had a significantly greater chance than those without such an infection of developing bacteriuria in the puerperium. Patients having endometritis had twice the frequency of having concomitant bacteriuria than those without endometritis, but the numbers were small and the difference was not statistically significant. Eschenbach and Wager state that identical organisms are frequently isolated from the endometrium and the bladder in women having endometritis. They speculate that a high vaginal bacterial concentration in cases of uterine infection may be a factor in colonization of the bladder.[16]

Urinary tract infection confined to the bladder usually is not accompanied by fever. Common symptoms are dysuria, frequent urination, and urgency, but these can be confused by other pain of the puerperium and the normal increase in voiding caused by diuresis in the early puerperium. Contact of urine with an episiotomy site or laceration can cause pain or burning while voiding. Careful questioning, however, can often elicit information to distinguish the "external" pain felt in such cases from the "internal" pain associated with cystitis. If there is any suspicion of infection, a urinalysis and urine culture and sensitivity should be done. It can be difficult to obtain an uncontaminated voided specimen during the puerperium, but catheterization for the specimen should be avoided. Since most postpartum women would have difficulty cleansing themselves properly to obtain a clean-catch specimen, this should be done by the nurse. Washing the vulva and periurethral area should be done with the usual technique and solution, and sterile gauze should be gently placed at the introitus after cleansing, to retain the lochia while the urine specimen is obtained.

If the infection ascends from the bladder to infect the upper urinary tract, fever, costovertebral angle tenderness and chills are seen. Nausea and vomiting are also frequent symptoms in pyelonephritis.[45]

As in most urinary tract infections, the majority in the puerperium are caused by coliform bacteria. *Escherichia coli* can be isolated from about 95 percent of women having their first UTI, but the percentage is somewhat less in repeated infections, where organisms such as *Klebsiella, Enterobacter, Proteus,* and *Pseudomonas* may be present.[16]

Medical treatment consists of appropriate antibiotics, administered orally in the case of a bladder infection and given intravenously for pyelonephritis. Frequent voiding and high fluid intake also are important.[45]

Preventive measures for UTI in the puerperium include detection and treatment of antepartum bacteriuria, attention to frequent voiding and adequate hydration during labor, avoidance of catheterization if possible, prevention of trauma by having the bladder empty during delivery, and frequent voiding and adequate fluids in the immediate puerperium.

Mastitis

Mastitis, seen in 1−5 percent of nursing mothers, is an occasional cause of morbidity in the puerperium.[16] This infection is more frequent in primiparous women and is rare in women who are not nursing.[45,50]

The causative organism of mastitis is almost always *Staphylococcus aureus*, quite likely acquired from a hospital reservoir.[16] Evidence suggests that, in many cases, the organism is passed from the infant's nasopharynx to the mother's milk while nursing. Nipple fissures can be a portal of entry. The newborn acquires the infection from other infants in the nursery, hospital personnel, and equipment. Even infants without clinical infection are colonized by *S. aureus* in the hospital environment. Epidemics of mastitis have occurred in hospitals, although not recently. A constant endemic infection rate is present today.[16]

Besides the presence of *S. aureus*, another factor encouraging the development of breast infection is milk stasis. This frequently occurs when engorgement is found, typically during the establishment of breastfeeding or at weaning.

The usual onset of mastitis is in the third or fourth week postpartum, with engorgement followed by painful inflammation of a lobule in the outer quadrant of the breast most commonly seen. Infection has been found as early as the fifth day postpartum. Rapid development of fever up to $39.8°C-40.6°C$ ($102-105°F$) can occur, and the pulse rate is elevated. If not treated, mastitis can proceed to breast abscess. If the area of inflammation is fluctuant or has pitting edema, abscess should be suspected.

Specimens should be obtained for culture and sensitivity before initiating antibiotic treatment. In simple mastitis the breast should be washed with hexachlorophene, then with sterile water, and milk from the affected area should be expressed onto a sterile swab. In cases of suspected abscess, the fluctuant area should be aspirated by needle, and culture and sensitivity of any pus should be obtained.[16]

Measures to prevent breast infection focus on avoiding milk stasis and preventing contact with the causative organism. Minimizing engorgement by frequent nursing, expression of milk when necessary, use of warm packs, wearing a supportive brassiere, and gradual rather than abrupt decrease in the frequency of nursing at weaning are important. Good breast care to help prevent nipple fissures is essential. Exclusion of hospital personnel with staphylococcal infections and isolation of any infant with skin or cord infection will help decrease spread of the organisms. Meticulous handwashing technique by nursery personnel cannot be overemphasized.

In simple mastitis without extensive nipple fissures, the infant should continue to nurse at both breasts. Eschenbach and Wager state that nursing during simple mastitis is not associated with infection or gastrointestinal upset in the newborn from either *S. aureus* or the antibiotics.[16] Since nursing in the presence of breast abscess has been associated with infant deaths from lung abscess, they recommend that breastfeeding be suspended until the abscess is cleared. The breasts can be pumped to maintain lactation.

Wound Infection

Wound infection is another source of postpartum morbidity. Only episiotomy and laceration infections, not abdominal wound infections, will be considered here.

Perineal wound infections are not common, despite the difficulty in keeping the area clean. Reported episiotomy infection rates range from 0.09−0.3 percent, but these figures may not include mild or late cases.[16] A variety of organisms may infect an episiotomy or laceration.

Daily assessment of the episiotomy site with adequate visualization is essential in the early puerperium. Edema is common in the first day or two, but this should soon subside and the incision should remain approximated with minimal erythema. Any purulent discharge should be cultured, and obvious infection requires physician consultation. The mother should be taught to evaluate her perineum by using a mirror. This will aid in identifying infections and help to dispel ideas about trauma to the perineum that may be worse than the reality.

In any perineal wound infection, it is vital to assess the depth of the infection, since early and accurate assessment of the spread of the infection is necessary to prevent serious morbidity or even mortality. Several cases of fatal perineal cellulitis from an episiotomy site have been reported.[59]

In a simple episiotomy infection, edema and erythema should be confined to the skin and superficial fascia immediately adjacent to the episiotomy. Necrosis of the skin and systemic manifestations such as fever, chills, and malaise are not present in a localized infection. Since the superficial fascia in the perineum is continuous with fascia of the legs, buttocks, and abdominal wall, the infection may spread along these planes. Edema and erythema spreading out from the episiotomy site are signs of an intermediate-depth infection. Most of these infections are without necrosis and respond to antibiotic therapy within 24−48 hours. A more serious form has been called necrotizing fasciitis, which has a 21−76 percent mortality rate. In these cases necrosis spreads along the superficial fascial layers, often onto the abdomen, buttocks, and thighs. The skin over the infected area becomes blue or brown, but rather late in the infectious process. Toxic systemic manifestations, including shock, appear as the condition progresses.[16,59]

Medical management of a simple episiotomy infection includes opening, exploration, and debridement, with antibiotic therapy sometimes used. The wound is not resutured, but is left to heal by secondary intention. Extensive surgical exploration and debridement along with antibiotic therapy are required for intermediate-depth infections.[59]

Preventive measures for episiotomy infections can be instituted before the postpartum period. Good nutrition, correction of anemia, and treatment of vaginal infections can help assure optimal tissue integrity and capacity for healing at the time of delivery. Careful management of the second stage of labor to prevent lacerations and the need for episiotomy will obviously reduce the infection rate. Meticulous attention to sterile technique when repairing episiotomies or lacerations is essential. In the postpartum period the mother should be taught how to cleanse the perineum after voiding and defecation. Use of a sitz bath several times daily will aid cleanliness and hasten healing.

Instructions to clean the sitz bath adequately after use are often overlooked. Mothers should be taught that applying home remedies for wounds, such as petroleum jelly, may interfere with healing. Exposure of the site to air as often as possible, careful use of a heat lamp, and adequate vitamin C and protein intake will aid the healing process.

Iffy and colleagues reviewed 9 years' experience at a major teaching institution and found that rigidly enforced preventive measures led to a dramatic decrease in wound infections and endometritis, even without the use of prophylactic antibiotics.[29] These measures included handwashing, good sterile technique for dressing changes, isolation of infected patients, and different personnel for care of infected and uninfected patients.

Preventing and Detecting Puerperal Infections

The nurse-midwife has an important role to play in the prevention of puerperal infections. All of the preventive measures previously mentioned can be initiated by the nurse-midwife. Teaching mothers about good nutrition and hygiene practices may positively affect the health of every family member. Instructions should be given in writing, as well as verbally.

Dectection of developing infection is another function of the nurse-midwife. Careful interpretation of vital signs and careful daily physical examinations for the first two or three days postpartum are important for early assessment of problems. Complaints of pain should be thoroughly investigated. Since infections can develop after hospital discharge or after a series of home visits is over, mothers need to be taught to take their own temperatures, evaluate lochia and fundal height, check for episiotomy and breast infection, be aware of signs of urinary tract infection, and to report suspected problems to their nurse-midwife promptly.

Assessment of temperature elevations is often difficult. The guidelines in Table 5-1 may be useful, although protocols may differ among practitioners and services.

Table 5-1
Guidelines for Assessing Temperature Elevations

Symptom	Action
Within first 24 hours:	
1. single temperature of 38.2°C (100.8°F) or less	push fluids implement measures to promote uterine drainage repeat temperature in 4 hours review chart for predisposing factors
2. single temperature of more than 38.4°C (101.1°F)	measures as in (1) but be aware ensuing infection is more likely physical exam for signs of infection

3. two or more readings ≤ 38.2°C,   measures as in (1)
    4 hours apart   physical exam for signs of infection

4. two or more readings > 38.4°C,   measures as in (1)
    at least 4 hours apart   clean-catch urine specimen for urinalysis,
                                             culture and sensitivity
                                         blood cultures—aerobic and anaerobic*
                                         endometrial cultures†
                                         consult physician for antibiotic therapy
                                         possibly start IV
                                         CBC
                                         breast pump for mother isolated from
                                             baby

After the first 24 hours:

5. single temperature of < 38°C   measures as in (1)

6. single temperature > 38°C   measures as in (1)
                                         physical exam

7. 2 or more temperatures in range   measures as in (1)
    of 37.6°C−38.0°C (99.6−   physical exam
    100.4°F) with normal pulse   if no obvious cause for low-grade temp
                                             such as breast engorgement or subinvo-
                                             lution and elevation continues for 24
                                             hours, get cultures as in (4) and consult
                                             physician
                                         if engorged or subinvoluted, treat, contin-
                                             ue temperatures every 4 hours

8. 2 or more elevations in range of   measures as in (1)
    37.6−38°C   with   elevated   physical exam
    pulse (> 100)   cultures as in (4)
                                         consult physician

9. 2 or more elevations > 38°C   management as in (8)

---

*If the woman is having chills, the best time to get blood cultures is at the beginning of a chill be-
cause organisms are most likely to be in the bloodstream at that time.
†Culturing of lochia as it comes from the vagina is almost useless. Endometrial cultures should be
obtained during a sterile vaginal exam by use of a sterile swab inside a sterile sheath to protect it
from contact with organisms in the vagina and cervix. Be aware that even with this technique
many specimens are contaminated with cervical flora, and that many women without infection have
organisms cultured from the lower part of the uterine cavity after delivery.[16]

When an infection has been diagnosed and is under treatment, the patient
may be transferred to the medical service or may be co-managed by the nurse-
midwife and physician, depending on the protocols of a particular nurse-
midwife or service. Even in cases of transfer of management responsibility, the
nurse-midwife has an obligation to provide emotional support and teaching for
the mother and family.

Another important role of the nurse-midwife is to be the mother's advocate in preventing unnecessary separation from the baby when the mother's temperature is elevated or when an infection has been diagnosed. If the fever is high (>38.4°C) and efforts are still underway to diagnose the problem, it is wise to separate the baby until it is determined that the condition is not communicable. The nurse-midwife should inform the pediatrician when an infection is suspected or has been diagnosed and encourage him or her to allow mother−baby contact whenever this would not endanger the baby's health. With most puerperal infections under treatment, especially if the mother is feeling relatively well, separation is not necessary, even if she is still febrile.

Interpretation of Blood Values

Although most blood components return to their nonpregnant values a few weeks following delivery, considerable variance from these norms may be seen in the immediate and early puerperium.

Hematocrit

Hematocrit values seen in the postpartum period are a reflection of two processes. One is the decrease in plasma volume, which expanded during pregnancy, to nonpregnant levels by the third week postpartum. A third of this decrease occurs shortly after delivery, and another third by the end of the first week postpartum. If the red blood cell mass remained constant, this contraction of plasma volume would lead to an increase in the hematocrit, and such an increase is often seen 3−7 days after a normal vaginal delivery. The second process, blood loss at delivery, may cause a decrease in hematocrit if blood loss is sufficiently large to counteract the normal contraction of plasma volume. A decrease in the hematocrit in the early puerperium indicates that the woman has had a considerable blood loss at delivery, at least 20 percent of her circulating volume, according to Novy.[45] In women who have a minimal blood loss at delivery, a marked increase in the hematocrit may be seen in the puerperium. The gradual normal destruction of excess red blood cells may help to increase iron stores in the postpartum woman.[42,45]

Opinions vary about the best time to do a hematocrit to most accurately reflect blood loss during delivery. Varney states any determination before 3−4 days postpartum is not useful.[68] For convenience, the hematocrit is often drawn on the second or third day, although the fifth day may yield more useful information. Novy thinks that if the hematocrit on the fifth to seventh day postpartum is equal to or more than a normal predelivery value, iron supplementation is not necessary in the postpartum period.[45] Nelson and colleagues, after doing serial hematocrits in 23 postpartum women who had at least a 10 percent decrease in hematocrit, found the biggest drop was at 8 hours in four women, at 16 hours in nine women and at 24 hours in 10 women.[42] They did not extend their study beyond 24 hours or attempt to correlate estimated blood loss with the hematocrit changes seen. Even in women experiencing a large blood loss at delivery, doing the hematocrit before 8 hours postpartum can be misleading. Nelson and colleagues recommend that the first hematocrit be done at 16 hours. If the decrease is less than 10 percent of the baseline determined at the beginning of the intrapartum period, no further hematocrit need be drawn. If more than a 10 percent decrease is seen, the hematocrit should be repeated at 24 hours. If the value at 24 hours is the same or more than at 16 hours, no further determination need be done. If there is a further drop, the hematocrit should be repeated every 8−24 hours until it is stable.

A reasonable plan of management for the nurse-midwife would be to do the hematocrit on the third to fifth (preferable) day postpartum, if the woman has had a normal or small blood loss at delivery. If this value is less than the immediate predelivery value, iron and folic acid supplementation should be given. For women suffering from a large blood loss (>600−700 ml), the scheme advocated by Nelson and colleagues could be used.[42] Physician consultation is required whenever the hematocrit is less than 30 percent or when a woman is symptomatic for large blood loss (tachycardia, hypotension, pallor, vertigo after the first 24 hours, extreme fatigue, cold clammy skin, and impairment of mental functions).

A subclinical folate deficiency in pregnancy may manifest itself as megaloblastic anemia in the postpartum period, especially in lactating women with poor dietary folate.[36] It is important, therefore, to investigate symptoms of anemia during the first year postpartum to rule out this or other causes of anemia. Complaints of fatigue in new mothers are easily attributed to lack of sleep and the rigors of child care, but need to be carefully assessed to eliminate a physical cause.

Reticulocytes

Because the sudden drop in red blood cell mass at delivery stimulates bone marrow activity, even though the total mass may be greater than prepregnancy levels, a CBC drawn in the early puerperium may show a reticulocytosis. This will be maximal on the fourth day and will return to normal a few days after that.[45]

Leukocytes

The leukocytosis of pregnancy continues and increases in the intrapartum and postpartum periods. Total leukocytes increase to an average of 15,000/mm^3 during labor and remain elevated in the puerperium, gradually decreasing to normal levels by the sixth postpartum day.[36] Prolonged labor may result in levels up to 25,000/mm^3 without pathologic cause, but values in this range need to be investigated to rule out infection.

The increased leukocyte count seen in pregnancy and the puerperium is due to an increase in polymorphonuclear neutrophilic leukocytes, so that values above the average nonpregnant levels of 62 percent can be normal. Circulating eosinophils fall during labor and are virtually absent at delivery, but return to normal nonpregnant levels (average 2.3%) by the third day postpartum. The numbers of monocytes and lymphocytes apparently do not alter significantly in pregnancy and the puerperium.[36] All of these changes from normal nonpregnant values need to be considered when interpreting the results of a CBC in the postpartum period.

Resumption of Menses and Ovulation

Considerable variation exists in the time of resumption of menses and ovulation in postpartum women. Different studies reported in the literature have varying results. In nonlactating women Novy states that ovulation will occur in 10–15 percent by 6 weeks postpartum and in 30 percent by 90 days.[45] Information obtained from a series of 400 endometrial biopsies on 92 women, both lactating and nonlactating, indicated that the earliest evidence of ovulation was at 44 days.[56] Edelman and colleagues report that by 12 weeks 40 percent of nonlactating women will be ovulating.[15]

Novy states that ovulation is rare in lactating women before the tenth week.[45] By the 12th week, 25 percent are ovulating.[15] Monheit reports that the probability of ovulation in the first 9 weeks in women who are nursing without supplementation is 0.08 percent.[41] If lactation lasts less than 28 days, ovulation returns at times comparable to those who did not breastfeed.

The first menses is usually preceded by an anovulatory cycle.[45] Generally, the longer menses is delayed, the greater the chance it will be associated with ovulation.[41] By 12 weeks postpartum menstruation will have returned in 65 percent of nonlactating and 45 percent of lactating women.[15] Women who are poorly nourished have a longer duration of postpartum amenorrhea.[13]

One possible explanation for the effect lactation has on delaying ovulation is that the ovaries may be refractory to the influence of gonadotropins during lactation. This is suggested by the finding that FSH returns to nonpregnant levels in lactating women, but estradiol levels are decreased longer.[41]

Contraception

Contraception is considered in detail in Chapter 7, but a few comments regarding contraception in the postpartum period will be offered here. As can be seen from the foregoing information it is unlikely that a nonlactating woman will be able to become pregnant before 6 weeks postpartum, and it is unlikely that a woman breastfeeding without supplementation, will be able to become pregnant before 10 weeks postpartum. The decision about when and what kind of contraception to initiate should be made by the woman and her partner after thorough counseling by the nurse-midwife. This discussion may begin in the prenatal period. Besides considering the earliest possible date of ovulation when deciding how soon to initiate contraception, the access of the couple to contraceptive services needs to be determined. Many practitioners believe the new mother should have some contraceptive method to use as soon as she resumes coitus. In addition, although pregnancy is not likely before 6 weeks postpartum, a couple may wish to initiate contraception as soon as they resume coitus in order to make it routine.

Oral contraceptives generally are considered to be contraindicated for lactating women, but the use of low-dose, progestin-only pills has some support.[15] The association of oral contraceptives with increased risk of thromboembolic disorder, coupled with the hypercoaguable state of the postpartum period cause many practitioners to recommend delaying initiation of oral contraceptives for at least 2, and preferably 6, weeks postpartum.[20] Although data do not appear to exist regarding post-pill amenorrhea following early postpartum use, some practitioners prefer to have normal menstrual cycles reestablished in postpartum women before recommending initiation of oral contraception.[15]

Contraceptive foam and condoms, used together at coitus, are a good choice for early postpartum contraception. Although not preferred methods by many people because of their inconvenience and interference with spontaneity, many couples are willing to use them until it is possible to begin a more long-term method.

There are some problems with use of the diaphragm in the postpartum period. Because of the time it takes for involution to occur, fitting a diaphragm should be delayed for 6 weeks.[20] The atrophic vaginal changes associated with breastfeeding may lead to difficulty with insertion of the diaphragm. Because introduction of supplementary feedings for the baby, resumption of frequent coitus or discontinuation of breastfeeding are likely to be associated with changes in the dimensions of the vagina, reevaluation of the size of the diaphragm should be made at these times.[20]

Involution has generally proceeded sufficiently for safe insertion of an intrauterine device at 6 weeks postpartum. Some practitioners think an IUD is the best contraceptive choice for breastfeeding mothers.[20] Immediate postpartum insertion has been advocated by some, but such a procedure has been associated with a high expulsion rate. Recently, efforts have been made to increase retention rates following immediate postpartum IUD insertion by tying biodegradable No. 2 chromic suture extensions to both the Lippes Loop D® (Ortho Pharmaceutical Corp., Raritan, N.J.) and the Copper-T 220C® (Searle Pharmaceuticals Inc., Chicago, Il). In preliminary studies the expulsion rate following insertion of these modified devices approximates the rates in nonpuerperal women.[35]

Postpartum sexual adjustment

The traditional prohibition of coitus following childbirth has been for a 6-week period. There is no evidence, however that an earlier resumption of sexual activity is harmful, providing that vaginal bleeding has ceased and any episiotomy or lacerations are healed.[53] Psychological readiness may take longer than physical readiness because the woman may fear pain, and the man may fear hurting his partner. Fatigue, especially of the new mother, may also inhibit sexual desire. In a study of 42 postpartum couples, Hames found that the mean time for resumption of coitus following delivery was 4.4 weeks.[25] Fuller states that a high percentage of couples resume sexual activity by 3—4 weeks postpartum.[20] Many couples obviously do not adhere to the traditional 6-week period of abstinence. When health-care practitioners place such limitations, they may induce feelings of disturbance and guilt in couples who do not follow them.

Couples need good counseling and anticipatory guidance by the nurse-midwife to facilitate resumption of a satisfactory sexual relationship after childbirth. Many couples are not adequately prepared for the difficulties they may encounter during this time. Counseling and teaching should be individualized for each couple, based on their needs, wishes, and circumstances. An understanding of normal postpartum physiology is important. Nursing mothers should be informed that milk may leak during sexual arousal. Mothers for whom this is a problem can nurse the baby before intercourse or wear a bra.[25] Couples should know decreased libido and less vaginal lubrication are normal in many women during the puerperium, especially in lactating mothers. Use of a water-soluble lubricant may be advised to alleviate the problem of vaginal dryness. Above all, couples should be counseled that the physical problems of the puerperal woman are temporary, and that the potential exists for a sexual relationship that is as good as or better than that before pregnancy. It is extremely important, however, that couples take time from their many activities as new parents to work on all aspects of their relationship if a good sexual relationship is to be resumed. The nurse-midwife should be available to answer questions about sexuality. Unless she is a qualified sex therapist, however, she should make referral to such a practitioner in cases of serious problems.

ISSUES IN NURSE-MIDWIFERY MANAGEMENT OF PSYCHOLOGICAL AND BEHAVIORAL ASPECTS OF THE PUERPERIUM

Normal Adaptation to Parenthood

In standard obstetric texts little, if any, attention has been given to the processes of adaptation to parenthood and how health care personnel might best foster a healthy transition to the new role. The little that is written about psychological and behavioral aspects of the puerperium focuses on maladaptation.[50,53] Often overlooked is the fact that all the time and resources devoted to attaining a good physical outcome to a pregnancy may be negated by parents failing to establish a healthy relationship with the infant and failing to successfully integrate him into the family. The potential for psychiatric disturbance in the mother, child abuse, and marital difficulties is high if these tasks are not accomplished.

Views differ about the nature of the events of childbirth and the transition to parenthood. There is no doubt that these are among the most profound experiences of life for women and men. This author has observed that, even in these times of expanded career opportunities for women and societal changes in role expectations, most adults view attainment of family life with children as a desirable goal.

One view of adaptation to pregnancy and motherhood comes from psychoanalytic theory. In this view the adaptation is largely an intra-psychic task that is a necessary component of healthy ego development and full maturity.[23] A loving and nurturing relationship with the woman's own mother is seen as crucial to allowing a woman to accept her femininity and to become a loving and nuturing mother.

Another concept is that pregnancy and transition to parenthood is a crisis with dual potentials: increased integration of the personality, or failure to cope and consequent disequilibrium. Sheehan describes the puerperium as a period when a woman's identity and self-confidence are in crisis, requiring a reordering of all the roles that are integrated into a woman's self-concept.[57] If there is conflict between role perception and self-image, there is identity confusion, which complicates the crisis state.

Doering and Entwisle use Janis' work on the coping behavior of people facing surgery to devise a theoretical framework for understanding women's reactions to the birth experience.[14] Janis divided the surgical experience into the following three phases: the "threat phase" (preoperative), the "impact phase" (surgery), and the "post-impact" phase (convalescence). Patients who prepared themselves by admitting that they were facing a crisis, by doing the "work of worrying," and by seeking information about what would happen to them coped most successfully with the surgical experience and had a more rapid recovery than those who did not prepare themselves. In the childbirth experience Doering and Entwisle view pregnancy as the threat phase, labor and delivery as the impact phase and the postpartum recovery period as the post-impact phase. Women who seek information and prepare themselves during the threat phase cope better with the crisis of the impact phase and with establishing a relationship with the infant during the post-impact phase than those who do not carry out such activities. In considering the view of childbirth as crisis it is important to determine just what is meant by "crisis." Data gathered by Shereshefsky on first pregnancies, do not support the view that pregnancy is a stress involving threat or loss or that requires resources beyond the ordinary.[58] Some families were found to be in this kind of crisis, but these families were already burdened with serious stress aside from the pregnancy or were suffering some loss or threat. Shereshefsky thinks that a definition of "crisis" as a turning point or transitional phase is appropriate to describe the experiences of first-time parents.[58]

In order to make the role change to motherhood, Mercer thinks it is necessary for the new mother to review the childbirth experience and to integrate her expectations with her actual behavior.[40] Relinquishing pregnancy fantasies about the infant and accepting the reality of her newborn are also important. The phase of relinquishing expectations and fantasies and adapting to reality is called "grief work." Mercer also views this process of "grief work" as applicable to the mother's reconciliation of her postpartum body with her ideal body image. Failing to complete postpartum "grief work" can interfere with adaptation to the motherhood role.

Rubin's views about puerperal changes in women are well known.[54] She describes the labor process as a progressive withdrawal of energy from surroundings to increasing focus on events within the laboring woman. During the postpartum period, a reverse process takes place. Rubin calls the initial two- or three-day period the "taking-in" phase, in which the passive new mother sleeps, eats a great deal, and assimilates what has happened. The second phase, "taking-hold," finds the new mother initiating actions, asserting her independence, and beginning to take hold of some of the tasks of mothering. Considerable anxiety can be found in this phase as she reestablishes control over her bodily functions and as her sphere of attention widens from self, to self-and-baby, and self-and-immediate family. This is a vulnerable time, when frustrations and failures make the new mother intolerant of her inadequacies, but also a time of maximum readiness for learning.[54]

Because people have been having babies, and presumably adapting to parenthood, since the human species evolved, it is logical to view the process as a normal developmental or maturational stage, a "rite-of-passage" experience. As with all developmental stages, there is the potential for emotional growth and maturity or for disturbance and psychiatric illness. This developmental turning point is accompanied by changes in physiology, roles, values, and relationships.[23] Each parent brings to this stage of development her or his own personality, set of life experiences, cultural, ethnic, socioeconomic, and educational background, and coping mechanisms which equip the parent well or poorly for making the role transition to parenting.

Until recently, little consideration had been given to the father's experiences of becoming a parent. His role had been seen primarily as that of providing emotional and financial support to his wife. Little research has been done in the area of the father's adaptation to parenthood, but there are indications that this experience is a major life event in his adult development. Grossman and colleagues speculate that many of the same factors that influence women also affect men during this stage of development—factors such as general psychological health, capacity to manage anxiety, comfort with his masculinity, and feeling of having been well-nurtured as a child. They identified several adaptive tasks of the puerperium for the first-time father, such as coming to see himself as a father; working out a balance between devoting time to his family and time for himself and his job; supporting his wife and helping to minimize her anxieties; working with his wife on their relationship; and developing a relationship with the new infant.[23] From her study of 60 normal, middle-class married couples, Shereshefsky concluded that pregnancy and parenthood are crucial for the male as well as the female.[58]

Not to be underestimated is the influence of the individual infant on the adaptation the family achieves. Recently we have come to appreciate the role an infant's behavior plays in eliciting responses from its parents. The baby's individual temperament interacts with its parents' personalities to determine the unique relationship a family achieves.[23]

Psychological Disturbances in the Puerperium

Psychological disturbances in postpartum women have been noted and written about for centuries. Hippocrates thought that retained lochia could be carried to the head and result in attacks of mania.[26] In spite of all that has been written, few prospective studies have been done. Most of the literature concerns women admitted to psychiatric hospitals in a psychotic state. Brown and Shereshefsky think that we are not close to understanding "the interaction between experience, physiology, and psychopathology in the postpartum period." They pose three important questions that remain unanswered, "1. Are there one or more unique psychiatric syndromes for which childbirth is a necessary precipitant? 2. What is the nature of the relationship between parturition and contiguous psychiatric disorder? 3. Can the woman who is prone to a severe postpartum disturbance be identified during pregnancy?."*

Even a mild, short-term psychological disturbance of the mother in the crucial period when the infant is being integrated into the family unit has the potential of interfering with this adjustment. Thus anything that can be done by the nurse-midwife to help reduce the incidence and severity of psychological disturbance in the postpartum woman may profoundly affect the whole family. In order to intervene effectively, it is necessary to have a thorough understanding of the phenomena involved.

Definitions

Standard definitions for the various forms of postpartum psychological disturbance (PPD) have not been utilized consistently in the literature, making meaningful discussion and comparison difficult. A spectrum of illness from "blues" to psychosis appears to exist. Brown has divided postpartum disturbance into three levels which seem to encompass the various types that have been described. (1) Postpartum "blues"—the short-lived emotional lability which generally occurs in the first week postpartum; (2) postpartum depression or chronic depressive syndrome—illness of a neurotic degree of intensity, with onset commonly from 2 to 8 weeks postpartum, which may last for a few months to more than a year; (3) postpartum psychosis—a relatively rare

---

*From Brown W, Shereshefsky P: Seven women: A prospective study of postpartum psychiatric disorders, in Shereshefsky P, Yarrow L (eds): Psychological Aspects of a First Pregnancy and Early Postnatal Adaptation. New York, Raven Press, 1974, p 182.

disorder with symptoms of schizophrenia, manic-depressive illness or primary depression, with onset most often in the first to third month postpartum.[6]

Incidence

The short-term postpartum blues seem to be very common, with an incidence of 50–80 percent found by various investigators.[4,62] Stein discovered that 76 percent of 37 normal postpartum women had episodes of weeping in the first week after delivery.[61]

The longer, neurotic-type depression occurs with less frequency. Usual estimates vary from 3–12 percent, although one prospective study found an incidence of 13 percent in 120 women evaluated during pregnancy and the puerperium.[4] Most of the researchers have included only white, middle-class women in their samples, and there may well be cultural variations that remain to be discovered.

There is general agreement that psychotic reactions have an incidence of 0.1–0.2 percent similar to that of schizophrenia in the general population.[49] Vandenbergh, however, thinks that these figures may be too low since they are based on hospitalized patients and that the real incidence may be closer to 12 percent.

Symptoms

Postpartum blues are characterized by seemingly inappropriate and unpredictable episodes of weeping. The affected woman often feels mildly depressed or anxious and especially vulnerable.[62,67] She may recognize that her behavior is inappropriate but not be able to control it. Occurring during the first week postpartum, these symptoms usually disappear in 2 or 3 days, but may last as long as 1 or 2 weeks. Although considered to be self-limiting and even "normal," such reactions can be miserable experiences for the new mothers suffering through them.

Brown's second level of disturbance, postpartum depression or chronic depressive syndrome, may be preceded by postpartum blues. In this case, however, the symptoms persist or worsen. It is also possible for the onset of symptoms to occur later, frequently 2 or 3 weeks after delivery, when full-time support from the husband or other relatives has ended, and the mother is faced with major responsibility for care of the baby and the household. The problem may persist for months to more than a year. Although this illness is not well defined, frequent symptoms are despondency, feelings of inadequacy, listlessness, apathy, inability to concentrate, irritability, fatigue, insomnia, and weight loss. The last two symptoms may be masked by normal postpartum weight loss and sleep disturbances due to meeting the needs of the infant which occur during the puerperium. While these symptoms may be similar to those of depressive illness in general, the difference lies in the specific content of the depressive thoughts. The depressed postpartum woman is faced with a great demand on her ability to love, both by the new infant and by other family members. Frequently her feelings focus on her inadequacy to love or love sufficiently. She may also have feelings of ambivalence toward the infant, which can be reflected in refusal to feed it or little interest in its welfare. Women whose disturbance falls into this category are of particular concern because their problem may not be correctly identified or appropriate help may not be given. Symptoms may be dismissed by the health care provider as being of the blues type or may not be revealed at all by the woman. Consequently, a minimally functioning mother may suffer through a moderately severe depression without receiving help for many months.[67]

Psychotic disturbances may resemble schizophrenia, manic-depressive illness or primary depression, and are relatively easy to identify. Delusional thoughts, changes in time sense, indecision, rapid alterations in mood, feelings of worthlessness, and auditory hallucinations may be found. Hyperactivity and rapid speech are sometimes seen. Deep depression may be accompanied by suicidal thoughts, paranoid thinking, and threats or actual violence directed at the infant. The severity of these symptoms usually assures that medical attention is sought by the family and diagnosis is rapid.[67]

In the late nineteenth and early twentieth centuries, the psychotic types of puerperal disturbance were viewed as syndromes unique to pregnancy. This idea has more recently given way to the concept that the psychiatric syndromes occurring in the postpartum period are indistinguishable from those occurring at other times of life.[7] However, this belief is not well grounded in clinical research, and it is being challenged by some investigators. Brockington and co-workers, in a retrospective analysis of the symptoms of 135 psychotic patients, 50 of them postpartum psychotic women, found four symptoms to be significantly more common in the postpartum group.[5] These were agitation, lability of mood, loss of social reserve, and being clouded or confused. Preliminary results of a prospective study being conducted by the same investigators show a large number of differences between the postpartum group and the controls. They propose that there is strong evidence against the prevailing view that postpartum psychosis is indistinguishable from recognized types of psychotic illness.[5] Other authors who view postpartum psychosis as an entity unique to the puerperium have described a clinical picture resembling a mild acute organic brain syndrome. The symptoms include labile mood, confusion, inability to sustain attention, poor recent memory, and transient delirious states.[62]

Etiology

Theories about the causes of postpartum psychological disturbances fall into three general categories: biogenic, psychogenic, and environmental or cultural. Several authors have proposed theories that combine etiological factors from more than one of these areas. Following is a review of theories from these three categories and an evaluation of their application to the three levels of postpartum disturbance previously described.

Biogenic etiology. Although studies are not conclusive, there seems to be some genetic influence on the occurrence of postpartum psychotic reactions of the schizophrenic or affective type.[62] In one controlled, longitudinal study the researchers found that the incidence of these disorders in daughters of women who had been treated for postpartum psychosis was 47 percent. The incidence increased to 58 percent when granddaughters were considered.[65]

Since endocrine changes occurring during pregnancy and after childbirth are unusual in their magnitude, complexity, and the speed at which they occur, attention naturally has focused on these changes as a possible cause for PPD. Mental changes including psychoses have been seen in other states of hormonal change, such as adrenal and thyroid disorders.[21]

It has been suggested that withdrawal of estriol, the estrogen secreted mainly by the placenta, may play a role in the development of PPD. Estrogen is thought to be involved in regulation of serum prolactin, and changes in prolactin levels have been associated with a variety of mental disorders.[62] Another possible mechanism for estrogen to affect the mental state is through its inhibitory action on the enzyme monoamine oxidase (MAO). In premenopausal depressed women, increased plasma MAO activity has been reported.[32] The rapid drop in estrogen levels after delivery might allow for increased MAO activity in postpartum women.

Progesterone levels drop suddenly between the first and second stages of labor, giving rise to the suggestion that, in some women, a greater drop or rate of drop than is normal might lead to PPD. Studies have failed to produce any good evidence of such a correlation, however.[70,44]

Prolactin, which rises after delivery, has been proposed to be involved in a variety of mental disorders, including depression and schizophrenia. Such an association has not been confirmed, however.[62] There is better evidence for the involvement of prolactin in premenstrual tension syndrome. Results of studies have shown that prolactin levels are significantly higher during the luteal-premenstrual phase than at other times in the menstrual cycle in women with severe premenstrual tension syndrome. Such women also have higher basal levels of prolactin throughout the cycle than do controls.[8] Dalton suggests that women who have difficulty in adjusting to the hormonal changes of the menstrual cycle might have even more problems adjusting to the greater hormonal changes in the puerperium.[12]

Various other hormones, including ACTH, cortisol, FSH, and LH change during pregnancy, childbirth, and the puerperium. There is no reliable evidence, however, about the effect of these hormones on human mood and behavior or an association of these hormones with PPD.[62]

Numerous investigations have been conducted to determine the role of the central nervous system neurotransmitters in mental illness, including depression. The monoamine hypothesis of depression proposes that a deficiency of the CNS monoamines norepinephrine, dopamine, and serotonin (5-hydroxy-ryptamine) in the synaptic cleft leads to decreased neurotransmission and that this is related to depression. The enzyme monoamine oxidase (MOA) is present in the synaptic cleft and will catalyze the breakdown of monoamines released into the cleft. A category of antidepressant drugs known as MOA inhibitors blocks the action of the enzyme, thus increasing the concentration of neurotransmitter in the synaptic cleft. Another group of drugs, the tricyclic antidepressants, block reuptake of monoamines into the neuron, which also results in increased concentration of neurotransmitter in the synaptic cleft. The effect of these drugs in reducing clinical depression in many people suffering from such illness would suggest a role for CNS neurotransmitters in the development of depression. [55]

Evidence linking neurotransmitters to PPD is scanty and inconclusive. The complexity of the action of CNS monoamines and their role in regulation of reproduction via the hypothalamic-pituitary-ovarian axis make cause-and-effect relationships difficult to determine. One study demonstrates a significant correlation between decreased urinary norepinephrine excretion and the severity of PPD. [66] Although the involvement of prolactin in the pathophysiology of PPD remains to be proved, monoamines are known to be involved in prolactin secretion. Dopamine inhibits prolactin release, and norepinephrine may promote it. [62] Thus there are numerous possible ways neurotransmitters could be involved in the genesis of PPD.

The role of 5-hydroxtryptamine (5-HT) in depressive illness has been the subject of much research, and there is evidence of a disturbance in 5-HT metabolism in such mental illness. The amino acid tryptophan is the substrate for 5-HT synthesis in the brain. In the bloodstream, some tryptophan is bound to plasma proteins, and only free plasma tryptophan is available for transport into the brain. A reduced level of free plasma tryptophan has been found in depressed patients, including in depressed postpartum women, in several studies. [10,27]

Pyridoxal phosphate (vitamin B_6) functions as a coenzyme for many chemical reactions relating to amino acid and protein metabolism. It is also believed to act in the transport of some amino acids across cell membranes. Although some investigators have found a vitamin B_6 deficiency in postpartum depressed women, [43] others have not found a difference in vitamin B_6 status between postpartum depressed women and controls. [37]

From the foregoing discussion it is obvious that the role of biological factors in the development of postpartum depressive disturbances is complex, but not clear. Some physiological factors have been found to be associated with PPD, but cause-and-effect relationships have yet to be demonstrated.

Psychogenic etiology. Postpartum depression may be viewed as ego decompensation, triggered by pregnancy and birth. The stresses surrounding childbirth weaken the ego so that earlier, repressed conflicts surface and are reactivated. Many of the conflicts center on the woman's relationship with her own mother, involving intense dependency needs or great hostility. Symbiotic ties to her mother result in interference with the woman's development of self-identity. The demands of an infant are perceived as a drain on her emotional resources. [38]

A number of factors have been identified as important in the psycho-pathology of postpartum disturbance. These include overidentification with or hostility toward the infant, unresolved sexual identification, ambivalent identi-fication with the woman's own mother, low tolerance to pain, marital conflict, and an ambivalent attitude toward the pregnancy.[62] It should be noted, howev-er, that these factors may occur without psychological disturbance. Many normal women, for example, have an ambivalent attitude toward pregnancy.

Varney views postpartum disturbance of the blues type as a result of grief for losses occurring during the puerperium.[68] The physical loss of intimate contact with the baby that the mother has been experiencing for months, along with loss of center-stage status to the baby, result in a mild grief process. Varney also views the rapid hormonal changes taking place as physiologic factors contributing to the labile emotions of the early postpartum period. She says that avoiding separation from the baby and increased attention from family and friends will decrease the incidence and severity of postpartum blues.

Environmental and cultural etiology. Examples of environmental fac-tors that may affect a woman's postpartum adjustment are financial problems, marital difficulties, limited living space, and death or illness of a family member. Even an emotionally healthy woman may have difficulty coping with the responsibilities of caring for a new infant if one or more significant environmental stressors are added.

Cultural attitudes and practices surrounding the childbearing experience can play a major role in a new mother's postpartum adaptation. Traditional societies often have rituals that honor the new mother instead of the infant, and prescribe patterns of behavior that must be followed in the puerperium. Extended families form support systems and provide role models for childbear-ing and childrearing. For example, among the Ibibio of Nigeria a special hut is built for the new mother and infant where they live for 2 or 3 months, cared for by the mother or mother-in-law. At the end of the stay, a feast takes place honoring the mother and baby, and the mother receives special gifts from her husband. A palm tree is planted as a legacy for the child. Postpartum depression is rare among the Ibibio.[30]

Pillsbury has described the period of convalescence following childbirth in traditional Chinese culture. Called "doing the month,"[48] there are many prescriptions and proscriptions for the new mother during this 30-day period of relative isolation. These include not bathing or washing her hair, not going outside, not eating any raw or cold food, consuming a chicken every day, not reading or crying, and not having sexual intercourse, among many others. Adhering to the prescribed behavior will lead to restoration of health and prevention of misfortune and ailments in the future. During the month the woman is usually attended by her mother-in-law. She is expected to stay in bed as much as possible, and the infant is usually cared for by another family member. Far more attention is lavished on the mother than on the baby, and new mothers do not appear to experience postpartum depression.

In modern Western societies many new parents live in isolation from other family members. There is a lack of clear cultural models for behavior during childbearing and the postpartum period. Career-oriented, middle-class women may feel that interrupting a career for childbearing is not a culturally-approved practice. Such women also may view discussion of the problems of bearing and raising children as stereotypic behavior to be avoided, thus cutting off possible support from other women.

In contemporary nuclear families the father's emotional support and involvement in the childbearing and rearing process becomes critically important, as does his practical help with the chores of child care and housework.[62] Since other female family members are often not available for long-term support and assistance, much of the burden assumed by them in extended families falls on the father in a nuclear family. If adequate help and support from the father are not forthcoming, the new mother's postpartum adjustment may be very difficult.

Other characteristics of a culture may be related to events in the childbearing experience. Cross-cultural studies have shown that in societies with more positive attitudes toward sexuality in general, there is an easier postpartum adjustment for new mothers.[62]

Modern obstetrics often includes practices that may make postpartum adjustment more difficult for new mothers. Separation of the infant from the mother after delivery may disrupt normal maternal behavior patterns and provide another stressor that could contribute to the development of postpartum depression.[33]

Tentoni and High conducted a survey of 49 primigravidas and found three culturally-determined factors which they propose to be precipitating agents in the postpartum depression syndrome.[64] All related to a loss of self-esteem, the three factors are changes in body proportions, changes in public attitudes, and changes in social life. Negative societal attitudes toward being overweight or blemished cause a loss of self-esteem when the pregnant woman gains weight or has stretch marks. These investigators also state that public attitudes toward pregnant women are largely negative, and that glances and stares when in public may lead to a loss of self-esteem. A tendency for those around her to overprotect the pregnant woman may lead to a withdrawal from social situations. Changes in social life can affect how a woman views herself and her pregnancy, again resulting in possible loss of self-esteem. Tentoni and High propose that these three factors, acting in the latter part of pregnancy, can have a gradual and deleterious effect on how a woman views herself, her pregnancy, and her baby and may make postpartum adjustment more difficult. In this study no attempt was made to follow women who exhibited concern about the three factors mentioned to see if they did, indeed, develop postpartum depression.[64]

Combining elements from all three categories of etiological factors, McGowan has reviewed postpartum disturbance in terms of a stress response.[39] Physiologic, psychic, and environmental factors serve as stressors during the childbearing experience. The number of stressors and their intensity will vary for each woman, but for all childbearing is a stressful time. A woman's constitutional traits and her acquired methods of coping with stress will determine if mental disturbance or emotional growth will be the outcome.

Summarizing the etiology of postpartum psychological disturbance. It is likely that the etiology of the various postpartum depressive states is multifactorial and complex. Even in women having the same level of depression, it is improbable that a common cause will be found for all their illnesses.

Since postpartum blues occur during the time of dramatic endocrine changes, it is reasonable to assume there is some physiologic basis for this response. This does not explain, however, the 20−50 percent of women who do not experience postpartum blues. Presumably they are undergoing similar hormonal changes, but perhaps their reaction to the changes is different. It is also possible that the underlying physiologic changes provide a potential basis for the blues that cultural, environmental, or psychic factors enhance or modify.

There is no clear explanation for the origin of the mid-level disturbance or postpartum depression. A physiologic basis related to hormonal changes is less likely than in postpartum blues, although the physiologic bases proposed for depression occurring separately from the childbearing process may apply. A combination of psychogenic and environmental factors may be at work. Vandenbergh states that the woman's own internal conflicts toward motherhood play the key role, while environmental factors serve as triggers that may cause these conflicts to be exhibited in the form of depression.[67]

Psychotic forms of postpartum depression may be severe manifestations of a disturbance unique to the childbearing process, as some authors have claimed. The evidence is not conclusive, however, for the existence of a postpartum syndrome separate from other forms of psychotic illness such as schizophrenia, manic-depressive states or primary depression. The stress of childbirth may trigger these illnesses in otherwise predisposed individuals.

Many unanswered questions remain about the origin of postpartum psychological disturbances. It is important that research continue in this area so that ways to prevent or cure such illnesses may be found.

Prediction of Postpartum Disturbance

If effective and practical ways to predict postpartum depression could be found, the nurse-midwife would be able to intervene or refer the woman with a potential problem so that illness might be prevented or decreased in severity. A number of factors have been shown to be associated with postpartum adjustment or maladjustment. It should be kept in mind that these are not demonstrated cause-and-effect relationships.

Various authors disagree over whether age, parity, and socioeconomic status are related to postpartum depression. Some studies have found primiparas to be more at risk than multiparas,[67] but others have not found parity to be important.[2] Kumar and Robson found women over 30 years old were more likely to be affected,[34] while others state that age is not related.[2] Higher socioeconomic status leads to better postpartum adjustment, according to Grossman and co-workers,[23] but was found not to be related by Ballinger.[2]

Anxiety during pregnancy has been found by several investigators to have a high positive correlation with depression in the postpartum period. This is true for anxiety measured in the first trimester[23] and at 36 weeks.[28] Hostility during the first trimester was also found in one study to be positively associated with postpartum depression.[23]

A negative life adaptation or chronic maladaptive responses to new maturational tasks by the woman have been associated with increased postpartum disturbance.[23,58] Increased life stresses not associated with the pregnancy and lack of coping with them increases the risk for postpartum depression.[47,58] Denial by the pregnant woman of the approaching childbirth crisis also makes a woman more vulnerable to difficulties in puerperal adjustment.[14]

Previous postpartum depression or psychosis apparently places a woman at high risk for another such illness.[4,67] Disrupted or poor family relationships in childhood also have been implicated as risk factors.[2,34] Shereshefsky found a recall of a woman's own mother as being warm, empathetic, close, and happy in her own mothering role to be associated with more positive adaptation to a first pregnancy.[58]

Carrying an unwanted pregnancy has been found by numerous authors to be highly related to difficulties in postpartum adjustment.[4,34,67] At the opposite extreme, women who had been trying to conceive for 2 or more years also were found to be at higher risk for a postpartum depression.[34] Perhaps their long-term desire for a pregnancy led to unrealistic expectations of childbirth and parenthood which, when not met, contributed to development of a postpartum depression.

The more aware a woman is during childbirth and the more she views herself as having done well during the labor and delivery experience, the less likely she is to have difficulty in postpartum adjustment.[14,23] One study found women who were breastfeeding at 5 weeks postpartum to be considerably less emotionally distressed, including less depressed, than similar women who had been given lactation suppressants.[52]

A major factor associated with postpartum adjustment is the amount of social support the new mother has and especially the amount of support from the baby's father. Feeling unloved by the partner or having marital difficulties have been shown to be associated with postpartum depression in a number of studies. Single or separated women are also at increased risk for postpartum depression.[2,4,34,67]

As can be seen from the foregoing discussion, although there is some disagreement among investigators, several factors seem to be highly associated with postpartum depression and can help the nurse-midwife to formulate guidelines for assessing prenatal patients.

Postpartum Psychological Disturbances in Fathers

Emotional problems may also be found in new fathers. Feelings of jealousy and uselessness are not uncommon, and depression is sometimes seen. The problems men experience may not result in painful feelings, but are demonstrated in behaviors such as lack of support, noninvolvement, and negativism, or in psychosomatic illness.[31]

Cavenar and Butts reviewed studies concerning psychiatric disturbances in new fathers that required hospitalization, and found several different theories of etiology:

1. presence of oedipal rivalry with the man's father, with the illness as a defense against identification with his father now that he was expected to assume a fathering role;
2. unconscious envy of the reproductive capability of the woman;
3. marked dependency on the wife with conflict resulting from her attention to an even more dependent family member.[9]

Cavenar and Butts present four case studies to support a different explanation for neuroses in new fathers who were being treated on an outpatient basis. In each case sibling rivalry was an important factor in the development of conflict over the wife's pregnancy. The threat of the pregnancy brought out many unresolved feelings associated with the birth of a sibling at some significant point in the patient's life. These feelings, primarily rage, were manifested in the following different ways: acute anxiety, severe obsessional thoughts related to the child, ambivalence, desire not to father a child, and fleeing from the pregnant wife in a phobic manner. This explanation somewhat parallels the psychoanalytic view of postpartum depression in women—the stresses surrounding childbirth weaken the ego and earlier repressed conflicts are reactivated.

Role of the Nurse-Midwife in Detecting, Treating, and Preventing Postpartum Psychological Disturbances

Nurse-midwives, as primary health-care providers, have a vital role in the prevention and detection of postpartum emotional disturbance.

Screening for those at risk. During a routine history obtained on a woman's first prenatal visit, the following factors predictive of postpartum psychological disturbance should be elicited: being single or separated, previous or family history of postpartum depression or psychosis, unwanted or unplanned pregnancy, severe premenstrual tension syndrome, poor relationship with the father of the baby or the woman's own mother, a feeling of having been unloved as a child, financial problems, death or illness of a family member or other environmental stresses. If risk factors are present, a more detailed psychiatric history may be obtained including information about the woman's abilities to cope with stress and previous adaptive or maladaptive responses to new maturational tasks. Women identified as having multiple risk factors are especially vulnerable, and should be noted as needing special counseling, teaching, and support during pregnancy and the puerperium. If the potential for problems is high, the nurse-midwife might utilize psychiatric and social service consultations.

A tool found to be reliable in predicting or detecting emotional distress is the Hopkins Symptom Checklist (HSCL), a self-administered questionnaire (See Appendix following this chapter). Besides providing an overall assessment of emotional distress, distress is measured in the five symptom areas of somatization, obsessive-compulsive traits, interpersonal sensitivity, depression, and anxiety.[62] This tool could be used to screen all women at their initial prenatal visits and again at 36 weeks of gestation, when anxiety has been shown to be highly correlated with PPD. If use of the Hopkins Symptom Checklist is not practical for all patients, it could be selectively used prenatally and postpartum to detect actual emotional distress in those women identified as having one or more risk factors for PPD.

Assessment of postpartum psychological disturbance. It is important to identify psychological problems as early as possible in the postpartum woman, not only for her benefit, but also for that of the infant and the family. Early initiation of treatment may prevent the development of more serious illness. The nurse-midwife should plan sufficient time during postpartum visits to evaluate carefully for depression. The new mother may not be willing to admit negative feelings because she may view them as a sign of failure to become a good parent. The Hopkins Symptom Checklist might be used as a less-threatening method than direct questioning to elicit information on depression or other emotional distress.

A careful history of the antepartum, intrapartum, and postpartum periods should be taken. Waletzky recommends that the evaluation be done with the father and infant present.[69] She says areas of questioning should include the following:

1. emotional reactions during the childbearing experience
2. emotional reactions following previous births
3. previous personal and family psychiatric history
4. feelings of attachment to the infant
5. feelings about taking care of the infant
6. feelings about breast or bottle feeding
7. information about the mother's relationship with the husband and his involvement with the baby
8. relationship with other children and any differences in the feelings toward this baby and the others
9. relationship with her mother

10. style of living before pregnancy and reaction to role changes since the baby's birth
11. financial, emotional, or environmental problems
12. emotional supports available
13. whether she has ever felt this bad or worse
14. whether she thinks she needs help with her emotional problems

Observation of the mother's interaction with the infant is also important.

Once as much information as possible has been gathered and psychological disturbance has been identified, it is important to evaluate the level of the disturbance. If the primary feelings are mild depression or anxiety, if weeping is a major symptom, and if the problem occurs within the first 2 weeks postpartum, the most likely diagnosis is postpartum blues. Indifference or hostility toward the infant would be a sign of a more serious disturbance. Even when the evaluation of blues is made, careful follow-up is necessary to ensure the problem does not continue or worsen.

Psychological disturbance continuing after 2 weeks generally is postpartum depression or psychosis. Despondency, feelings of inadequacy, fatigue, irritability, insomnia, apathy, and inability to concentrate may be seen in postpartum depression. Suicidal or delusional thoughts, paranoid thinking, changes in time sense, rapid alterations in mood, and threats or violence directed at the infant would indicate the psychotic level of postpartum disturbance.

Nurse-midwifery management. If postpartum blues have been identified, the major roles for the nurse-midwife are support and anticipatory guidance. When the new mother knows that her feelings of distress are likely to be brief, they may be easier to tolerate. Other family members need to know that weeping or other unusual behavior do not mean that the mother is seriously ill. Promotion of contact between the mother, baby, and other family members during the early postpartum period will often reduce or prevent postpartum blues.

Identification of postpartum depression or psychotic disturbance requires psychiatric consultation and referral. Acting as an advocate for her patients, the nurse-midwife should try to ensure that the symptoms of postpartum depression are not dismissed as blues by a therapist unfamiliar with the different levels of postpartum disturbance. If hospitalization is necessary, every effort should be made to find a hospital with facilities to accommodate the baby as well as the mother.

Prevention. The most important nurse-midwifery management function for postpartum psychological disturbance is prevention-directed effort before childbirth. In this country people generally come to the tasks and joys of parenting woefully unprepared. In their local communities nurse-midwives can initiate or support programs in high schools that teach parenting skills and child development. This author believes that such courses should be a requirement for graduation, since the skills and knowledge acquired have the potential for being as, or more, important in the individual's personal life and for the welfare of society as traditional academic requirements. Nurse-midwives might become active participants in teaching such courses and would have much of value to offer.

During the prenatal period the whole spectrum of the nurse-midwife's activities to promote emotional well-being and adaptation to pregnancy and parenthood are important in preventing postpartum psychological problems. In general, these activities include providing factual information, anticipatory guidance, ego-strengthening, mobilizing environmental resources, and promoting physical health and well-being. In addition, if identification of risk factors indicates a high risk for postpartum problems, special counseling or psychiatric referral may be offered.

Besides the obvious usefulness of providing factual information and dispelling myths, enlarging the store of knowledge also increases ego strength. During the prenatal period the woman's readiness for learning postpartum information may not be maximal, since she is more apt to focus on adapting to pregnancy and on the labor and delivery experience. In the immediate and early puerperium, she is likely to have good receptivity for learning. At that time classes or video tapes on infant care and feeding, postpartum restoration and nutrition, postpartum marital and sexual adjustments, and contraception should be available. Classes involving only demonstrations of infant care are not adequate. To develop confidence in her abilities to care for her infant, a new mother needs "hands-on" experience. If she receives the impression that health-care personnel do not consider her capable of caring for her baby in the hospital or birthing center where skilled assistance is available, she will be unlikely to feel confident when she is on her own with the infant at home. Fathers and other family members need to be involved in prenatal and postpartum learning experiences as much as possible.

There are a number of areas in which anticipatory guidance will be of use to new parents. Parents, especially first-time parents, need to know that they may not feel a great deal of love for the baby at first. Maternal and paternal feelings often take some time to develop, and they should know that not having strong feelings right away is perfectly normal and does not mean they are unnatural parents. Articles and books portraying the childbirth experience as a totally joyful, mystical, or perhaps a religious experience may lead new parents to have unrealistic expectations of what the experience will be like. Hopefully, the experience *will* be joyful and rewarding, but prospective parents need to know that even if they do not have the "perfect" birth experience, they are not failures and they are capable of bonding with the baby and of being good parents. Promoting the benefits of and helping the parents to plan for a traditional "lying-in" period, when social and household tasks are not expected, will be helpful to many people. Parents should be encouraged not to plan too many activities too early.

Ego-strengthening and support can come directly from the nurse-midwife or indirectly through support groups in which she encourages parents to participate. Actions of the nurse-midwife, which help the woman to feel a sense of mastery about her labor and delivery experience and satisfaction with her behavior during that time, can help to reduce postpartum problems. Review and discussion of labor and delivery with the nurse-midwife in the early postpartum period can be very useful in helping the new mother come to terms with her intrapartum experience. Unresolved conflicts about that period have the potential to interfere with postpartum adjustment.

Postpartum support group programs have much to offer new parents. Such groups may be composed of mothers or couples who were participants in prenatal classes. Cronenwett investigated the outcomes of one program.[11] Questionnaires were sent to 90 women from 15 groups and there was a 73 percent response rate. About one-third of the groups had met for 5 months or less, one-third had met for 6−11 months and the remaining one-third a year or more. Members of the support group were drawn from those who had participated in Lamaze classes. Postpartum groups were started with the assistance of volunteer leaders who withdrew when the group was sufficiently organized to continue on its own. At the first meeting each group decided how it would function. One of the decisions made was whether to include babies and fathers at the meetings. The groups in the study were almost evenly split between infants and no infants, but none elected to include fathers. Reasons for which mothers initially joined the groups varied, with "desire to talk to other persons in my situation," "desire to meet new people with children my child's age," "desire to talk with people about childbearing and parenting issues," and "desire to get out of the house regularly" most frequently mentioned. Over 80 percent of the respondents felt all their initial needs had been met by the groups. Some of the topics discussed were negative feelings since the birth of the baby, feelings about working outside the home, feelings about the labor and delivery experience, changes in the marital relationship since the baby, sleep-related problems of the infant, changes in husband−wife roles, and infant feeding problems. Women in the study identified discovery of the universality and normality of their feelings as the key reason group discussions were important to them. More than 70 percent of the women said they would highly recommend the experience to others and more than 60 percent said they would seek out similar group experiences in the future. The nurse-midwife could be instrumental in initiating postpartum support groups for women or couples within her practice.

Nurse-midwives also may facilitate postpartum adjustment by assisting parents to mobilize environmental resources. The nurse-midwife can inform parents of prenatal and postpartum classes, support groups, and community resources for child and nursing care and household assistance. In addition, the nurse-midwife can encourage parents and other family members who will assist in the postpartum period to make contracts to agree in advance on the role and function of each person. Clearly specifying roles in advance will help prevent misunderstanding and conflict after childbirth. Family members should be prepared to make arrangements for the new mother to get adequate sleep, which is essential to her physical and emotional well-being.

Promotion of physical health and well-being is important for good emotional health. Obviously, a woman who feels well during her pregnancy is more likely to have a positive attitude than one who has been miserable much of the time.

The preceding discussion on postpartum psychological disturbances might lead to the conclusion that childbirth leaves women in an especially unstable emotional condition. However, Paschall and Newton evaluated the results of the Neuroticism Scale Questionnaire administered to 97 new mothers and found women 2 or 3 days postpartum to have scores for neuroticism similar to the national norms.[46] These authors state, "despite radical hormonal changes, the strange environment and schedule of the hospital, the adjustment of the new baby, the recent experience of labor which frequently involves medication of several types, appreciable blood loss, and an incision cutting deeply into one of the most sexually sensitive areas of the body ... ."[46] the conclusion could be drawn that new mothers are unusually stable individuals. Nurse-midwives, while always doing our best to promote good psychological and physical health and to identify problems in childbearing women and their families, must also convey our belief in the normalcy of the process and our faith in the family's ability to attain a positive outcome.

REFERENCES

1. Anderson A: The genital system, in Hytten F, Chamberlain G (eds): Clinical Physiology in Obstetrics. Oxford, Blackwell, 1980, pp 328–380
2. Ballinger B, Buckley D, Naylor G, et al: Emotional disturbance following childbirth: Clinical findings and urinary excretion of cyclic AMP (adenosine 3'5' cyclic monophosphate). Psychol Med 9:293–300, 1979
3. Bowes W: The puerperium. Clin OB Gyne 23:971, 1980
4. Braverman J, Roux J: Screening for the patient at risk for postpartum depression. Obstet Gynecol 52(1):731–736, 1978
5. Brockington I, Schofield E, Donnelly P, et al: A clinical study of postpartum psychosis, in Sandler M (ed): Mental Illness in Pregnancy and the Puerperium. Oxford, Oxford University Press, 1978, pp 59–67
6. Brown WA: Psychological Care During Pregnancy and the Postpartum Period. New York, Raven, 1979, pp 119–134
7. Brown W, Shereshefsky P: Seven women: A prospective study of postpartum psychiatric disorders, in Shereshefsky P, Yarrow L (eds): Psychological Aspects

---

*From Paschall N, Newton N: Personality factors and postpartum adjustment. Primary Care 3(4):748, 1976

of a First Pregnancy and Early Postnatal Adaptation. New York, Raven Press, 1974, pp 181−207

8. Carroll BJ, Steiner M: The psychobiology of premenstrual dysphoria: The role of prolactin. Psychoneuroendocrinology 3:171−180, 1978

9. Cavenar JO, Butts N: Fatherhood and emotional illness. Am J Psychiatry 134(4):429−431, 1977

10. Coppen A, Stein G, Wood K: Postnatal depression and tryptophan metabolism, in Sandler M (ed): Mental Illness in Pregnancy and the Puerperium. Oxford, Oxford University Press: 25−33, 1978

11. Cronenwett L: Elements and outcomes of a postpartum support group program. Res Nurs Health 3:33−41, 1980

12. Dalton K: Prospective study into puerperal depression. Br J Psychiatry 118:689−692, 1971

13. Delgado H, Brineman E, Lechtig A, et al: Effects of maternal nutritional status and infant supplementation during lactation on postpartum amenorrhea. Am J Obstet Gynecol 135:303−307, 1979

14. Doering S, Entwisle D: Coping mechanisms during childbirth and postpartum sequelae. Primary Care 3:727−739, 1976

15. Edelman DA, Goldsmith A, Skelton JD: Postpartum contraception. Int J Gynaecol Obstet 19:305−311, 1981

16. Eschenbach D, Wager G: Puerperal infection. Clin OB Gyne 23(4):1003−1037, 1980

17. Evrard JR, Gold EM: Cesarean section and maternal mortality in Rhode Island: Incidence and risk factors, 1965−75. Obstet Gynecol 50:594, 1977

18. Filher R, Monif G: The significance of temperature during the first 24 hours postpartum. Obstet Gynecol 53:358−361, 1979

19. Friedman C: Maternal infections: Problems and Prevention. Nurs Clin N Am 15(4):817−824, 1980

20. Fuller W: Family planning in the postpartum period. Clin Obstet Gynecol 23(4): 1081−1085, 1980

21. Gelder M: Hormones and postpartum depression, in Sandler M (ed): Mental Illness in Pregnancy and the Puerperium. Oxford, Oxford University Press, 1978, pp 80−89

22. Gibbs R: Clinical risk factors for puerperal infection. Obstet Gynecol 55(5):1785−1835, 1980 Suppl

23. Grossman FK, Eichler LS, Winiehoff SA: Pregnancy, Birth and Parenthood. San Francisco, Jossey-Bass Publishers, 1980

24. Gruis M: Beyond maternity: Postpartum concerns of mothers. MCN 19:182−188, 1977

25. Hames CT: Sexual needs and interests of postpartum couples. JOGN Nurs 9:313−315, 1980

26. Hamilton J: Postpartum Psychiatric Problems. St. Louis, Mosby, 1962, p 126

27. Handley S, Dunn T, Waldron G, et al: Tryptophan, cortisol and puerperal mood. Br J Psychiatry 136:498−508, 1980

28. Hayworth J, Little B, Carter S, et al: A predictive study of postpartum depression: Some predisposing characteristics. Br J Med Psychol 53:161−167, 1980

29. Iffy L, Kaminetzlry H, Maidman J, et al: Control of perinatal infection by traditional preventive measures. Obstet Gynecol 54(4):403−411, 1979

30. Kelly JV: The influence of native customs on obstetrics in Nigeria. Obstet Gynecol 30:608−612, 1967

31. Ketai R, Brandwin M: Childbirth-related psychosis and familial symbiotic conflict. Am J Psychiatry 136:190−193, 1979

32. Klaiber EL, Broverman DM, Vogl W, et al: Effects of estrogen therapy on plasma MAO activity and EEG driving responses of depressed women. Am J Psychiatry 128:1492−1498, 1972

33. Klaus MH, Trause MA, Kennell JH: Does human maternal behavior after delivery show a characteristic pattern: Parent−infant Interaction Ciba Foundation Symposium 33:69−85, 1975

34. Kumar R, Robson K: Neurotic disturbance during pregnancy and the puerperium: Preliminary report of a prospective survey of 119 primiparae, in Sandler M (ed): Mental Illness in Pregnancy and the Puerperium. Oxford, Oxford University Press, 1978, pp 40−51

35. Laufe L, Cole L, Wheeler R: Modification of the CUT 220C for immediate postpartum use. Am J Obstet Gynecol 137(1):151−152, 1980

36. Letshy E: The haematological system, in Hytten F, Chamberlain G (eds): Clinical Physiology in Obstetrics. Oxford, Blackwell, 1980, pp 43−78

37. Livingston J, MacLeod P, Applegarth D: Vitamin B_6 status in women with postpartum depression. Am J Clin Nutr 31(5):886−891, 1978

38. Markham S: A comparative evaluation of psychotic and non-psychotic reactions to childbirth. Am J Orthopsychiatry 31:565−578, 1961

39. McGowan M: Postpartum disturbance: A review of the literature in terms of stress response. J Nurse-midwif 22:27−34, 1977

40. Mercer RT: The nurse and maternal tasks of early postpartum. Maternal-Child Nursing J 6:341−345, 1981

41. Monheit A, Cousins L, Resnik R: The puerperium: Anatomic and physiologic readjustments. Clin Obstet Gynecol 23(4):973−983, 1980

42. Nelson G, Donnell S, Griffin G, et al: Timing of postpartum hematocrit determinations. Med J 73(9):1202−1204, 1980

43. Nabbs B: Pyridoxal phosphate status in clinical depression. Lancet 1:405, 1974

44. Nott PH, Franklin M, Armitage C, et al: Hormonal changes and mood in the puerperium. Br J Psychiatry 128:379−383, 1976

45. Novy M: The puerperium, in Benson R (ed): Current Obstetric and Gynecologic Diagnosis and Treatment. Los Altos, Lange Medical Pub, 1980, pp 781−806

46. Paschall N, Newton N: Personality factors and postpartum adjustment. Primary Care 3(4):741−749, 1976

47. Payhel E, Emms E, Fletcher J, et al: Life events and social support in puerperal depression. Br J Psychiatry 136:339−346, 1980

48. Pillsbury B: ''Doing the month'': Confinement and convalescence of Chinese women after childbirth, in Kay M (ed): Anthropology of Human Birth. Philadelphia, FA Davis, 1982, pp 119−143

49. Pitt B: Introduction, in Sandler M (ed): Mental Illness in Pregnancy and the Puerperium. Oxford, Oxford University Press, 1978, pp 1−6

50. Pritchard J, MacDonald P: William's Obstetrics (ed 16). New York, Appleton-Century-Crofts, 1980

51. Rehu M, Nilsson C, Haukkamaa A: Significant bacteriuria in the puerperium: A prospective study of the risk factors. Ann Clin Res 12(3):112−115, 1980

52. Rickels K, Garcia CR, Lipman R, et al: The Hopkins Symptom Checklist: Assessing emotional distress in obstetric gynecologic practice. Primary Care 3(4):751−764, 1976
53. Romney S, Gray M, Little AB, et al: Gynecology and Obstetrics: The Health Care of Women (ed 2). New York, McGraw-Hill, 1981
54. Rubin R: Puerperal change. Nsg Outlook 9:753−755, 1961
55. Sandler M: Some biological correlates of mental illness in relation to childbirth, in Sandler M (ed): Mental Illness in Pregnancy and the Puerperium. Oxford, Oxford University Press, 1978, pp 9−21
56. Sharman A: Reproductive Physiology of the Postpartum Period. Edinburgh, E and S Livingstone, 1966
57. Sheehan F: Assessing postpartum adjustment: A pilot study. JOGN Nurs 10:19−22, 1981
58. Shereshefsky P: Summary and integration of findings, in Shereshefsky P, Yarrow L (eds): Psychological Aspects of a First Pregnancy and Early Postnatal Adaptation. New York, Raven Press, 1974, pp 237−251
59. Shy K, Eschenbach D: Fatal perineal cellutis from an episiotomy site. Obstet Gynecol 54(3):292−298, 1979
60. Sibai B, Schneider J, Morrison J, et al: The late postpartum eclampsia controversy. Obstet Gynecol 55:74−78, 1980
61. Stein G: The pattern of mental change and body weight change in the first postpartum week. J Psychosom Res 24(3−4):165−171, 1980
62. Steiner M: Psychobiology of mental disorders associated with childbearing. An overview. Acta Psychiatr Scand 60:449−464, 1979
63. Sweet RL, Ledger WJ: Puerperal infectious morbidity. J Am Obstet Gynecol 117:1093−1100, 1973
64. Tentoni SC, High KA: Culturally induced postpartum depression: A theoretical position. JOGN Nurs 17:246−247, 1980
65. Thuwe I: Genetic factors in puerperal psychosis. Br J Psychiatry 125:378−385, 1974
66. Treadway C, Kane F, Jarrahi-Zadeh A, et al: A psychoendocrine study of pregnancy and puerperium. Am J Psychiatry 125:1380−1386, 1969
67. Vandenbergh R: Postpartum depression. Clin Obstet Gynecol 23(4):1105−1111, 1980
68. Varney H: Nurse-Midwifery. Boston, Blackwell, 1980
69. Waletzky L: Emotional illness in the postpartum period, in Ahmed P (ed): Pregnancy, Childbirth and Parenthood. New York, Elsevier, 1981, pp 337−357
70. Yalom ID, Lunde DT, Moos RH, et al: "Postpartum Blues" syndrome. A description and related variables. Arch Gen Psychiatry 18:16−27, 1968

APPENDIX 5-1

Hopkins Symptom Checklist (HSCL)*

To obtain the total score, sum all the HSCL items rated and divide by the number of items rated. Mean scores thus obtained will range from 1 to 4 with higher scores indicating greater emotional distress. To obtain a score for each of the 5 symptom dimensions, use the above method, but sum only those items listed in Table 5-2 after each symptom.

Symptom checklist
Name: _____
Date: _____

Please read each symptom carefully and decide how much the complaint bothered or distressed you during the past week, including today. Then put a checkmark (   ) in one of the four spaces.

	How much were you bothered			
	1	2	3	4
	not at all	a little	quite a bit	extremely

DO NOT LEAVE OUT
ANY ITEMS

1. Headaches	_____	_____	_____	_____
2. Nervousness or shakiness inside	_____	_____	_____	_____
3. Being unable to get rid of bad thoughts or ideas	_____	_____	_____	_____
4. Faintness or dizziness	_____	_____	_____	_____
5. Pains or butterflies in the stomach	_____	_____	_____	_____
6. Loss of sexual interest or pleasure	_____	_____	_____	_____
7. Feeling critical of others	_____	_____	_____	_____
8. Bad dreams	_____	_____	_____	_____
9. Difficulty speaking when you are excited	_____	_____	_____	_____
10. Tired or fatigued during the day	_____	_____	_____	_____
11. Trouble remembering things	_____	_____	_____	_____

(continued)

*Reprinted with permission from Rickels K, Garcia CR, Lipman R, et al: The Hopkins System Checklist: Assessing emotional distress in obstetric gynecologic practice. Primary Care 3(4):751–764, 1976.

Appendix 5-1 (continued)

| | How much were you bothered | | | |
	1 not at all	2 a little	3 quite a bit	4 extremely
12. Worried about sloppiness or carelessness	___	___	___	___
13. Feeling easily annoyed or irritated	___	___	___	___
14. Pains in the heart or chest	___	___	___	___
15. Thoughts of ending your life	___	___	___	___
16. Itching	___	___	___	___
17. Feeling low in energy or slowed down	___	___	___	___
18. Sweating	___	___	___	___
19. Trembling	___	___	___	___
20. Constipation	___	___	___	___
21. Feeling confused	___	___	___	___
22. Crying easily	___	___	___	___
23. Feeling shy or uneasy with the opposite sex	___	___	___	___
24. A feeling of being trapped or caught	___	___	___	___
25. Loose bowel movements	___	___	___	___
26. Suddenly scared for no reason	___	___	___	___
27. Temper outbursts you could not control	___	___	___	___
28. Blaming yourself for things	___	___	___	___
29. Pains in the lower part of your back	___	___	___	___
30. Poor appetite	___	___	___	___
31. Feeling that you can't get anything done	___	___	___	___
32. Feeling lonely	___	___	___	___
33. Feeling blue	___	___	___	___
34. Worrying or stewing about things	___	___	___	___
35. Nausea or upset stomach	___	___	___	___

36. Feeling no interest in things _____ _____ _____ _____
37. Feeling fearful _____ _____ _____ _____
38. Your feelings are easily hurt _____ _____ _____ _____
39. Having to ask others what you should do _____ _____ _____ _____
40. Sleepy during the day _____ _____ _____ _____
41. Feeling others do not understand you or are unsympathetic _____ _____ _____ _____
42. Feeling that people are unfriendly or dislike you _____ _____ _____ _____
43. Having to do things very slowly in order to be sure you were doing them right _____ _____ _____ _____
44. Heart pounding or racing _____ _____ _____ _____
45. Dry mouth _____ _____ _____ _____
46. Feeling inferior to others _____ _____ _____ _____
47. Soreness of your muscles _____ _____ _____ _____
48. Difficulty in falling asleep or staying asleep _____ _____ _____ _____
49. Having to check and double-check what you do _____ _____ _____ _____
50. Heavy feelings in your arms or legs _____ _____ _____ _____
51. Difficulty making decisions _____ _____ _____ _____
52. Wanting to be alone _____ _____ _____ _____
53. Trouble getting your breath _____ _____ _____ _____
54. Hot or cold spells _____ _____ _____ _____
55. Having to avoid certain things, places or activities because they frighten you _____ _____ _____ _____
56. Your mind going blank _____ _____ _____ _____
57. Numbness or tingling in parts of your body _____ _____ _____ _____

Appendix 5-1 (continued)

	How much were you bothered			
	1 not at all	2 a little	3 quite a bit	4 extremely
58. A lump in your throat	_____	_____	_____	_____
59. Feeling hopeless about the future	_____	_____	_____	_____
60. Trouble concentrating	_____	_____	_____	_____
61. Weakness in parts of your body	_____	_____	_____	_____
62. Feeling tense or keyed up	_____	_____	_____	_____
63. Having to repeat the same actions such as touching, counting, hand washing, etc.	_____	_____	_____	_____
64. Having impulses to hurt, injure, or beat someone	_____	_____	_____	_____

Table 5-2
HSCL Symptom Dimensions and Contributing Items

Symptom Classification	Symptom Dimension and Contributing Items
Somatization	Headaches, faintness or dizziness, pains in the heart or chest, sweating, pains in lower part of back, nausea or upset stomach, soreness of your muscles, heavy feelings in your arms and legs, trouble getting your breath, hot or cold spells, numbness or tingling in parts of body, a lump in your throat, weakness in parts of your body
Obsessive-Compulsive	Being unable to get rid of bad thoughts or ideas, trouble remembering things, worried about sloppiness or carelessness, feeling that you can't get anything done, having to do things very slowly to insure correctness, having to check and double-check, difficulty making decisions, your mind going blank, trouble concentrating, having to repeat the same actions such as touching, counting, hand washing, etc.
Interpersonal Sensitivity	Feeling critical of others, feeling easily annoyed or irritated, feeling shy or uneasy with the opposite sex, temper outbursts, feelings easily hurt, feeling others do not understand or are unsympathetic, feeling people are unfriendly or dislike you, feeling inferior to others, impulses to hurt, injure or beat someone

| Depression | Loss of sexual interest or pleasure, thoughts of ending your life, feeling low in energy or slowed down, crying easily, feelings of being trapped or caught, blaming yourself for things, poor appetite, feeling lonely, feeling blue, worrying or stewing about things, feeling no interest in things, difficulty in falling or staying asleep, feeling hopeless about the future |
| Anxiety | Nervousness or shakiness inside, trembling, suddenly scared for no reason, feeling fearful, heart pounding or racing, having to avoid certain things, places or activities because they frighten you, feeling tense or keyed up |

Total Score: _____

All items listed above as well as pains or butterflies in the stomach, bad dreams, difficulty speaking when you are excited, tired or fatigued during the day, itching, constipation, feeling confused, loose bowel movements, having to ask others what you should do, sleepy during the day, dry mouth, wanting to be alone

Sarah J. Naber

6

The Neonate

The nurse-midwife needs to be aware of infant-care options and alternatives that are currently under discussion in the literature and by consumer groups in order to provide families with sufficient information to make intelligent decisions regarding child rearing. Certain priorities for information sharing may be set by the nurse-midwife according to an assessment of individual family needs, but the family members should set priorities for their own actions.

There are two groups of issues in the area of early child rearing. The first includes "common-sense" issues such as the cost effectiveness of paper versus cloth diapers or liquid versus powdered formula ingredients. The second includes "value-laden" issues such as ecological considerations regarding the use of cloth diapers versus paper ones or the long-term benefits of breast- versus bottle feeding. Decision making by parents can be facilitated in both of these areas by a nurse-midwife who is well informed, but, more importantly, who has the ability to communicate effectively. It is easy to share information from the corner drugstore about the cost and brands of various infant-care products, but it is often not as easy to guide families in making decisions about circumcision or infant feeding methods.

Sharing the information families need regarding the more subjective and value-laden aspects of parenting is more difficult than sharing information on the practical aspects for two reasons. First, the clinician must recognize that her or his own biases and preferences need to be dealt with and separated from those of the consumer-family. One must be cautious and sensitive in proceeding to give information on certain topics; it may be acceptable to sway opinion when true ignorance or ambivalence about circumcision exists, but it is unfair to cause undue stress by making the woman who has demonstrated obvious discomfort in handling her own body feel guilty for not breastfeeding. Fortunately, most of the guidance and information needs fall somewhere between these extremes, but information needs can be rendered more complex by practitioner biases. Secondly, there is much more work for the nurse-midwife when helping the family to make decisions affecting the long-term health and welfare of an individual or of the family. Such decisions require a well-informed and dedicated practitioner who is willing to spend time and effort to educate or to find resources for families to obtain essential informational needs. More importantly, the practitioner must communicate effectively and provide continuity of care. It is difficult for parents to understand and accept that the benefits of what they are doing today may not be reaped for a generation or so unless we remind them and give ongoing positive feedback. All of us need some immediate gratification for our actions, and the remoteness of the idea that a baby who is breast-fed today could possibly suffer fewer adult health problems may not be powerful motivation for the mother with current social or health needs of her own. The practitioner must be considerate of such a mother and yet provide her with enough information and ongoing support to make decisions that could significantly affect future society.

INFANT CAPABILITIES

In the early 1970s the literature began to swell with articles about the newfound capabilities of the human newborn. "Of course," a lot of nurses said, "mothers have been telling us for years that they not only could recognize their unseen infants' cries but that their babies knew them, too." Unfortunately, the state of the art of nursing was such that, until recently, research on and records of such observations were limited to a few publications that were usually unrefereed, parochial journals. Once the ball started rolling in the non-nursing literature, however, nurse authors were quick to pick it up and to see the importance of expanding beyond clinical observations into the development of practical guidance for nurse and parent education.[1]

The Brazelton Neonatal Behavioral Assessment Scale[13] was developed to test and record the abilities of newborns to organize responses to their environments by using waking or sleeping state-related behaviors. The assessment scale consists of 20 neurological reflex items and 27 behavioral items used to measure the infant's interactive behavior, and it requires some training of the examiner in order to ensure reliable results for interpretation. It was designed as a clinical tool to investigate the individual personality of the newborn, and its secondary value was to convince clinical practitioners that babies were well equipped to react to their environments in distinctly different ways according to their personality makeups. The next step, of course, was to share this information about newborn capability with the parents so that their interactions with the neonate would be more in synchrony with the infant's abilities. The caregiver's interaction with the neonate perceived to be stimulated by the environment is likely to differ from interaction with the neonate perceived to be—as neonates had been described previously—unseeing, unhearing, and unfeeling.

The Brazelton Neonatal Behavior Assessment Scale has been used as a teaching tool for mothers (with the pinprick item omitted), and maternal−infant reciprocal interaction was shown to be enhanced in the group who received an assessment demonstration versus a group only told about the test.[4] The old reminder that "seeing is believing" appears to hold true here. Cognitive skills were enhanced in infants of teenage mothers who were given Brazelton demonstrations in one study.[40] It may not be possible to administer the assessment to every baby due to constraints on time and on the number of individuals prepared to do the testing, so the suggestion has been made that Brazelton films should be used as part of prenatal education.[22] Parent expectations regarding their infants can in this way be made more realistic, and parents can be prepared for the variety of newborn personalities and activities that have been documented. Films are easily obtained through distributors or, if one has access to a setting where standardized testing takes place, a videotape could be made. Since many nurse-midwives are parent educators, the inclusion of this information should be considered.

It should be stressed that the Brazelton scale probably has more value as a tool to teach about infant capability than as one to predict personality. There are many variables measured with the scale, as previously mentioned, and in at least one study, certain of these have shown little stability when followed over time.[23] More work will need to be done on infant capability, but parents should be taught about the variety of behaviors and should not be encouraged to expect that a limited number of responses regarding a particular variable is preferable or more in tune with normal infant personality development.

Consumers have been alerted to and bombarded with information about parent−infant bonding. Along with the idea that the infant is capable of participating in the bonding process as much as the parents has come the idea of a "critical period" during the first hours after birth when optimal parent−infant bonding may occur. Certainly, the undistressed neonate's quiet alert state, which is when she or he is most receptive to sensory stimuli, and the parents' eagerness and willingness to establish contact with their offspring during the first hours after birth make such a conclusion seem logical. Some studies have shown that extended contact between parents and infants after birth caused more positive interaction behaviors at a later testing, but others have not confirmed these findings.[31] Nevertheless, the research indications that affectionate behaviors between parents and infants and breastfeeding success are related to early contact opportunities have caused most clinicians to support the idea of providing initial bonding opportunities when the condition of the infant and the mother permits.[36]

One should always be sensitive to the desires of the parents and subtle in the promotion of bonding, however. A matter-of-fact approach such as asking the father *to* hold the baby rather than *if* he wants to hold the baby may enable a man to have early physical, verbal, and eye contact with his infant although he may feel uneasy about verbalizing his desire to do so; perhaps if the father had seen a newborn assessment demonstration and knew that the infant's eyes focus on objects or persons about 8–10 inches away, he would be eager to try out this principle. On the other hand, promoting the benefits of initial bonding to the point where parents will feel guilty if they do not desire this extended closeness may induce some stress. In addition, a clinical emergency at delivery may preclude or delay contact. It is important for the clinician to be aware that effective bonding opportunities or sensitive periods for forming human relationships extend over time (up to 6 months).[1] The clinician should therefore support and promote parent–infant interaction opportunities whenever they may occur. Helping parents to understand their rights, to gain entrance into a nursery, and to participate in newborn caretaking is not as hard today as it was a few years ago, but it is still an issue to be dealt with when one is working with an uninformed or unassertive family.

Whatever the situation regarding the birth and the opportunities for bonding with the neonate, the clinician should be aware that the degree of positiveness women feel for their infants during their first meeting has been shown to be associated with the amount of antepartum childbirth preparation.[10] This may be because the mothers were motivated persons who sought out prenatal education or because they learned about infant capabilities; in any case, this information can assist the nurse-midwife in her assessment and management of the prepared family and their neonate. Prepared families are shown to be more likely to demand participation in their own care,[10] but the hospitalized woman and her family may not feel free to ask questions or expect flexibility in routines. It has been shown, however, that prepared couples who undergo unexpected cesarean section deliveries may lose the positive effects of preparation,[10,23] and these families will need special reinforcement or reeducation regarding parent–infant interaction.

The recognition of infant capabilities and the sharing of this information with parents should lead to enhanced human interaction. It certainly cannot be detrimental in any way, and the inclusion of a film or of an assessment demonstration regarding neonatal behaviors seems justified in the prenatal education curriculum.

Significance of Newborn Assessments

The knowledge that the newborn has the capacity to respond to sensory stimuli can cause parents to be more eager and uninhibited in interactions with their infants. Families who have been prepared prenatally to expect the possibility of a mutually satisfying relationship with their infant and/or who have had early contact with their newborns have been shown to demonstrate more close or affectionate behaviors later.[2,19,35,40] Both fathers and mothers from certain studies have engaged in closer physical contact with their infants on follow-ups to one year, and there is a tendency for breastfeeding to be successful over a longer period of time.[2,19,35,40] These results make health care professionals feel good about having taught families about newborn responsiveness and about having interested parents in taking advantage of bonding and communication opportunities. The practical implications of these studies also should be shared.

Parents should know that, of the six infant behavioral states—deep sleep, light sleep, drowsy, quiet alert, active alert, and crying—it is the quiet alert state in which the most effective parent–infant communication takes place. Communication is a two-way process, and the caregiver must know that pausing and allowing the infant time for looking, listening, and unihibited motor activity is essential. Parents should be taught that babies can be brought to the quiet alert state by talking to them, uprighting them so they can see a human face in the same axis, giving physical stimulation by massage, or allowing grasp, rooting or sucking reflexes to operate. They should know that a crying baby does not always need to be picked up or fed, but that self-consoling behaviors involving visual or auditory responses or sucking on tongue or fingers are as important to the infant in regaining control of herself or himself as the help the parent can give.

In addition to behavioral assessment, physical assessment of the newborn is important for various reasons. Apgar scores of the infant at both 1 and 5 minutes of age should be obtained. Low 5-minute Apgar scores (6 or under) place an infant at risk for increased mortality or later neurologic problems.[29] Infants with low Apgar scores will require more intensive nursery observation and care, and the clinician will need to provide parents with opportunities for bonding by direct contact and caretaking. The perinatal team should share information regarding the infant's condition and risk status with the family so that realistic care plans and expectations may be set. If an infant must be transferred to a perinatal center, it would be logical to explore the possibility of also transferring the mother who may need to be hospitalized. (This has not been a customary practice, but there is no reason it should not become one if consumers and professionals decide to work assertively toward this end).

Apgar scoring is explained in most prenatal education programs, but the information may need to be retaught or reinforced for the family under unexpected stress with a sick infant. Every family should be aware of Apgar scoring and provided with the scores assigned to their infant. The Apgar scores need to become part of the family's personal health records, not data simply left to the hospital record room or the Bureau of Vital Statistics. Careful explanation of the scoring system and the possible later use of Apgar scores in pediatric follow-up is important.

Gestational age assessment has become routine in many clinical practice settings. The risks associated with small for gestational age (SGA) and large for gestational age (LGA) infants have justified this assessment procedure. Complete Dubowitz scoring using 10 neurologic criteria and 11 physical criteria sometimes is done, especially in facilities caring for high risk or sick infants. This extensive assessment may be difficult to carry out on a sick infant undergoing complicated therapy, however, and it requires skill to obtain reliable results. Most clinicians will use five or six of the Dubowitz physical criteria to confirm gestational age, especially when menstrual history is sketchy or unreliable or if uterine growth has been greater or lesser than expected. Another system, the Finnström method, has been developed for estimating gestational age by scoring only physical criteria, and one study has shown this method to be less invasive for distressed infants and equally as reliable as the more complicated and time-consuming Dubowitz method.[25]

The gestational scoring system and the reason for employing it must be shared with the family. This is also very important information to be made part of the family's health records, and the clinician needs to be sure that the family receives it.

Height, weight, and head circumference charts are included in most newborn clinical records or are easily obtained from infant product manufacturers who provide this information as a professional service. These are age-measurement grids with percentile curves superimposed. It is common not to see these filled out in the hospital until the record is completed for the medical records department, however, and valuable visual evidence for the clinician may be overlooked. Whether a baby is SGA, average for gestational age (AGA), or LGA, certain correlations between measurements can be used in estimating the prognosis for later infant growth and development. Of the three measurements—height, weight, and head circumference—head size is the most critical for judging the type of fetal compromise and the infant's potential for encountering later health problems.[29] An SGA infant whose weight, height, and head size are all below the 10th percentile has probably suffered intrauterine growth retardation from early on in pregnancy and is at greater risk than the SGA infant whose height and weight may be below the 10th percentile but whose head size is near the 50th percentile. The latter infant probably was compromised during the last part of pregnancy, and the brain development was largely spared. This infant is at much lower risk for subsequent health problems.

The nurse-midwife certainly will want to plan a different kind of follow-up or referral for the symmetrically small infant. Information should be shared with the family so that they respond seriously to the need for infant surveillance and the possible institution of special infant stimulation programs. Good communication and a relationship of trust between family members and the nurse-midwife is necessary to preserve an optimistic but purposeful attitude in the management of such an infant.

While studies regarding long-term follow-up of infants assessed as high risk during the intrapartum period are relatively few at this time, some results are particularly interesting. One small study of 12 children in which those with positive contraction stress tests (50 percent or more of the uterine contractions during a 10-minute period were associated with late heart rate decelerations) were followed for over 4½ years showed that no major neurologic abnormalities were detectable.[17] Three-fourths of these infants were delivered by cesarean section, and two-thirds of them were assessed SGA. The issue here is whether the surgical intervention was timely and saved them from further damage. If prenatal electronic monitoring is conducted on all antepartum patients, some percentage of intermittent or false-positive results will be obtained, and the tendency will be toward more obstetric intervention. Options for fetal monitoring are discussed in Chapter 4 and the intention here is to point out that infants who are frequently said to be at risk for death in utero have done well on developmental follow-up in one particular study.[17]

Another longitudinal developmental study involved over 500 children, most of whom were high risk either on the basis of birthweight or because their mothers were undergoing treatment for hypertension during pregnancy.[38] Fetal distress during labor, birth asphyxia, and emergency cesarean delivery were strongly associated with and occurred more often in the SGA and maternal hypertensive groups. These babies also had more problems in the neonatal period. However, there were no direct associations between any of the perinatal risk factors and later developmental scores, and the children generally were in good health. One child, moribund at birth due to a shoulder dystocia and delayed delivery, was achieving normally in all developmental areas while another infant whose delivery was uncomplicated and whose condition at birth was good had a stormy neonatal course and was grossly retarded at the age of one year.

Many more studies such as the foregoing are needed in order to establish convincing data bases upon which to make informed clinical judgments. Decisions must be made today, however, and it is a real challenge for the clinician to provide families with information which will be more helpful than confounding. Dealing with the quality of life of an entire future lifetime is very serious business, but it is the family who bears the ultimate responsibility and who will need to be involved in decision making regarding fetal monitoring and obstetric intervention. It is no exact or predictable science, and the decisions can be agnoizing, but they should be shared.

INFORMATIONAL NEEDS OF FAMILIES

Families are increasingly seeking out and are being bombarded with information regarding certain issues involved in childbearing and childrearing. Some issues such as location for birthing and infant feeding have been very popular while others such as personal hygiene and home environment have not received much attention. One must read and analyze a great deal in order to weed through the prevalent biases about the popular issues, but it is important for the clinician to be able to present "both sides of the coin" to families who are involved in decision making. It is essential for the nurse-midwife to recognize and admit her own biases here, and it is only fair to develop an attitude of respect for others with varying views.

Feeding

Breast-feeding

Much of the consumer-oriented literature has "why you should breast-feed" titles. This is in response to the heavy marketing of infant formulas and the formula company pamphlets with the "just in case you don't breast-feed" titles. For years the formula sample discharge packs with their tips for successful bottle feeding have been handed out to families, breast-feeding or not, as they leave the hospital. Physicians have not seemed to care very much, and only a handful of nurses have felt assertive enough to scrutinize the materials and proclaim them as nonsupportive to many new families regarding their infant feeding intentions. The formula companies have earned themselves a poor reputation with some professional and consumer groups by merchandizing in underdeveloped nations and to low-income women. The wave of resultant breast-feeding literature is extremely positive, and evidence of benefits to the mother and baby are certainly documented and convincing.[9,11,21,30]

Women who look for information about breast-feeding are likely to get the "hard sell" from many sources. It is a good idea for the nurse-midwife to ask the woman who needs to make a decision what she understands from the information she has heard or read so that any misunderstandings can be clarified. The woman should then be asked how she feels about what she knows. From her responses, it can be determined if she feels pressure from any source to feed her infant in a manner to which she cannot be totally committed. One analysis of the current literature about breast-feeding concludes that it includes some unrealistic and romanticized information which is not fitting and natural for all women but which allows little room for alternative action without guilt.[7,8] Some prevalent generalizations about good mothering, a part of which is supposed to be breast-feeding, may not permit a woman to work through an objective evaluation of herself and her situation, and there may be danger in this.

The main area of conflict in the breast-feeding controversy appears to be between the pro-baby and the pro-mother factions. When there are two primary subjects involved (some fathers will certainly see this as a three-way proposition), there are two persons' needs to be considered, and the tendency is for one side not to want to sacrifice expected gains to the other. One prominent pediatrician only accepts babies into his practice if their mothers are breast-feeding. He considers the infant the primary and most affected partner in the feeding process and has stated that it is worth social and psychological inconvenience to the mother to give the odds for a healthier lifetime to the infant. He is fair in identifying his strong biases, and anyone who does not want to follow the rules need not play his game. It would be sensible for any professional who simply cannot work under certain conditions to admit this, but it is also appropriate to respect other points of view and to have information on alternative resources available.

Major issues that will need to be considered by the breast-feeding family involve the posibility of neonatal jaundice, contraception decisions, management of physical or social inconveniences, and the introduction of other foods. A great deal of information on these subjects can be found in both lay and professional literature, and some families will be able to verbalize a plan of action for any or all of these without much professional guidance; others will need input so they can formulate those plans. Breast-feeding is not exactly free, and the family should know that the mother must consume 30 calories for every 20 calories she gives the infant in her milk.[6]

The fact that there is a documented "breastmilk jaundice" in about 2 percent of breast-fed infants has been recognized.[27] This appears to be an exaggerated form of so-called "physiologic jaundice of the newborn," and total serum bilirubin levels may reach as much as 25−30 mg percent between the age of 1−2 weeks of life. Of course, these infants become visibly jaundiced by the second or third day of life, and some mothers are likely to be pressured to interrupt or cease breastfeeding. Even if the condition is not one of the 2 percent which will become more severe, phototherapy and glucose water supplementation are often ordered by the pediatrician when total serum bilirubin levels reach 10−12 mg percent. Sepsis workups are even done in some settings after determining that the direct bilirubin level does not indicate biliary blockage or that red cell morphology does not reveal an abnormal hemolytic condition.

Some well-read and prepared women and their families are refusing medical intervention for newborn jaundice. They are finding sources of information which question the vigorous treatment for physiologic jaundice of the newborn, and they may have discovered that the 20 mg percent serum bilirubin level which is used as a decision line for exchange transfusion is a very conservative figure.[34] In addition, the long-range effects of phototherapy have long been questioned by consumer groups. The family can choose to refuse or accept medical intervention for jaundice, and it is the nurse-midwife's responsibility to provide the family with the necessary information. Breast-feeding and the associated jaundice is discussed by some prenatal educators. Women can also be referred to breast-feeding support groups who usually have the results of current studies.

When a breast-fed jaundiced infant's serum bilirubin level is being monitored and it reaches the 20 mg percent level, many clinicians will suggest a 48 hour cessation of nursing during which the baby's bilirubin level will almost always decline.[27] The mother may pump and discard her milk, and she needs to know that there is nothing "bad" in her milk which is going to damage the infant when she resumes nursing. Some women feel very strongly about avoiding the use of artificial nipples, and it may be possible to arrange for a friend or relative who is nursing a baby of her own to provide cross-nursing for this short period. This will not appeal to some women, but this practice apparently is increasing.[24]

The return of fertility in breast-feeding women is delayed, but variable. Up to 10 percent of lactating women in some studies have become pregnant before the resumption of menstrual periods when they were using no form of contraception.[20] There is no doubt that menstruation and ovulation return sooner in women who practice partial breast-feeding (supplementation of the infant with other milks or with solid foods) versus full breast-feeding (nursing on demand without supplementation of other foods).[18,37] Nevertheless, the critical time for continuous contraceptive protection is the time before the first menstrual period, as ovulation is unpredictable. The choice of a method can present problems, however.

The common practice has been to provide lactating women with barrier devices for postpartum contraceptive purposes. A usual plan prescribes vaginal foam and condoms until a diaphragm or cervical cap can be fitted at the later postpartum checkup. However, the nonoxynol-9 spermicidal ingredient used in most vaginal preparations has been shown in one animal study to appear in breast milk soon after application.[20] More documentation of this phenomenon will be necessary, and the effect on offspring must be investigated in order to know the danger of this substance.

The immediate postpartum woman does not have the signs of fertility she may have been used to monitoring before pregnancy—cervical mucus characteristics, basal body temperature changes, breast and abdominal signs—though it is a good idea to encourage her to resume checking these soon after delivery. Any hormonal contraceptive should be avoided because of the possible excretion into the breast milk and the unknown risk to the infant; breast milk volume also will be diminished with the use of female hormones. There is a high expulsion rate for intrauterine devices inserted in the immediate postpartum period, and indications are that increased risks of uterine perforation exist for as long as 8 weeks postpartum. (Currently, several intrauterine devices modified with biodegradable sutures attached to their upper arms are being tested;[20] the suture material is designed to impinge on the enlarged postpartum uterine walls and prevent displacement into the lower uterine segment from which the device may be expelled. This modified device may prove useful in the future for women, breast-feeding or not, who wish to avoid hormones and chemicals altogether.)

It appears that no temporary contraceptive method used in the lactating woman is without some risk. As at any other time, the choice must be based on informed consent and the risk-benefit ratio regarding subsequent pregnancy.

The woman who is breast-feeding for the first time may not really be prepared for the physical and social changes it will cause in her life. It is important to try to ensure that she has the support of someone who is lactating or who has breastfed in the past. Many common-sense suggestions about infant and self-care can come from such a contact.

A woman spends a great deal of time breast-feeding. Because breast milk is digested faster than cow's milk or formula, the breast-fed baby will want to eat about every 2 hours rather than at the 3–5 hour intervals of the bottle-fed baby. The woman who has had a hospital delivery and has been introduced to 4 hour nursery routines will not have been helped to anticipate the real infant feeding world which awaits her at home.

There is a diurnal fluctuation in milk production with early morning (6 A M.) volumes the greatest and dinnertime (6 P. M.) volumes the least.[6] Milk production also decreases as the mother tires from performing home and baby-care routines.[5] The baby is hungrier in the afternoon when less milk is available, and will want to nurse frequently then; this may be the time when the mother has planned to be most active with housework and evening meal preparation. These facts about milk production and activity should be explained to the lactating woman so that the idea of planning morning activities and preparing dinners in advance will make sense to her.

The use of any medication during lactation must be carefully considered because of the "shared" dose with the infant. There are certainly times when the mother's health and comfort, however, will warrant medication. She should be instructed to plan her medication schedule so that doses are taken at the beginning of a nursing period, resulting in the achievement of maximum drug levels at the end of a feeding when the breasts are empty.[6] In this way, there is less milk for the drug to pass into and milk is produced as the mother's drug level is falling.

Part of the treatment for breast infections has been cessation of nursing to protect the baby from illness. Now it is recognized that the causative organism most often comes from the infant's nasal or oral flora (probably picked up from hospital staff since it is foreign to the bacteriologically compatable family) and that the mother may continue to nurse. Although antibacterial proteins build up in the ductal system after nursing ceases entirely, the worst time to wean is during a breast infection. Antibacterial substance requires a 2–3 day period to build up significantly, and the infection may worsen as the static milk in the ducts provides a good culture medium during that time.

Vitamin and mineral supplementation of breast-fed infants has been under discussion for some time. Breast milk has been said to be deficient in vitamin D and in iron, but more recent research findings are changing opinions regarding this.

Vitamin D, a fat-soluble substance, has been found in a sulfated, more water-soluble form in breast milk.[30] The question is whether this form has adequate antirachitic properties, and some have claimed that rickets is more prevalent in breast-fed babies.[15] The American Public Health Association (APHA) currently recommends a 400 IU vitamin D daily supplement to breast-fed babies who are not exposed to sunlight or who are not "growing very rapidly."[3] Parents should be made aware of the natural vitamin D source from sunlight, especially if they prefer to minimize the use of artificial dietary supplements.

Iron is present in human milk in relatively low levels, but it has been shown to be in a highly utilizable form. Furthermore, the vitamin C level in breast milk is high, and this enhances iron absorption from the infant's gut. Studies have shown that the incidence of iron deficiency anemia is no higher in totally breast-fed babies than in infants fed iron-fortified formula.[30] Solid foods may interfere with iron absorption, and the APHA recommends supplementary iron drops or iron-fortified baby cereal to begin at the time other foods are introduced into the infant's diet.[3]

It has been confirmed that breast milk is an adequate total food for the first 6 months of human life. The APHA recommends that solid foods be introduced not before the fourth month but by the end of the sixth month of life.[3] Typically, the first food introduced is cereal, and this can be iron fortified as mentioned earlier. The parents should take care to introduce foods one at a time so that the infant's reactions and tolerance can be observed closely. If there are allergies in the family, it would be wise to suggest the keeping of a food diary so that episodes of skin eruption or nasal stuffiness can be investigated with regard to a food allergy cause. Lastly, if home-prepared instead of commercially-prepared infant foods are used, parents need to know that portions can be reduced as these tend to be higher in calories (except for fruit or juices prepared without sugar).[3]

Bottle Feeding

The family who decides that bottle feeding is best for them needs support and advice, but this is often left up to the formula can labels and the mother's intuition. Important topics for teaching and discussion include the choice of a formula, preparation techniques, and feeding suggestions.

Commercial formulas are closer in composition to human milk than is cow's milk and are more digestible for the newborn. Hence, the switch from evaporated cow's milk mixtures occurred, and a very large infant formula industry developed during the years that breast-feeding was on the decline in this country.

If families have adequate financial resources and can pay for the convenience of having ready-made, sterile, bottled, nippled feeding units to use, this is fine. They do need to know that the same commercial formula may be available in powdered form and that a lot of money can be saved if they have time to prepare their own bottles. Careful instructions must be given so that proper dilutions are used and cleanliness is ensured in preparing and storing the formula. The biggest danger in using commercially-prepared bottles is that the caregiver feels obligated to feed the whole amount (4 or 8 oz) or to save the leftovers for a later feeding; the amounts put into home prepared bottles can be varied according to the infant's needs for calories and fluids and parents can be taught to calculate this according to the baby's weight. Overfeeding of bottle-fed infants is thought to be related to obesity in later life, and this potential problem should be pointed out to parents.[29]

Feeding time for the bottle-fed baby should be one of physical closeness and interaction with another human being. Parents should be reminded of this and of the importance of taking the opportunity during feeding to communicate and to enhance to parent−child relationship.

The danger for development of dental caries in bottle-fed babies is greater than in breast-fed infants,[3] especially if the bottle is propped or left in bed with the baby and there is an opportunity for continuous drinking with milk laying in the mouth. Before the teeth erupt, the parents should be taught to start oral hygiene by giving the baby a drink of water after a feeding to clear the milk and to give drinks of water at bedtime to avoid oral milk stasis.

Hygiene

Recommendations for immediate newborn skin care have recently departed from long-standing practices. The most persistent idea from the early part of this century was that the vernix caseosa should be removed fairly soon after birth. It was recognized that the infant was susceptible to chilling during bathing, and a warm oil bath generally was used to remove the vernix and to prevent subsequent evaporation from the skin. By the 1960s, newborn thermo-regulation was better understood. Radiant heat sources and incubators had been developed for providing warmth and stable newborn environments, so soap-and-water bathing became the trend. At that time the use of hexachlora-phene for infant bathing became widespread, but demonstration of the presence of this chemical in human and animal bloodstreams caused the Federal Food and Drug Administration to warn against its continued use in 1971.[29]

The American Academy of Pediatrics recommended procedures for new-born "dry" skin care in 1975.[29] After temperature stabilization the gentle removal of blood and meconium with cotton and sterile water is advised. Then only water and possibly a gentle soap with rinsing need to be used to cleanse the infant at diaper changes or for other reasons of soiling. There is no mention of head-to-toes routine sponge or tub bathing.

Sponge baths at home routinely have been advised until the infant's umbilical cord has fallen off and the underlying tissue is healed.[29,39] Mothers hospitalized for delivery generally receive baby bathing instructions in the immediate postpartum period, and an actual tub bath may be demonstrated using a doll or an older infant whose umbilicus is healed. Often a sponge bath is demonstrated and the tub bath may or may not be discussed. Parents therefore can be left with little information which will make them feel competent in later infant care. There is no one standard or recommended procedure for cord care at this time, and iodine, alcohol, and triple dye are all being used in newborn nurseries and in parent instruction; no studies have shown one method to be significantly better than the others.

Recognition of the unhealed umbilicus as a potential entry point for infection has provided the rationale for special cord care and bathing of the neonate. No data can be found at this time regarding any increase in skin or umbilical infections in infants who have undergone LeBoyer baths at delivery. On the basis of this lack of data one obstetrical nursing staff known to the author has set up a tub bathing protocol for normal newborns. This procedure is thought to be more valuable not only as a teaching tool for parents, but as a practical means for learning to handle and to communicate with their new infant. In this particular obstetrical unit where sibling visitation is allowed, older sisters and brothers may also receive instruction and supervision regarding infant care. The practical and psychological benefits of such a program may be great, but its permanent establishment will depend on formal studies which can be replicated. This is an excellent area for nursing research in that it has implications for much future work.

Diapers

Diapering is a subject which has not received much attention from clinicians. Marketing professionals, on the other hand, have been very interested in the diapering practices of American parents. Many social and economic forces have influenced the move from the laundry to the supermarket as a source of diapers, but only a few of the practical aspects of cloth versus paper diapers will be taken up here.

The nurse-midwife should be aware of the family's financial and home circumstances in order to provide helpful and appropriate guidance. Even parents who are able to afford disposable diapers can be encouraged to compare the cost of disposables to laundry service in locations where this is an option. Parents with a concern for the ecological problems created by nonbiodegradable plastics may become aware of an alternative choice. Families who do not have washing facilities or hot water may have no choice but to use disposable diapers even though this cost can require tradeoffs in other essential areas such as food, clothing, or fuel.

Parents who choose to use disposable diapers need to know that they are very absorbant and efficient and that the tendency is to change them less often than cloth diapers. The plastic contains perspiration and excreta against the body in a more or less airtight condition and, with less frequent changing, skin breakdown can occur. The discomfort to the infant and the cost of skin creams and pediatrician visits could amount to more than the cost of more frequent diaper change. Parents should be advised that paper diapers which are saved over a long period of time will lose bacteriostatic properties,[26] and the infant may exhibit more diaper rash problems.

Plain petroleum jelly can be used to coat the infant's buttocks and perineal area and can be helpful in preventing skin irritation. Some find that corn starch also is good for this purpose. Parents can be told that it is unnecessary to buy special or medicated baby skin care products unless the home remedies are not satisfactory to them.

If the parents choose to use reusable cloth diapers, it is important that they know how to care for them properly. Cloth diapers should be sanitized (sterility is impossible to ensure at home and is probably unnecessary) with a very hot wash water and laundry bleach in quantities advised by the manufacturer. Cold-water detergents and cool or warm washing machine temperature settings should be avoided, and hot dryer settings are the best to use.

Circumcision

Circumcision of the newborn male has come under close scrutiny by both health care professionals and consumers in the past several years. Earlier strong arguments for circumcision claimed a lower incidence of carcinoma of the penis in the circumcised male and of cervical carcinoma in the female sexual partner. These arguments have been weakened as it has been shown that good penile hygiene is as effective a cancer deterrent as circumcision.[12] The incidence of true phimosis in the uncircumcised male to the point where urinary flow is obstructed is rare and may even be increased by the scarring which follows some circumcision procedures.[12] Many families elect to have male babies circumcised so that they will not "look" different from their fathers or brothers, but the risks associated with a surgical procedure which is done for a purely cosmetic reason may not be justifiable according to some medical practitioners.[38] Finally, the incidence of balanitis and venereal infections has not been shown to be higher in uncircumcised males if penile cleanliness is maintained.[12]

Circumcision is practiced for religious reasons by certain groups, and the nurse-midwife should be aware of the importance of this procedure to some parents; plans for circumcision in the event of the birth of a baby boy often will have been made before birth, and these generally should not interfere with hospital or birthing room procedures. Other families, however, may need to be provided with facts about circumcision so that they can make decisions based upon sound information. This should be done during the third trimester of pregnancy when the parents are developmentally ready to deal with the realities of parenting.

The American Academy of Pediatrics has recommended that circumcision should not be a routine newborn procedure,[12] and families should be so advised by the nurse-midwife. Information about research on the incidence of cancer and infection should be made available, and specifics about the care of the uncircumcised penis should be taught in order to increase awareness that an alternative choice is possible. Some nurse-midwives make a file of research and medical articles on circumcision available for loan to parents who want general information. In an information file, both sides of the discussion should be represented.

Hygienic care of the uncircumcised penis and teaching the youngster about later self-care have not always been accurately addressed in the past. A survey including 90 pediatricians and the mothers of 15 uncircumcised male infants revealed that retraction of the newborn foreskin was incorrectly advised in many cases.[32] Although the foreskin is retractable in only about 4 percent of newborns,[12] 7 of the above 15 mothers had been told to retract it and clean the penis daily whereas the remaining 8 had received no advice. Moreover, the majority of pediatricians surveyed in this study did not know at what age the foreskin should be expected to retract easily. Since 90 percent of males have foreskins which will retract readily by the age of 3 or 4 years,[12,32] parents of the uncircumcised newborn should be taught to wash the infant and periodically gently test foreskin retractability. Just as a youngster is later taught to bathe independently, he can be instructed to care for his penis as well as his ears and his fingernails.

Parents who choose to have their male infants circumcised find that this is often done in the hospital setting when the baby is 2 or 3 days old. Since this may coincide with the mother's day of discharge, careful teaching about care and complications must be done before the family is sent home. If the mother has delivered in a birthing room where early discharge (less than 24 hours postdelivery) is possible, the timing of circumcision needs to be considered. Disruption of bonding and/or the initial states of infant reactivity may occur if circumcision is performed on the first day of life, and it may be wise to schedule the procedure for a later time on an outpatient basis. For medical-legal reasons, it is not advisable for the nurse-midwife to obtain the parents' signatures on the surgical permit for circumcision unless she will perform the procedure; issues of informed consent may arise later, and it must be kept in mind that the incidence of circumcision-related complications may be as high as 2 percent with a mortality of about 2 per million procedures.[12]

ENVIRONMENT AND STIMULATION

Some instruction for parents regarding infant competencies, growth, and development has become available in childbirth education in the past few years, but formal courses for potential parents are still relatively few in number. Infant stimulation programs have usually been devised by psychologists and educators for babies at risk for developmental problems or delays, and pediatricians have not been overly active in referring parents to these groups.[14]

As information about infant capabilities becomes more widely disseminated, parents will need advice about providing environments for their infants which are appropriately interesting but not overstimulating. Parents who are aware of the differences in infant personalities and tolerances can learn to interact with their newborns in ways which delight both the child and parent. Parents should know that they can learn to be alert to the newborn's cues and the environment can be adjusted accordingly. Degrees of infant contentment, consolability, and cooperation can be used as signals to increase or decrease the amount of stimulation the infant is receiving.[16]

The newborn begins to learn early from her or his environment and needs a variety of experiences in order to develop according to potential. The infant prefers bright, colorful and contoured visual stimulation, lilting and soft auditory stimulation, and warm, gentle, and rhythmical tactile stimulation.[1] The sensory threshholds of infants vary widely, however, and these differences need to be respected in order to stimulate some infants but not overstimulate others.[16]

Infants with low sensory threshholds tend to be wakeful and appear to be ready for frequent play or diversion. The low–sensory-threshhold baby seems to naturally invite social interaction. However, these children need to be handled in a soft and gentle manner, and they must be shielded from excessive stimulation which will cause them to become tired and cranky. The caregiver should introduce environmental changes carefully and observe the infant for signals that the sensory threshhold has been reached; instead of "trying everything" to console the child who appears to be demanding attention, backtracking to less stimulating surroundings is appropriate.

On the other hand, infants with high sensory threshholds may sleep a lot or spend long periods in quiet states which do not invite social interaction. These babies may not be stimulated adequately and, in fact, may peacefully endure environments which are downright boring and uninstructive. Parents should be taught to gently introduce experiences which provide adequate stimulation; the baby simply may be moved about the house and spoken to even when she or he is not demanding attention.

The nurse-midwife should assess aspects of the infant's behavior and environment during an early postpartum contact with the parents. If there is no regular well-baby office or clinic visit, the baby should be brought in at the mother's regular postpartum appointment so that their interaction can be observed. It is essential to get a feeling for the fact that one may be dealing with an infant who is at either end of the sensory threshhold spectrum and to give some guidance if it is needed. Most infants, however, are of somewhat "average" sensory threshhold and are able to handle a variety of external experiences. Parents may be reassured that whatever activities and environments the baby appears to enjoy in good safety are good for her or him.

HEALTH SURVEILLANCE AND FOLLOW-UP

Before leaving the hospital or birthing center, parents should be encouraged to ask for summaries of clinical and laboratory assessments of the newborn, especially if there have been problems. It is a good idea to discuss a plan for compiling a file of such information for the purpose of maintaining a complete health record. In the case of a later medical or behavioral problem requiring systematic workup, the family may have moved or the record may not be available for a variety of reasons. Families under the care of private practitioners usually do not have too much difficulty in obtaining old medical records, but those who have used public clinical health services may not find their records very easily. Since dates and specific information are quickly and easily lost to simple recall, the importance of having recorded data to which one can refer cannot be overemphasized. Parents should be reminded to keep original records for their own files and to allow others only to make copies.

New parents frequently are confronted with unanticipated problems and responsibilities regarding newborn care once they are home and on their own.[28] Even second- or third-time parents are bound to find that aspects of infant care vary with each baby, and parents often require support in developing confidence and competence as caregivers.

Many nurse-midwifery services provide families with telephone numbers where they can reach a sympathetic ear during the early postpartum period. It is imperative to establish hours when telephone calls can be most conveniently taken by nurse-midwives in private or on-call practice settings. In large clinical services, however, where nurse-midwives are on duty 24 hours a day, constant availability of a resource person can be reassuring to parents as many anxieties about infant care and behavior loom large during the wee hours of the morning.[28] Routine postpartum telephone calls to the family can help to decrease anxiety and elicit questions before a situation becomes problematic.

The nurse-midwife should ask the parents about plans for infant health surveillance. If the newborn has had problems, arrangements for follow-up of some sort should have been made. Even so, there are cases in which parents may question the nature of a treatment regimen, and they should be encouraged to seek a second opinion from an appropriate source.

The parents of normal newborns should be informed about alternative sources for well-baby care. Some individuals will prefer to use private physicians, but all families should be aware of the fact that tax-supported health centers or nurse-practitioner run clinics are available in some locations. These may be good sources not only of free or low-cost baby shots but also of practical information about infant care, growth, and development. Encouraging new parents to develop a focus toward health maintenance and problem prevention rather than one of crisis intervention regarding pediatric illnesses is an important issue to be addressed by the nurse-midwife.

Available Resources

Many resource and support groups, both lay and professional, are available for families of infants with specific medical or genetic problems. These groups tend to be concentrated in urban areas, however, and they may be available only by letter or telephone to some families with limited finances or time for travel. In addition, many consumer support groups are not especially oriented toward the needs of minority cultural or lower socioeconomic groups, and satisfactory, supportive relationships will be difficult to achieve under such circumstances.

Support groups that assist families in adapting to "normal" circumstances such as breastfeeding, postpartum adjustment or multiple births, are also generally not geared for minorities. Middle-class families in urban or suburban areas will have little trouble finding resources for information and group sharing to which they can relate, but minority populations currently need help in finding or forming such groups. Nurse-midwives practicing in settings which serve minority or lower socioeconomic families should look for mechanisms to facilitate the organization of family group activities and support. Nurse-midwives who are in administrative positions or who are seeking funding through grant proposals should seriously consider including personnel, equipment, and space to meet the needs for information and group support.

REFERENCES

1. Affonso D: The newborn's potential for interaction. JOGN Nurs 5:9−14, 1976
2. Ali Z, Lowry M: Early maternal−child contact: effects on later behaviour. Dev Med Child Neurol 23:337−345, 1981
3. American Public Health Association Policy Statements: Infant feeding in the United States. Am J Public Health 71:207−211, 1981
4. Anderson CJ: Enhancing reciprocity between mother and neonate. Nurs Res 30:89−93, 1981
5. Bachrach S, Fisher J, Parks JS: An outbreak of vitamin D deficiency rickets in a susceptible population. Pediatrics 64:871−877, 1979
6. Bertino JS: The pharmacology of human milk. Birth Fam J 8:237−243, 1981
7. Blachman L: Dancing in the dark I. Romanticized motherhood and the breastfeeding venture. Birth Fam J 8:271−279, 1981
8. Blachman L: Dancing in the dark II. Helping and not-so-helping hands. Birth Fam J 8:180−286, 1981
9. Blackwell AG, Salisbury L: Administrative petition to relieve the health hazards of promotion of infant formulas in th U.S. Birth Fam J 8:287−296, 1981
10. Blehar MC: Preparation for childbirth and parenting, in Science Monographs, Families Today, Vol 1. Dept of HEW, Division of Scientific and Public Information, Washington, DC, US Government Printing Office, 1981, pp 143−170
11. Bloom M: The romance and power of breastfeeding. Birth Fam J 8:259−269, 1981
12. Boyer DB: Routine circumcision of the newborn: reasonable precaution or unnecessary risk? J Nurs Midwif 25(6):27−31, 1980
13. Brazelton TB: Neonatal Behavioral Assessment Scale. Philadelphia, JB Lippincott Co, 1973
14. Browder JA: The pediatrician's orientation to infant stimulation programs. Pediatrics 67:42−44, 1981
15. Cerutti ER: The management of breastfeeding. Birth Fam J 8:251−256, 1981

16. Clark AL, Affonso DD: Infant behavior and material attachment: two sides to the coin. Am J Mat Child Nurs 1:94−99, 1976

17. Crane J, Anderson B, Marshall R, et al: Subsequent physical and mental development in infants with positive contraction stress tests. J Reprod Med 26:113−118, 1981

18. Cronin TJ: Influence of lactation upon ovulation. Lancet 2:422−424, 1968

19. deChateau P: The first hour after delivery—its impact on synchrony of the parent−infant relationship. Pediatrician 9:151−168, 1980

20. Edelman DA, Goldsmith A, Shelton JD: Postpartum contraception. Int J Gynaecol Obstet 19:305−311, 1981

21. Hartmann PE, Kulski JK, Rattigan S et al: Breastfeeding and reproduction in women in western Austrialia—a review. Birth Fam J 8:215−226, 1981

22. Jones C: Father to infant attachment: effects of early contact and characteristics of the infant. Res Nurs Health 4:193−200, 1981

23. Kestermann G: Assessment of individual differences among healthy newborns on the Brazelton scale. Early Hum Dev 5:15−27, 1981

24. Krantz JZ, Kupper NS: Cross-nursing: wet nursing in a contemporary context. Pediatrics 67:715−717, 1981

25. Latis GO, Simionato L, Ferraris G: Clinical assessment of gestational age in the newborn infant, comparison of two methods. Early Hum Dev 5:29−37, 1981

26. Livesay RP: Principles in good diapering for parent education. JOGN Nurs 5:25−27, 1976

27. Maisels MJ: Breastfeeding and jaundice. Birth Fam J 8:245−249, 1981

28. Mercer RT: The nurse and maternal tasks of early postpartum. Am J Mat Child Nurs 6:341−234, 1981

29. Moore ML, Davis OS: Realities in Childbearing. New York, WB Saunders, 1978

30. Pittard WB: Special properties of human milk. Birth Fam J 8:229−235, 1981

31. Pridham KF: Infant feeding and anticipatory care: supporting the adaptation of parents and their new babies. Mat Child Nurs J 10:111−126, 1981

32. Osborn LM, Metcalf TJ, Mariani EM: Hygienic care in uncircumcised infants. Pediatrics 67:365−367, 1981

33. Ounsted M, Scott A, Moar V: Delivery and development: to what extent can one associate cause and effect? J Soc Med 73:786−792, 1980

34. Ramer CM: Letter to the editor. Birth Fam J 8:37−38, 1981

35. Rodholm M: Effects of father−infant postpartum contact on their interaction 3 months after birth. Early Hum Dev 5:79−85, 1981

36. Saigal S, Nelson NM, Bennett KJ, et al: Observations on the behavioral state of newborn infants during the first hour of life. Am J Obstet Gynecol 139:715−719, 1981

37. Salber EJ, Feinlaub M, McMahon B: The duration of postpartum amenorrhea. Am J Epidemiol 82:347−358, 1965

38. Scanlon JW: Routine neonatal procedures: risk/benefit calculations and informed consent. Birth Fam J 7:218−224, 1980

39. US Department of Health, Education and Welfare: Infant care (DHEW Publication No 78-30015). Washington, DC, US Government Printing Office, 1978

40. Widmayer SM, Field TM: Effects of Brazelton demonstrations on the development of preterm infants. Pediatrics 67:711−714, 1981

Virginia Michels

7

Conception Planning and Gynecologic Health Care

For more than 50 years certified nurse-midwives have successfully provided maternity care. Family planning services, however, were not instituted until the 1950s. Nurse-midwives originally began offering family planning care in eastern Kentucky where they were stimulated by the region's poor physician–population ratio of 20:100,000, as compared to the national ratio of 150:100,000.[4] Since the area attracted few physicians because of its depressed economy and its isolation, certified nurse-midwives offered desperately needed care by providing health assessment, education, counseling, and follow-up.

Nurse-midwives were among the first nonphysician primary care providers to participate in federally funded maternity and infant care projects and family planning services.[58] Organized family planning service programs increased in number from 863,000 in 1968 to 4,083,000 in 1976.[53] Because of this rapid growth in services and a corresponding inability to provide sufficient physician staffing, nurse practitioners were utilized with very positive results.

Several researchers recently reported on the substantial contributions made by nurse practitioners who provide family planning services.[6,54,86] These researchers described the positive outcomes in terms of patient satisfaction, new and varied services, nurturant and efficient care, increased patient volume, and more appropriate use of physician time.[6,54,86] With the expanding role of nurse practitioners, it is likely that nurse-midwives will be called on to provide a significant and increasing portion of primary care, not only in family planning clinics but also in private practice.

241

Common management issues that the nurse-midwife confronts when assisting a patient in the selection of a satisfactory contraceptive method include not only the patient's age but also her ethnic and religious background. Nurse-midwives must also address the informational needs of women as they self-monitor their health status, identify their own problems early, and utilize health care information resources. Some of these issues touch on sensitive areas, and it is important for the nurse-midwife not only to be well informed about different contraceptive methods or the techniques of gynecologic examination but also comfortable talking about other factors that affect a woman's choices.

FACTORS INFLUENCING OPTIONS FOR CONCEPTION PLANNING

Religion

Religion is an important variable that greatly influences sexual behavior and contraceptive practices. The Judeo-Christian heritage of combined religious and legal authority continues to affect human sexuality in Western society.

In Judaic teachings the sexual drive is considered a divine gift to be utilized within controlled boundaries, that is, within marriage. The instincts of the libido should thus focus on establishing a family.[68,91]

The Protestant and Roman Catholic churches struggle with this same issue of sexual ethics. A culture, society, or religion that supports the concept of procreative sex frowns on contraceptive activity employed for the improved enjoyment of intercourse. In this context birth control is taboo because of its disruptive effects on child production and rearing, and until the 1950s the use of contraceptives was forbidden by most Prostestant denominations. Generally, Protestantism today focuses on the value of human relationships as its sexual ethic,[95] and currently contraceptive practices are permitted by most Judeo-Christian religions, with the exception of the Roman Catholic church. In the Catholic church ecclesiastical law demands chastity of unmarried women and, as do most religious groups, sexual fidelity after marriage. Many Roman Catholics, while attempting to maintain the biblical concept of man, are ambivalent about attempting to personalize the ethics of sexuality.[84] The essential Roman Catholic argument against the use of contraceptives is based on the belief that any unnatural act is sinful. Since the natural purpose of intercourse is procreation, contraceptives interfere with this natural purpose.

In the 1968 encyclical Pope Paul VI reconfirmed the church's stand against the use of contraceptives to avoid not only unwanted pregnancy but also other deleterious effects of promiscuous sexual activity.[47] This stand supports a presumed inhibitory force of fear of pregnancy, particularly among the young, as the primary inhibitor of premarital or extramarital sexual relations.

While the Catholic church has made few exceptions to the prohibition of contraceptives in recent years, the popes have been careful to rationalize contraceptive use in terms of the concept of natural law. Women suffering from particular health problems such as dysmenorrhea or endometriosis, for example, may take oral contraceptives as a curative method. This practice is accepted even though inhibition of ovulation is the side effect, since the belief is that it is lawful to correct defects of nature.

The rhythm methods of birth control do not interfere with any natural processes, and rhythm methods are therefore the only approaches to contraception, in the true sense of the word, that the Roman Catholic church accepts. The rhythm methods are controversial, though, and recent findings indicate poor results. Failure rates with the use of the calendar method range from 14.4−47/100 woman years, largely because menstrual cycles tend to be more variable than the theoretical model.[69] The temperature method also offers women a similar lack of reassurance because it tends to be inaccurate and difficult to interpret even when the measurements are correct.[50] Although the basal temperature chart will indicate ovulation in most women, it does not do so in approximately 20 percent of all ovulatory cycles.[57]

In counseling and instructing the woman who intends to use the rhythm methods, the nurse-midwife must direct her in considering pre- and postovulatory phase intercourse. Apparently when intercourse occurs both before and after ovulation, the failure rates of these methods are approximately 10−20/100 woman years. Yet when intercourse is restricted to the postovulatory phase only, the failure rate drops to 0.3−6.6/100 woman years.[69]

In view of these statistics, and despite the ban on contraceptive devices and techniques by the Catholic church and a few fundamentalist Christian sects, contraceptives are still thought to have a positive value in marital and family relations. Marriage experts, as well as religious leaders from most denominations other than Roman Catholic, support this position.

The rhythm methods, also known as natural family planning, offer the nurse-midwifery patient not only a religiously acceptable method of contraception but also an opportunity to learn more about her body. Since many women seek this type of educational experience from nurse-midwives, a complete understanding of these methods by the nurse-midwife and a comfortable teaching approach are of paramount importance.

Ethnicity

The term *ethnicity* is used in sociology to describe both cultural and racial differences among people. The members of each ethnic group share the same heritage, subjective identification, and often the same language or dialect. In order to understand patients' needs more fully, nurse-midwives must consider their patients' ethnicity because ethnicity may play a significant role in the choice of a contraceptive method or whether contraception will be used at all.

Here in the United States several ethnic groups are quite visible and frequently utilize family planning clinics. Of these, the most prominent are the black and Hispanic populations, and our discussion will be limited to them since there are more data available on these two groups.

Hispanics

When an ethnic group is transplanted into a society where the norm for family size drastically differs from its own, the ethnic group is placed in a period of transition. The individual's inherited and shared beliefs, norms, and values are questioned and challenged; the woman's ethnic identity with respect to childbearing and family size differentiates her from the social mainstream. Nurse-midwives practicing in urban areas, where a large number of Latin American immigrants seek family planning services, need complete bilingual skills. If this is not possible, a working knowledge of Spanish and the local dialect would be acceptable in order to completely evaluate and treat these women.

For the woman of Latin American heritage, the social role of motherhood generally is mutually exclusive of other social roles. If her opportunity for childbearing is artificially limited, she may be forcing herself to minimize her only effective social role or activity.[2] Compared to all other ethnic minorities, the United States Census of 1950, 1960, and 1970, identified women of Spanish origin as having the highest fertility rate.[92]

Birth control methods are still not widely accepted in the Mexican-American community, perhaps because of a traditional orientation to family life and early religious influences.[2] Most of these women are Catholics, yet may not actively practice the faith. The religious orientation nevertheless still influences many of their contraceptive choices.

In this author's clinical experience, the Hispanic woman frequently rejects, or at least does not place importance on, the medical profession's definition of high-risk category of care, and this may be a factor in her motivation to successfully use birth control. For example, a grand multipara may not understand that she has been referred to the sterilization clinic because she is at risk for complications in future pregnancies. Temporary contraception may be an option for such a woman as well as for the Hispanic woman who feels that her family is complete.

Sterilization of the woman may be more readily accepted rather than a prolonged interruption of fertility by oral contraceptives. With sterilization she has a one-time decision to make, and therefore has a one-time confrontation with religious and moral conflicts.

The Hispanic woman generally does not make a choice of this nature without her spouse or significant other. Often the decision is made solely by the mate. Working knowledge of the language will aid the nurse-midwife in explaining, discussing, and eliciting informed consent, or in supporting the patient's decision not to elect the method suggested by the medical community.

A Chicano is an American of Mexican and southwest-Hispanic descent. The results of a study in 1973 of 1129 Chicanos from Los Angeles between the ages of 15–44 years who were married to Chicanos prove to contradict the popular stereotype about Chicano family planning. The findings suggest that, when considering determinants of fertility planning success, ethnicity and type of health-care facility for the last pregnancy are more important variables than age, age at pregnancy, socioeconomic status, and religiosity. The data presented also suggest that high fertility rates of Chicanos are due to the desire for larger family size rather than unsuccessful family planning.[71] Sabagh reports, in a review of recent studies, that contraceptive practices among Chicano couples are modern. In 1973 the pill, intrauterine device (IUD), and condom accounted for 78 percent of the contraceptive methods used by Chicanos.[71]

The Chicano population must not be confused with women who were born and raised in Mexico and then moved to the United States, as these two populations differ in several respects. For example, in their choice and use of birth control, women reared in Mexico appear to be more affected than Chicanos by religious influences. Most Mexican immigrants are more likely to live in poorer circumstances than the Chicano couples who are at least first or second generation Americans. The ghettoization of a neighborhood, with its economic and social deprivations, may hamper successful family planning.

The following are recommendations for nurse-midwifery family planning counseling for Hispanic women:

1. Bilingual nurse-midwives should serve non-English-speaking Hispanic women.
2. Qualified Hispanics should be recruited for nurse-midwifery education programs.
3. Nurse-midwives should be aware of cultural variations existing in these populations.
4. Small community clinics, rather than impersonal, large institutions, should be fostered and promoted. Small clinics provide easy access and have been shown to increase family planning success rates.[71]
5. Bilingual health education materials regarding birth control methods should be improved and available in greater quantity. The safety and long-term effects on fertility of each method should be addressed.
6. The use of female nurse-midwives should be considered when dealing with health assessment and provision of services to Hispanic women. This may promote patient comfort and avoid the collection of incomplete or inaccurate information.
7. Good interpersonal communication skills should be developed since, in this author's experience, Hispanics prefer a personal, conversational rapport with their care provider.

8. The women's value system and the significance of fertility in that system should be considered when counseling.
9. The mate should always be afforded the opportunity to participate in this visit and decision making, to the degree the woman wishes his participation.

Blacks

As is true for any ethnic group, ethnically acceptable health care providers may be more sensitive to the specific needs of the black patient. The nurse-midwife who is skilled in establishing a working and productive rapport with this patient and her significant others may learn more about the patient's family relationships and the pressures on the woman to conceive or not to conceive.

In the clinical experience of this author, the black female's selection of a contraceptive is influenced not only by her boyfriend or husband but also by her mother. Particularly with the lower socioeconomic group, the sexually active single female usually lives with her mother or aunt. A disproportionate number of households headed by females in the United States are headed by black females.[12] In many African societies, the matrilocality, or residence with or near the mother, is a common cultural pattern.[12] To imply that this pattern is bad is to denigrate all but male-dominated or patriarchal family models.

The female elders in the Afro-American family relate their family planning experiences to the young and may suggest birth control methods. Including the matriarch, with the patient's permission, in the discussion or educational session often greatly reduces tension and misinformation. It will also offer more support for the patient's assisted selection of birth control and its proper use.

Black women appear more likely than black men to be influenced in their attitudes toward premarital sex by the affectionate or love-quality of the relationship.[13] Premarital sexual relations for black women are not stigmatized with as much of a double standard as they are for white women.[12] Social class, however, does influence attitudes and sexual practices among blacks as well as whites; middle class blacks function similarly to middle class whites in attitudes and sexual practices.[13]

Black sexuality, family size, structure, member roles, and relationships all have two historical factors that greatly influence fertility control—slavery and the heritage of African culture. These issues greatly affect today's black society and continue to be the focus of much debate.

After blacks were uprooted from their culture in Africa, many ethnic groups were deprived of their languages and customs and were transplanted into a vastly different society. Their new family life and sexual relationships resulted from forced white, Southern patterns and fragments of their lost culture. Furthermore, the effects of slavery additionally altered this culture. A stable family structure was forcibly deteriorated, and promiscuity was encouraged to increase the production of new slaves. Perhaps these circumstances promoted the concept of black women raising their families and shouldering the brunt of the family's burden.

Sensitivity to the cultural heritage and socioeconomic factors that influence the health care needs of black women may improve the quality of nurse-midwifery care of these patients. The results of increased awareness of the ethnic patient's needs may be fewer missed appointments, improved communication between the caregiver and the patient, increased patient motivation for using contraceptive methods correctly, and positive role modeling.

Nutrition

The nurse-midwife is well aware of the importance of good nutrition during the prenatal period. Good nutrition is one significant factor which increases the woman's chances of an improved pregnancy outcome. The outcome of each pregnancy is also dependent on the eating habits and nutritional status of each woman before conception. Problems are reduced if the woman and her nurse-midwife are able to begin her pregnancy without having to correct nutritional inadequacies.

Approaching each patient as an individual, we see that the age at first pregnancy, the duration of interconceptional periods, and life circumstances each present unique influences on a woman's nutritional status. The nurse-midwife must aid patients during and after the childbearing years to recognize the importance of good nutrition not only to enhance the quality of human reproduction but to prevent health problems and thus improve the quality of life.

Planning family size, timing each pregnancy, or avoiding pregnancy are major concerns of sexually active women of childbearing age. Two popular and highly effective contraception methods used today, the pill and IUD, affect nutritional status. Consequently, some nutritional problems of women are directly related to the use of these two contraceptives.

Oral Contraceptives

It is believed that numerous alterations occur in the metabolism of nutrients when oral contraceptives are ingested routinely.[67,104] (see Table 7-1). The significance and long-term effects of these changes are not completely understood. Thus, no absolute guidelines for nutritional supplementation have been outlined. However, the nurse-midwife may choose to use this information when providing nutritional counseling as a part of the health maintenance regimen. Table 7-1 lists the observed effects of oral contraceptives on nutrients and the suggested food sources.

Intrauterine Device

Among family planning health care providers it is commonly known that the IUD may cause increased blood loss during or between menstrual periods. Other than the potentially increased need for iron caused by iron

Table 7-1
The Effects of Oral Contraceptives on Nutritional Status

Nutrient	Need	Observed Changes Induced By Oral Contraceptives	Suggested Dietary Sources
Lipids	Decreased	Increase in plasma triglycerides No consistent changes in plasma cholesterol concentrations	Avocado, animal fats, cakes, cookies, lunch meats, dairy products
Proteins	Increased	Increase in plasma alpha and beta globulins and fibrinogen Increase in conversion of tryptophan to nicotinic acid Decrease in plasma albumin	Animal protein foods, legumes, nuts
Carbohydrates	Unchanged	Increase in blood glucose and insulin levels — small	Fruits, enriched breads and cereals
Minerals	Increased	Decrease in circulating levels of calcium, phosphorous, magnesium and zinc	Yellow cheeses, Wheat germ
	Decreased	Increase in serum iron and iron binding capacity with diminution of menstrual blood loss	Beef, pork, lamb, liver, kidney, peanut butter
	Decreased	Increase in serum copper and ceruloplasmin and no changes in urinary copper excretion	Nuts
Vitamin A	Decreased	Increase in circulating levels of vitamin A	Carrots, sweet potatoes, spinach, turnips, liver

248

Vitamin			
Vitamin B₆	Increased	Increase in metabolism of amino acid, tryptophan; vitamin B₆ required cofactor for several enzymatic reactions in metabolic pathway for tryptophan	Liver, meats, cabbage, banana, eggs, corn, whole wheat, fish, rolled oats, broccoli, brussels sprouts, sweet potatoes
Vitamin B₁₂	Increased	Decrease in serum concentration of B₁₂ possibly due to an increase in tissue affinity for B₁₂	All animal proteins
Riboflavin B₆	Increased	Possible interference with metabolism of riboflavin	Milk, cheese, eggs, meats, dark green leafy vegetables, lettuce, green peas, whole wheat, oats, rice
Vitamin C	Increased	Possible increase in rate of Vitamin C destruction	Oranges, grapefruit, tomatoes, raw cabbage, dark green leafy vegetables, strawberries, green pepper
Foliacin (folate, folic acid)	Increased	Possible increase in plasma clearance and urinary excretion of folate	Dark green leafy vegetables, lettuce, lima beans, liver, cauliflower, meats, eggs, nuts

Adapted from tables constructed by Kerwin DR: Nutritional concerns for women in Kerwin DR: Maternal Infant and Child Nutrition. North Carolina, Health Sciences Consortium, 1981 pp 1–38 and by Worthington B: Nutrition during pregnancy, lactation and oral contraception. Nurs Clin N Am 14:281, 1979.

loss with increased bleeding, the IUD has little effect on the nutritional status of the woman. Iron supplementation should be suggested only for those women who demonstrate evidence of anemia (hemoglobin less than 12g or hematocrit less than 37%), a drop in the hemoglobin or hematocrit, or a marked increase in menstrual blood flow (double the loss before insertion of the IUD).[48] This dietary supplement should be in the form of iron salts such as ferrous sulfate or foods rich in iron and vitamin C. Vitamin C along with iron is encouraged because it promotes the absorption of iron in the small intestine.

Prior to selecting an IUD, the nurse-midwife should consider several points in safeguarding the nutritional status of the woman. First, the nurse-midwife should assess the woman's menstrual history, determining the absence of anemia and blood dyscrasias. Second, the practitioner should evaluate the patient's ability to understand danger signs and reliability in seeking professional assistance when indicated. Additional considerations are the accessibility of care to ensure yearly evaluations of menstrual changes, screening for anemia, and dietary counseling. The woman with a hemoblobin below 10 gm, a history of menorrhagia, metrorrhagia, or blood dyscrasias is not a candidate for the IUD because of the potential for developing anemia secondary to increased or excessive blood loss or the potential for the aggravation of pathologic bleeding disorders.[98]

Recent studies have demonstrated the need for a more in-depth evaluation of the nutritional education and counseling component of family planning services.[79] The nurse-midwife, understanding the importance of nutritional counseling during the interconceptional period, may wish to utilize the team approach by enlisting the services of a nutritionist in her patient's care. This is not generally necessary in normal cases. When working in a clinic setting with a full complement of health team members, it is expected that nutritional needs are discussed. If this is not the case, or if the effects of contraception on nutritional status as well as general nutrition and weight control are not discussed directly, then the system should be evaluated further. Perhaps the nurse-midwife may offer to participate on a committee to explore the correction of potential stumbling blocks such as time limitations, personnel shortages, heavy client loads, funding, burnout, poor theoretical knowledge base, or lack of effective counseling skills.

Age Influences

Adolescence

By 1975 it was estimated that 11 million adolescents in the United States were sexually active. This increased teenage fertility led to 600,000 births.[70] In 1976 an estimated 400,000 legal abortions were performed on adolescents.[34] Today, one in five new mothers is an adolescent.[27] (See Chapter 1 for additional statistics.) Parents, health professionals, and governmental agencies have made considerable efforts to define the causes and arrest the problem of adolescent pregnancy.

Adolescent pregnancy is a national health problem. Nurse-midwives frequently deal with the physical, mental, educational, and social problems of the pregnant adolescent. Studies show a significant relationship between maternal age and complications of pregnancy. For mothers 15 years old and younger, infant mortality is much higher than for older adolescents. The causes most frequently cited are poor nutrition, inadequate prenatal care, and incomplete biologic maturation. These etiologic factors may lead to the major complications of anemia, toxemia, premature birth, and cesarean delivery. By failing to successfully complete their education, these women may experience lives of poverty, dependence on others, failure to establish stable family lives, and possibly repeated high-risk pregnancies.

Adolescents of both sexes are reported to begin using contraceptives approximately one year after initiation of sexual activity.[24,74,108] Because of this critical delay, one-half of all initial adolescent pregnancies occur in the first 6 months of sexual activity.[105]

The nurse-midwife is responsible for counseling adolescents about sexuality and for prescribing birth control methods when indicated. Consequently, the nurse-midwife's role as a primary care provider is critical in assisting young people to make decisions that affect not only their physical well-being but also possibly their entire lives.

Factors to consider when assisting a young woman in selecting the most appropriate contraceptive method include safety, effectiveness, benefits, medical desirability, risks, convenience, cost, personal feelings, acceptability to the sex partner, reversibility, alternatives, protection of future fertility, protection from sexually transmitted diseases, and frequency of coitus.

As a parent of three adolescents this author would suggest abstinence first. If sexual activity does occur, however, protection against pregnancy is warranted.

Condom.   Although condom sales have increased over the past decade, adolescent use has dropped.[22] Of all available and reliable methods, the condom is the only method that may aid in protection against sexually transmitted diseases. Sexually active 15–19 year olds are responsible for 25 percent of all reported cases of gonorrhea in the United States.[22,93] It is truly a shame that this form of contraception is not more frequently suggested to and accepted by adolescents. Perhaps the adolescent feels that the condom gets in the way, is a nuisance, inhibits spontaneity, is messy, or decreases sexual intimacy or pleasure.

Studies have shown that condoms, when used properly, are 97 percent effective and significantly effective in preventing gonorrhea and other sexually transmitted diseases.[7] This method has many other advantages for adolescents. It is sold over the counter without a costly or planned office visit and prescription. Condoms, unlike the popular pill and IUD, have no dangerous side effects. Condoms are conveniently small and may be carried by either partner. This method involves the male partner in a more active role in the responsibility for contraception. It is easily discontinued and fertility immediately returns. Finally, it may be used as a back-up method for inconsistent use of oral contraceptives and IUD problems.

Diaphragm. The diaphragm has a perfect-use rate of 96–98 percent effectiveness and an actual-use rate of 80–97 percent effectiveness.[63] This barrier form of contraception is regaining popularity yet not among adolescents. This may be because diaphragm use:

1. requires an office visit
2. is more costly than condom use
3. requires more user motivation than the pill or IUD
4. may be contraindicated in some women due to size or dislodgement problems
5. may require refittings
6. requires self-touching and genital manipulation
7. is messy
8. may cause allergic reactions to spermacidals or rubber
9. may cause recurrent bladder infections due to urethral or bladder trauma.

Before enumerating the advantages of diaphragm use, it is important to discuss the anatomic characteristics of women who should not use a diaphragm. Women with the following characteristics cannot use a diaphragm: inadequate pelvic muscle support; a short or unusually long anterior vaginal wall; a damaged pelvic floor, perhaps because of previous surgery; no palpable notch behind the symphasis pubis; a very small cervix; severe displacement of the uterus or adjacent organs such as cystocele or rectocele; anteflexion or retroversion of the uterus; uterine prolapse; and inability to reach into the vagina and palpate the cervix.[51]

The diaphragm may be considered a good choice for the adolescent because it does not threaten future fertility or general health. It is a good method when sexual intercourse is infrequent, and daily coverage, such as the pill and IUD provide, is not needed. Spontaneity is added to the sexual encounter because the diaphragm may be inserted several hours before intercourse. There are no physical discomforts, the cream or gel may provide additional lubrication, and the method does not interfere with any pleasurable sexual sensations for either the male or female.

It is often difficult to fit a diaphragm in a nulliparous woman who has had limited exposure to sexual intercourse or has never used tampons. Perhaps the flat spring diaphragm may work best for these women especially in the case of a shallow pubic arch.[51]

Whichever type of diaphragm is selected, careful instruction in insertion, practice during the fitting, home practice, and a return visit in one week while wearing the diaphragm are suggested to check not only fit and placement but to assess comfort and method acceptability. Since nurse-midwifery care generally is known to be longer and perhaps more focused on patient education, the adolescent wishing to use a diaphragm may benefit by receiving the care and instruction from a nurse-midwife.

Intrauterine device.   Because the incidence of gonorrhea among adolescents is extremely high, the IUD may not be considered the most desirable method for conception control. Known links between gonorrhea, the IUD, pelvic inflammatory disease, and the potential for future infertility have made many nurse-midwives, as well as other health care providers, cautious about suggesting this method for the nulliparous adolescent. Since adolescents generally have little money, limited access to transportation, and may be using this contraceptive device without parental knowledge, they may be less likely than older women to seek medical attention when danger signs present. These poor use factors may be reason enough to discourage the use of the IUD in this age group. Furthermore, IUD users experience increased menstrual flow with subsequent decrease in mineral stores and tend to suffer more from anemia than other groups. The IUD therefore is not recommended for adolescents, as well as adult women, who have either a poor dietary history, hemoglobin less than or equal to 10 gm, menstrual bleeding disorders, or hemoglobinopathies.

The IUD is attractive for some women since it requires only one-time motivation, at the time of insertion. It is also attractive to the adolescent who does not wish her parents or male partner to know that she is using a contraceptive or who has one or very few sexual partners. The adolescent most likely to benefit from using the IUD is reliable in seeking health care when indicated and considers asking or requiring her partner to use a condom to avoid sexually transmitted diseases and their sequelae.

Oral contraceptive.   When adolescents come to an office or clinic seeking a birth control method, they usually ask for the pill. Oral contraceptives are simple to take, very effective, require no genital manipulation, and no interruption of foreplay. Perhaps these are a few of the reasons for the pill's popularity with adolescents.

When counseling adolescents about birth control methods, caution must be taken before selecting the pill. In addition to assessing for absolute and relative contraindications for the pill, the nurse-midwife must consider the following:

1. Does the adolescent have a history of regular menses or at least 6−12 regular cycles before initiation of the pill? (Avoid the risk of prescribing the pill to an amenorrheic adolescent for whom the pill can cause more severe amenorrhea and infertility.)

2. Is the daily pill-taking regimen too demanding for this adolescent's lifestyle?
3. Does she have a poor history of pill usage?
4. Is she too young considering the disadvantage of beginning at an early age with the prospect of many years of use and increasing risks of heart disease, thromboembolic disease, and cancer?[89]
5. Is she willing to use a back-up method when problems arise, such as taking other medications that may interfere with pill effectiveness, incorrect usage, or untimely discontinuation of the pill?
6. Can she verbalize correct pill-taking instructions and course of action when pills are forgotten, when nausea and vomiting occur, and when there are dietary and medication considerations that may alter pill protection?
7. Does she understand why friends should not share oral contraceptives?
8. Is she able to verbalize danger signs and appropriate actions?

Natural family planning. Education regarding contraception should begin, in the opinion of this author, with the topic of natural family planning. There is perhaps no better opportunity to inform women about the basics of their anatomy, the physiology of reproduction, and about the physcial signs of fertility. This information should be taught to both men and women. Signs of ovulation should be well known. The alteration of the basal body temperature, the sensation of mittelschmerz, and the changes in the cervical mucus should be common knowledge among all women. In one study, of the 98 percent of adolescents who claimed to know when the fertile period in women occurred, only one-half were correct.[36]

Natural family planning may not be the method considered most desirable for adolescents because of lifestyle, immaturity, irregular menses, periodic abstinence, and sporadic sexual activity. Yet it provides an excellent opportunity to teach young people about fertility.

Abortion. Since 1970, approximately one-third of all legal abortions in the United States were performed on adolescents. The moral decision to abort or not is just as difficult for the adolescent as for any woman. Often the decision is very heavily influenced one way or the other by the girl's parents or boyfriend as she seeks assistance in dealing with this dilemma. Professional abortion counseling for all women, especially the adolescent, is critically important.

Adolescents frequently wait longer for help when suspecting pregnancy and consequently place themselves at greater medical risk when abortion is eventually performed. Termination procedures later in pregnancy, after 12 week's gestation or more, are associated not only with higher morbidity rates but also increased cost. Abortion, whether performed once or repeatedly, also is suspected of adversely affecting future fertility and pregnancy outcome.[37]

Women Aged 30 Years and Over

An increasing proportion of women in this country delay childbearing until after they are 30 years old. A woman may delay childbearing because she fears change in role and lifestyle, does not wish to interrupt educational and professional pursuits, has financial restrictions, has delayed marriage, or has been unable to find a suitable partner.[46] In 1970 the birth rate to women 30–34 years old was 7.3/1000 total pop. In 1976 that rate rose to 8.9/1000 according to the National Center for Health Statistics.[59] The number is still rising.

Because these women have avoided pregnancy until after they are 30 years old, they are often well informed and selective in choosing their care provider. It is hoped that this selection occurs before pregnancy.

If the nurse-midwife is confronted with an increasing number of gynecologic and family planning patients who have not yet made the decision to begin a family and are approaching or are in their 30s, certain factors should be considered during the counseling portion of the visit. Certainly all women who wish to have children wish to produce healthy children whether this goal is verbalized or not, and we know that babies born to mothers who are between the ages of 21–29 appear to be the healthiest. The likelihood of Down's Syndrome occurring in mothers less than 35 years old is 1/1000–2000 births; in women 35–40 years old it is 1/300; and in women 45 years old the risk is 1/30–35.[44]

Women between the ages of 20–35 tolerate pregnancy better than younger or older women. Physical maturation is associated with fewer complications of pregnancy, and improved nutritional and economic status may also be factors. This author feels it is only reasonable that nurse-midwives encourage patients to bear children before they are 35 years old, because of the lower risks of hypertension, thyroid dysfunction, kidney complications, hemorrhage, related delivery complications, and genetic disorders.

The nurse-midwife must inform each patient of the best approach to take to protect fertility and to avoid future birth defects while delaying childbearing. These include the careful selection of a birth control method, screening for susceptibility to particular infections or familial genetic disorders, and the detection of symptoms suggestive of potential infertility problems.

Oral contraceptives. Women who have irregular menstrual periods should not use oral contraceptives since this medication will only exacerbate the problem. In long-term pill use, about 3–10 percent of women are anovulatory when the method is discontinued.[46] The nurse-midwife must counsel women with normal menstrual cycles to discontinue use of oral contraceptives at least 3 months before planned conception. Discontinuation is a safeguard against pill-related fetal anomalies and possible multiple gestation.[46] In the event that the menstrual cycle does not become reestablished within 3 months after the medication is discontinued, an evaluation of the ovulatory-menstrual cycle is indicated.

Another concern about the use of oral contraceptives by women more than 30 years old is the possibility that these women may have already been on the pill for a number of years. Sexual activity along with long-term oral contraceptive use is under investigation for possibly having a combined influence on the development of cervical carcinoma.[77,89]

Since 1962 there have been reports of health-related risks associated with oral contraceptives. Partly because of these reports, the number of oral contraceptive users has decreased over the years, despite the pill's superb contraceptive effects. Approximately 10 million American women used the pill in 1974, but this number decreased to 8 million by 1978, according to Kistner.[49]

It is believed that the initial popularity of the IUD was partly responsible for the decline in pill use; the increased knowledge of major and minor complications caused by oral contraceptives, however, is also to blame. Results of a questionnaire circulated by Flekstein et al. to 591 previous pill users indicate that 127 women discontinued the pill because of side effects and an additional 78 stopped because they feared the potential adverse effects.[23] The purpose of this review is to discuss the management issues of pill usuage in women at risk for major complications.

Family planning health care providers are well aware of the potential ill effects of oral contraceptives and the need to weigh the risks as well as the benefits of this method when counseling each woman before prescribing any oral contraceptive. It is our obligation to discourage the use of oral contraceptives in women who demonstrate physical or historical findings suggestive of increased risk for this method of contraception.

The incidence of thromboembolic disease, one of several major side effects of the pill, appears to be linked with the dose of estrogen. Even the lower-dose estrogen pills, however, cause an increased risk of thromboembolic disease. The exact relationship between the oral contraceptive and this disease is unknown at this time. It has been suggested, however, that the use of oral contraceptives may be associated with certain abnormalities in blood clotting factors.[102] The risk of pulmonary embolus is 112/100,000 high-dose users each year and 81/100,000 low-dose users each year.[78] Research by Stolley and associates demonstrates an increased incidence of leg deep-vein thrombosis in women on oral contraceptives with estrogen doses greater than 100 μg.[87]

In identifying a patient appropriate for oral contraceptive use, the nurse-midwife must review with the woman her potential for risk. In doing so, it is recommended that the patient sign a consent form acknowledging risk. Those factors that would place a woman at risk for thromboembolic disease and, therefore, warrant not taking an oral contraceptive may include hypertension, diabetes, history of thrombophlebitis, cancer, suspected pregnancy, varicose veins, anticipation of surgery, and limb immobilization.[72]

Myocardial infarction is another major complication of oral contraceptive usage. Women at risk for this complication smoke cigarettes, are diabetic, hypertensive, obese, have abnormally high beta cholesterol levels, or have a family history of arterial disease.[73] According to Jick and associates, acute myocardial infarction appears to be a disease exclusively of cigarette smokers.[45] Their statistics indicate that among women who smoke and take the pill, the myocardial infarction rate for those women between 27−37 years old is 1/8400 each year, and for those 38−45 years old the rate increases dramatically to 1/250.[45] Present information suggests, however, that the risk of nonfatal acute myocardial infarction is greater in pill-using women 38 years old and older, even when they do not smoke, than in women of this age who do not take the pill.[45]

Stroke or cerebrovascular accident may also be added to the list of potential major complications attributed to use of oral contraceptives. Even though stroke is rare in young women of childbearing age, the risk of thromboembolic or hemorrhagic stroke is a distinct threat when oral contraceptives are used. As early as 1970 the literature indicated that oral contraceptive use increases the risk of stroke sixfold.[16] Inman writes that the incidence of stroke, unlike myocardial infarction, does not appear to be affected by the estrogen content of the pill.[42]

The development of liver cell adenoma is a rare disorder which Edmonson and associates found to have a positive correlation with the duration of pill use.[18] It is a benign growth, and the actual cause and effect relationship between the development of liver cell adenoma and the pill is currently unknown. It is believed, however, that the amount of estrogen in the pill and long-term use could have a major influence on the development of this growth. In addition, long-term pill use is being considered in the evaluation of hypotheses concerning a positive correlation with the development of cancer.[21]

Oral contraceptives in higher estrogen doses are appropriate when treating endometriosis and hypermenorrhea.[78] Again, lower doses of estrogen may decrease a woman's chances of developing major side effects yet do not eliminate these potential complications.

Intrauterine device. Certain women concerned about protecting their fertility are not candidates for this method. According to Kapstrom, an infertility specialist, women at risk for infertility with IUD use are those with a history of pelvic inflammatory disease, multiple mixed vaginal and cervical infections, cervical erosions requiring cauterization, frequently inserted devices rather than those that remain in place for 2−3 years, ectopic pregnancies, or surgery leaving only one fallopian tube, and those who are nulliparous.[46]

Intrauterine devices have the possible short-term side effects of syncope, perforation, expulsion, cramping, bleeding, pregnancy, and pelvic inflammatory disease. A potential long-term side effect of the IUD is a possible decrease in fertility, most likely as a result of an increased incidence of pelvic inflammatory disease.[26] An estimated 3 million women in the United States wear the IUD, and the incidence of pelvic inflammatory disease is about 600,000/year with or without the presence of an IUD.[26] The risk of pelvic inflammatory disease in the IUD user is 1−2.5 percent overall, but up to 7 percent in selected populations are prone to this disease.[94] The woman and her nurse-midwife must pay attention to early symptoms of this disease and begin immediate treatment in order to safeguard fertility.

Abortion. In the opinion of this author, abortion should not be relied on as the sole method of contraception. In the 1980s health care providers will see more and more women who have received elective abortions. As a result of one or several abortions, it is speculated that the woman may later experience postabortion infection or scar tissue development, both of which can cause infertility; a weakened or damaged cervix with the potential for spontaneous abortion; premature birth; dysfunctional cervical dilatation in labor; intrauterine growth retardation due to scarred uterine tissue, or poor placental perfusion.[37] Recent advances in perinatology have improved maternal and fetal outcomes for pregnancies with complications related to previous abortions. However, the cost of care for these pregnancies is increased, and the choice of birthing style and of practitioner is limited. These factors may prove disappointing to the woman in question.

Sterilization. An increasing number of women are seeking sterilization as a reasonable approach to permanent contraception. Most frequently this surgery occurs immediately following the last pregnancy desired. Results of several surveys show this to be the most commonly used method of fertility control in the United States for married couples over 30 years old.[38,63] During 1970 the national figure of tubal ligations performed was estimated at 201,000, and that figure rose to 550,000 in 1975.[76,103] According to the Population Research Center at Princeton, New Jersey, in 1975 approximately 6.8 million couples worldwide elected sterilization for contraception, and over half of these were female sterilizations.[88] It is Siegler's belief that liberalized laws, greater availability, lower cost of the procedures, and changing lifestyles are contributing to this trend.[76]

This method has become popular most likely because there is no need to use a back-up method, no disruption of sexual foreplay, genital manipulation is not required, sexual response is not affected, and no repeated contraceptive decisions and costs are required. However, certain religious, racial, and cultural groups do not consider permanent loss of childbearing capacity acceptable.

A woman may choose to become sterilized for several reasons. It is helpful if the nurse-midwife, while discussing options for conception control, assists the woman in identifying her reasons for sterilization. As Stone suggests some of the following reasons may be verbalized:

1. Desired family size has been achieved.
2. Medical contraindications for future pregnancies are demonstrated.
3. Other methods of contraception are considered undesirable.
4. A family history of serious genetic defects has been demonstrated.
5. There is financial inability to support more children.
6. There is family, peer, or social pressure to cease childbearing.[88]

When counseling each woman or couple, the nurse-midwife must always provide adequate information regarding the law, alternative methods, benefits, explanation of the procedure, mechanism of action, and recovery instructions. Along with this information all of the patient's questions should be answered, and the patient should know that she may change her mind at any time before the initiation of the procedure.

Most misunderstandings regarding sterilization deal with legal concerns and return of fertility.[88] The legal concerns may require clarification with the following comments:

1. The spouse's permission is not required for sterilization.
2. Federal funds only reimburse women who are over 21 years old and are mentally competent.
3. In order for federal funds to be collected, an institution or physician must have the woman sign the consent papers at least 30 days before surgery.[38]

Each woman seeking a tubal ligation must be informed that this method should be used by women who do not plan to have children in the future. The woman may not have fully understood the procedure and, through friends, relatives, and lay-group discussions, was lead to believe that the tubal ligation method is easily reversible. Prudent health professionals educating women before securing consents for sterilization certainly are not promising easy reversibility.

Breast-Feeding

Breast-feeding women who do not wish to conceive soon after pregnancy should be well informed of their options. As always, the choice of a contraceptive method ultimately is made by the woman as long as the method is not medically contraindicated.

If for personal or religious reasons the woman does not wish to use either barrier or mechanical methods of contraception while lactating, she must be well instructed in the external signs of ovulation. The nurse-midwife should then carefully review practices of identifying ovulation by means of cervical mucous testing and basal body temperature evaluation.

Vorherr reports that by 3 months after delivery 33 percent of lactating women have had a menstrual period as compared to 91 percent of nonlactating women. This researcher also projects, in accordance with collected data, that at 9 months postpartum more than half of the lactating women who are not using an additional means of contraception will become pregnant.[101]

Early in the postpartum period, during the first 3 months, lactation does provide some protection against pregnancy. Controversy exists as to whether the initial menses occurs before the onset of ovulation.[60] The risk of pregnancy during this time of lactational amenorrhea is about 5 percent.[60]

The onset of menstruation in a breast-feeding mother marks the clinical return of fertility. This return of reproductive function is greatly dependent on the amount and frequency of suckling. A token breast-feeder who begins solid food early, spaces out feedings, encourages supplementation, and uses a pacifier for non-nutritive sucking gratification will experience a shorter period of amenorrhea. On the other hand, the woman who feeds 24 hours on demand, avoids supplementation and early introduction of solid foods, and puts the baby to breast for nonnutritive sucking will experience a longer period of lactational amenorrhea. This approach will require a highly motivated mother who also has sound family, peer group, and nurse-midwifery support.

Oral contraceptives are not prescribed by the nurse-midwife or any other primary care provider for breast-feeding mothers because of the concern that any hormone combination used to inhibit ovulation may be of potential long- or short-term risk to the infant. Curtis has documented the experience of breast enlargement in a breast-fed male infant whose mother ingested less than one pack of oral contraceptives.[10] The issues revolving around oral contraceptive usage in breast-feeding mothers include ill effects on milk production, composition of the milk, and uterine involution, as well as growth and development of the breast-fed infant in terms of bone maturation, genital development, or impaired fertility.[90,101]

For those women interested in barrier, mechanical, or chemical means of contraception there does not appear to be any problem. Since there is no evidence of contraindications during breast-feeding, any of these methods may be prescribed when medical contraindications are absent.

Desired Family Size

It is hoped that every women has the opportunity to decide whether or not to have children, when, how many, and with whom. These decisions are perhaps some of the most important and exciting of a life-time. Proper education and counseling of both women and their partners are critical in avoiding unplanned and unwanted pregnancy. Parenthood should be preceeded by learning about the changes that frequently occur in a couple's lifestyle, emotions, and possibly careers. According to the Population Institute, it is believed that over 90 percent of Americans will marry at some time in their lives and will have 2 children.[64]

Before any of these decisions regarding parenting are made, the woman must first make the decision to become involved in sexual activity. If she does not wish to begin a family, then the appropriate contraceptive method should be sought. Today the responsibility of contraception still falls most heavily on the woman. Women appear to be more highly motivated to control fertility than men do. This may be due to the woman's concern for the physical changes and events of pregnancy and birth. Since it is the woman who conceives, the largest number of effective contraceptives have been developed for the woman's use.

Even though contraceptive methods are widely available to women, not all women choose to take measures to avoid pregnancy. The decision to use contraception is a very important step in the sexual development of the individual. It confirms acceptance of planned sexual intercourse. For some people sexual pleasure is heightened by taking risks. Planned readiness for sexual intercourse may project a social image of loose morals, especially among singles. Among married couples, however, sexual intercourse without contraception is foolish unless a pregnancy is desired.

Research indicates that couples who desire a pregnancy have a greater chance of failing at contraception than those who do not want a pregnancy. Vaughn writes that from 1970–1973, 7.3 percent of married couples wishing to delay a desired pregnancy failed the first year as compared to 3.7 percent of those wishing not to have children.[100] This indicates that motivation plays a significant role in the success of contraceptive method use.

There also exists evidence of a racial difference with respect to the number of children born into a family. Zelnik and Kantner report that most blacks do not want more children than whites, yet they appear certain to have more because of factors such as earlier sexual activity, preference to marry earlier, diminished use of contraceptives, and less access to abortion.[107]

Certain societal influences appear to contribute to the increase in the number of pregnancies a woman may experience. First, there is an increase in the frequency of sexual intercourse among married couples today when compared to couples of a generation ago. According to Hunt, the median frequency of intercourse among the youngest age groups evaluated increased from 2.45/week in the 1940s to 3.25/week in 1972, and in the oldest group from 0.50/week to 1.00/week.[41] This increase in frequency may be caused by societal influences, improved general health, and achievement of higher educational levels. The movement toward a more urban and industrialized lifestyle also may be a contributing factor, despite the agrarian family's requiring many children to help support the family farm.

Sociologically it is reported that the importance of the woman's family role compared to that of her husband affects family size; when the wife's position is more equal to the husband's, fewer children are desired and planned.[72]

One of two styles of married life may be selected. The newer concept of a woman achieving satisfaction, recognition, and monetary gain outside the home may be attractive to the couple. The alternative would be the more traditional approach of bearing children and the woman remaining home to care for them. More and more women are faced with a combination of both styles. In fact, many women must, with today's economic problems and high divorce rate, raise children and work outside the home. With a change in women's roles, society is more accepting of women functioning in the work force, pursuing higher education, and limiting family size. Working women are documented to have higher success rates with contraception than women who do not work outside the home.[72]

Today, the woman of childbearing age who wishes to have children may be influenced to limit the number. When considering finances, she finds that it is easier to support and educate fewer children. Having fewer children also increases the amount of money available to maintain a higher standard of living for the family. Part of the pleasure and joy of parenting is spending time with the children. By having fewer children, the woman may find that she is more accessible to each individual child. It is hoped that this circumstance would lead to improved parent–child communication.

The amount of stress a woman experiences often increases as the number of children she has increases. This may be related to continuous responsibility for daily care and parenting, demands that continue over a long period of time.

An increasing number of women find it economically and professionally necessary to increase the family's financial income and to develop a stable professional career. Women with a career outside the home find limitation of family size convenient. Fewer children make babysitting arrangements easier. If professional growth and development concern her, she may find that having fewer children leads to a greater amount of time and money to pursue higher education and successfully meet career responsibilities.

Biologic influences have been found to cause a potential increase in the number of pregnancies experienced. There is a trend in the decline of the age of menarche. In 1940 the average age at menarche was 13.5 years, whereas in the 1960s that age dropped to 12.5 years and continues to fall.[106] According to Cutright, adolescent girls become fully fertile one year earlier than their mothers did.[11] In addition, with improved economic, medical, and nutritional circumstances, the rate of spontaneous abortions has declined.[11] Advancements in perinatal medicine and an era of improved maternal health care have led to greater newborn salvage.

The most appropriate contraceptive method for the woman limiting the size of her family should embody the characteristics listed in Table 7-2.

The nurse-midwife may also encounter the woman who does not wish to have any children; after all, marriage and parenthood are not for everyone.

Women who wish never to have children for personal, social, or medical reasons may desire a more permanent form of contraception, and voluntary sterilization is the most effective. As discussed previously, the woman must be counseled to realize that sterilization is permanent and, in the majority of cases, irreversible.

Table 7-2

Factors to Consider when Selecting the Appropriate Contraceptive Method.

Characteristics of the Appropriate Contraceptive	Characteristics of the Woman Prepared for Contraception
Not medically contraindicated	Demonstrates correct method usage
Affordable	Verbalizes danger signs and plans for seeking medical assistance when indicated
Acceptable to the woman and her partner	
Does not compromise future desired fertility	Selects and verbalizes correct usage of appropriate back-up method
Easily reversible	
Acceptable for either short- or long-term contraception	Verbalizes circumstances when the method may become ineffective and a consequent, appropriate course of action
	Verbalizes method risks
	Has access to follow-up health care when indicated
	Signs an informed consent form for the pill or an intrauterine device.

All young women should be encouraged to develop as individuals before becoming parents. The responsibilities of functioning well in a meaningful relationship, marriage, family, and society will be better accomplished if the young woman matures first.

Pregnancy may occur before it is desired. The following factors contribute to the occurrence of undersired pregnancy:

1. pressure from the male partner to prove his virility
2. contraceptive method failure
3. submission due to fear of physical violence
4. rape
5. loneliness
6. validation of sexual identity
7. act of anger or hostility toward parents, spouse, partner, or society
8. lack of contraceptive use due to guilt feelings over planned sexual activity

Family size currently is controlled by more than just the technology and availability of a contraceptive method. The couple's view of each other's roles within the marriage, the appreciation of and desire to parent, the educational and professional aspirations of the woman, as well as societal and biological influences, all have a direct effect on method selection, its successful use, and desired family size.

Subfertility

Family planning services provided by the nurse-midwife and other health professionals must include care and counseling for those couples who wish to delay conception, as well as those who wish to conceive. The term *subfertile* is used to describe couples who are not yet diagnosed as infertile and are having difficulty conceiving. McCusker describes subfertile couples as those who are still trying to achieve pregnancy after 6–18 months of unprotected intercourse.[55] Women in their 20s may not be upset when asked to continue trying to conceive a while longer. On the other hand, women more than 35 years old may consider 18 months of waiting to be impractical and injudicious.

Couples who suspect subfertility to be their problem may experience symptoms of tension, feelings of inadequacy, and a sense of loss of control over their lives. The nurse-midwife should cautiously take a positive, supportive, and educational approach to their dilemma. Neither partner is at fault.

Inform a couple suspecting subfertility that society may be a powerful influence in promoting subfertility problems. The influence may include popular use of certain contraceptive methods which, in some cases, have caused fertility reestablishment problems when discontinued. The IUD and oral contraceptives fall into this category.[20,26] In addition, a decrease in the popularity of condoms and an increase in the incidence of sexually transmitted diseases have led to more cases of pelvic inflammatory disease. This disease is linked with diminished subsequent fertility. Furthermore, a delay in childbearing due to marrying late or pursuing educational or professional goals pushes women into ages beyond peak fertility. Kistner reports that peak fertility occurs in women aged 24 years and rapidly falls after age 30.[49]

The nurse-midwife should make complete detailed psychosocial and physical assessments of the couple seeking assistance for subfertility. These assessments should include information about desired family size, religious orientation, cultural influences on childbearing, general health, menstrual history, contraceptive usage, emotional and marital status, coital frequency and timing, medications taken regularly, and use of drugs or alcohol. Next, evaluate the couple's knowledge of fertility-awareness techniques. Review the correct steps to follow when employing the basal body temperature method, calendar methods, and the Billings ovulation method, as well as the detection of other physical symptoms of ovulation. These methods are described in great detail in other readings.[8,19,97] It is important to begin with fertility-awareness techniques because these determine whether or not ovulation is occurring.

If ovulation is occurring, provide the couple with concrete suggestions to enhance the possibility of conception. The tips listed in Table 7-3 may be helpful.

If the woman is not ovulating she should be referred to the gynecologist or infertility specialist for pharmacologic induction of ovulation. It is also possible that her partner may require evaluation by a urologist with interest

Table 7-3
Suggestions to Promote Conception

Woman	Man
Practice good nutrition.	Practice good nutrition.
Get enough rest.	Get enough rest.
Maintain a suggested normal weight.	Maintain a suggested normal weight.
Avoid running very long distances (i.e., >25 miles/week)	Avoid excessive alcohol.
Abolish unnecessary stress in your life.	Quit smoking marijuana or taking psychotropic drugs.
Quit smoking marijuana or taking psychotropic drugs.	Consider decreasing heat exposure to the testicles (hot tub).
Avoid excessive alcohol consumption.	
Seek consultation with the nurse-midwife if excessive uterine cramping, abnormal vaginal discharge, or bleeding occur.	
Know how to use the symptothermal and basal body temperature methods of fertility awareness.	
Time intercourse appropriately Ovulation occurs at the end of mittelschmerz.	
Optimal frequency of intercourse is 4/week.	
Intercourse should occur no more than every second or third day after menstruation while awaiting the fertile-type mucus.	
Intercourse should take place during the presence of the fertile type mucus.	
Avoid using vaginal lubricants sprays, or douches and perfumed tampons, pads, or toilet paper as they may cause irritation and alter cervical and vaginal secretions.	

in subfertility problems. The man should first, however, have semen analysis as a screening method to determine whether referral and further testing are indicated. Semen analysis in the fertile male should show a sperm density of no less than 20 million/ml and volume of greater than 1 ml. The normal volume ranges from 2−6 ml, and the normal progressive motility is 50 percent average. Morphology also must be considered; if there is a question of an abnormal semen analysis, at least three specimens should be evaluated before this diagnosis is made.[83] The consulting gynecologist should enter into the process of evaluating the semen analysis and initiating the appropriate referral.

The Effect of Health Status on Contraceptive Method Selection

The nurse-midwife, when counseling a woman in the selection of a contraceptive method, must consider the woman's personal, psychological, and social health-status characteristics which may influence successful and safe method usage. A systematic review of certain health-status characteristics and the acceptability of some of the more popular contraceptive methods are presented in Appendix 7-1 (p 296).

Each woman's health status dictates the most appropriate contraceptive method for her; yet the contraceptive that may be contraindicated in one circumstance may be the method of choice in another. Furthermore, it is unlikely that a woman will use only one method of contraception throughout her fertile years. Women therefore need to be educated about all contraceptive options so that they may participate fully in the selection of appropriate back-up and alternative methods. Having selected a safe, effective, and readily available back-up method diminishes anxiety and decreases the chance of contraceptive failure. The woman who understands that at some future date an alternative method may be indicated is more prepared to make informed choices without undue stress and unprotected intercourse. The nurse-midwife's job is also easier when the woman is prepared and able to participate in the method selection.

INFORMATIONAL NEEDS

Self-Monitoring of Health Status and Early Identification of Problems

Vulvovaginitis

A large part of nurse-midwifery services to the normal gynecologic patient include discussion, diagnosis, treatment, and follow-up of vulvovaginitis. The infections discussed in this section are rarely serious; they may cause acute discomfort, however, resulting in severe distress. The nurse-midwife can provide the patient with the information necessary for self-assessment and consequent early treatment of vulvovaginitis; the use of printed material is a helpful adjunct to teaching during an office visit (see Table 7-4).

As a part of promoting the patient's increased knowledge of the body and self-monitoring of health status, the nurse-midwife should teach the patient to recognize normal from abnormal vaginal secretions and vulvovaginal sensations. That discussion will be an opportunity to teach the woman to be aware of fertility and to monitor cervical and vaginal secretions. The woman should be directed to note changes in the cervical mucus throughout the menstrual cycle. An explanation of the effect of estrogen and progesterone on the cervical mucus may be appropriate. Inform the woman that, at the time of ovulation, cervical mucus is clearer, stretchable, and increases in amount. The estrogenic effect on the mucus crypts in the cervix causes this change in the mucus. She may wish to test the mucus obtained from underpants, labia, or vagina by noting its stretchability between two fingers. Tell her that the character of the mucus aids the sperm in traveling up the cervix to promote fertilization. In contrast, describe the cervical mucus of the luteal phase affected by progesterone, causing the development of a thick and sticky mucus which prevents the sperm from passing up through the cervix. Of course, neither of these secretions is malodorous nor cause the discomforts of vulvo-vaginitis which will be discussed later. Call her attention to the fact that if for some reason she is not ovulating, possibly due to being pregnant, taking combined oral contraceptives, or experiencing anovulatory cycles, she may not recognize these changes in cervical mucus.

Introducing information about other experiences which may alter the amount, color, and odor of vaginal secretions may also be helpful in teaching patients about their bodies. For example, sexual arousal increases the amount of vaginal secretions and causes a slippery texture which aids in lubrication for intercourse. This secretion also causes no irritation or inflammation and has no foul odor.

Since a thorough history of any presenting problem is of paramount importance in arriving at a correct diagnosis, the nurse-midwife may inform the patient that many questions will be asked to evaluate abnormal vaginal discharge or vulvovaginal discomforts. Questions about symptoms may be followed by a review of sexual practices and related discomforts. The patient should also be asked about current or recent use of antibiotics, use of new soaps, detergents or feminine hygiene products, wearing binding slacks or nylon underpants, and about the type and frequency of douching.

The patient's ability to recognize abnormal vaginal discharge and the frequently associated discomforts is important for rapid and successful treatment of vaginal infections, as well as to control sexual transmission.

Urinary tract problems

The nurse-midwife can assist women in taking a preventive approach to health maintenance. During an office visit the nurse-midwife may wish to discuss measures for avoiding common problems associated with the urinary tract. Each woman should have access to information regarding urinary tract infections. The most frequently encountered urinary difficulties include infections and incontinence.

The manner in which information is disseminated may be dictated by the particular circumstance. Those women with no history of previous or current

Table 7-4

Discover Vaginal Infections Early — For Patient Information

This guide describes the most frequently encountered vaginal infections women experience. A normal, healthy woman has many bacteria growing in the vagina. At times these or other bacteria multiply greatly and cause an infection. This guide may help you to recognize a vaginal infection early, identify events in your life which help infections occur, know what to do if you think you have a vaginal infection, and follow suggestions for avoiding infection.

Infection	You May Notice	You May Feel	Why It Occurs	What To Do	Sexual Precautions
Candidiasis ("fungus, yeast, nomilia")	Vaginal discharge: small amount, thick, white, with cottage cheese appearance, smells like baking bread A mirror may show the perineum (skin between your legs) to be red and swollen.	Itching and/or burning around the lips and skin outside the vagina Discomfort usually happens before your period. Painful urination and/or sexual intercourse	Taking, or recently discontinued, antibiotics, birth control pills or steroids Having health problems: diabetes thyroid disorders Problems with immunity Pregnancy Menstruation	Make an appointment to see the nurse-midwife Reduce or eliminate sugar and refined carbohydrates in your diet. If it is difficult to cure, you may need to use another method other than birth control pills. Follow the "Suggestions for avoiding vaginal infections" listed below.	Chances of you giving this to your partner are very slim. You may wish to have your partner use a condom until the problem is diagnosed and successfully cured.

	Symptoms	Cause	What to do	
Trichomoniasis ("Trich")	Vaginal discharge: large amount of greenish-yellow-colored, thin, and foamy or bubbly liquid having a bad odor. Perineal swelling and redness. Your pap smear may show continuous irritation of the cervix.	Itching and/or burning around the lips and skin outside the vagina. Discomfort begins following your period. Painful urination and/or sexual intercourse. A feeling of fullness in the vagina and on the perineum because of swelling.	Probable cause: sexual intercourse with an infected partner. Possible cause: communal bathing; sitting on a contaminated toilet seat; or sharing contaminated towels, washcloths, clothes, or douche equipment.	Make an appointment to see the nurse-midwife. Take a vinegar and water douche. Use sanitary pads instead of tampons. Stop using ordinary douches and perineal feminine deodorant sprays. Follow the "Suggestions for Avoiding Vaginal Infections" listed below. Don't douche or put any creams, jellies or home remedies in the vagina at least 48 hours before your visit with the nurse-midwife.	This is passed sexually. Have your partner use a condom until this infection is diagnosed and successfully treated. If you were sexually active with your partner before you noticed the infection, request that he have his doctor treat him for this infection so that you do not catch it again.
Hemophilus	Vaginal discharge: thin, creamy white or grey and sometimes foul smelling	Slight itching or mild burning	Sexual intercourse with an infected partner	Make an appointment to see the nurse-midwife. Follow the "Suggestions for Avoiding Vaginal Infections" below.	This is passed sexually. Have your partner use a condom. Ask your partner to seek medical treatment before you resume sexual relations. *(continued)*

Table 7-4 (continued)

Suggestions for Avoiding Vaginal Infections

Follow good health practices:

Eat well-rounded meals, avoid extra sugar and refined carbohydrates.

Get enough sleep.

Bathe regularly.

Wash hands before and after using the bathroom, inserting tampons, or using contraceptive devices such as the diaphragm, foam, jelly or cream applicator.

Don't share towels or washcloths, bathing suits, underpants, douche equipment or contraceptive devices.

Don't use irritating soaps, sprays, douche liquids.

Wear clean, cotton crotch underpants.

Don't wear binding slacks or jeans.

After going to the bathroom wipe yourself from front to back.

Have new or infrequent sex partners use a condom to protect against sexually transmitted diseases as well as for contraception.

Request your partner to wash his penis and hands before having intercourse.

Avoid painful intercourse or the use of uncomfortable vaginal vibrators.

Avoid any activity which may irritate or scratch the lining of the vagina.

Use contraceptive jelly when added lubrication is needed during intercourse.

Avoid douching too frequently.

Certain vaginal douches aid in promoting comfort when vaginal infections are present, suspected, or are to be avoided. Talk with your nurse-midwife about good douching practice.

1–2 tablespoons white vinegar added to 1 quart of comfortably warm water will help kill trichomonas and promote an environment unfavorable for infections to begin.

2 tablespoons plain yogurt added to 1 quart of comfortably warm water will help restore normal bacteria to the vagina.

1–2 tablespoons baking soda and 1 quart of comfortably warm water will help remove odor and relieve itching.

urinary problems may be satisfied with printed material from the office or clinic, which she can review at a later time or keep handy in case problems arise. On the other hand a woman in distress with a current problem may require not only treatment but additional evaluation and counseling in the hope of successful prevention of recurrence. In either case, the information given may include a brief definition of each type of frequently encountered infection, a description of the characteristic symptoms, comfort measures, and general suggestions for avoiding or preventing these infections. Table 7-5 serves as an example of an information sheet.

Stress incontinence is a frequently encountered urinary tract problem. Urinary stress incontinence is the involuntary leakage of urine when coughing, sneezing, laughing, lifting, running, walking, or undergoing similar physical stresses.[32] This seems to occur most frequently when the woman is in an upright position. This problem is linked with relaxed pelvic support. It is suggested that poor pelvic support may occur following obstetric trauma. Stress incontinence is rarely a problem of nulliparas. According to Green, in multiparas, this occurs secondary to poor pubococcygeal muscle tone, congenital weakness, or inadequate innervation of the pelvic floor muscle supports.[32] This appears to be a more common problem among multiparas, hence the association with obstetric trauma.

The nurse-midwife, as a routine part of a gynecologic history, should inquire about symptoms of stress incontinence. It may be difficult for the woman to offer this type of information. Remind her that you are available to discuss any future problems that may occur and will assist her in instituting whatever treatment or referrals are indicated.

In order to avoid overlooking the possibility of a urinary tract infection and secondary urgency incontinence, the nurse-midwife should begin by requesting a urine specimen for culture and sensitivity evaluation. For overweight women experiencing stress incontinence, it may be helpful to suggest weight reduction to reduce the extrinsic forces that may aggravate weakened urethroversical supports. The treatment of a persistent cough or allergy causing chronic sneezing may prove helpful in reducing physical stress provoking urinary incontinence.

The Kegel exercise has become a popular item on the health education teaching list of nurse-midwives treating gynecologic patients. It is an exercise used to improve pelvic floor muscle support. This exercise may be taught during an office visit or in a women's health education class.

Teaching the Kegel exercise is easy. During an office visit, the nurse-midwife may find the pelvic exam provides an excellent opportunity to discuss this exercise. With two fingers inside the vagina, request that the woman squeeze your fingers, and then relax and stop squeezing. She may wish to practice this with her partner during sexual intercourse. If the teaching session takes place in a health education class, the nurse-midwife may suggest she begin her practice while seated on the toilet. Suggest that she will identify

Table 7-5

Frequently Encountered Urinary Tract Infections — For Patient Information

You may, at some time in your life, develop a urinary tract infection. Your nurse-midwife wants you to know the answers to some important questions:

What are the different kinds of urinary tract infections?

How will you feel if an infection is developing?

What should you do if you think you have a urinary tract infection?

What should you do to help avoid getting a urinary tract infection?

Infection	Definition	Symptoms
Cystitis	This is an infection or inflammation of the bladder. The bladder is the organ that holds your urine. During cystitis many bacteria and red blood cells are present in your urine.	You may feel that you need to urinate very suddenly and more frequently than usual. There may be a burning sensation at the end of urination. You may also feel an aching pain in your lower abdomen just above your pubic bone.
Acute pyelonephritis	This is an infection of the kidney(s). Bacteria have caused the irritation. Your urine now contains bacteria, white and red blood cells and protein.	You may have a fever of 100°F or above and shaking chills. A low backache and blood in your urine may be present. Nausea and vomiting may occur. You will not have an appetite. You may notice that you suddenly and frequently need to urinate. Pain is present at the urethra (the opening where the urine comes out). Pain may also occur in your lower abdomen.
Asymptomatic bacteriuria	This means there is a large amount of bacteria in your urinary tract and they are increasing in number.	This is a "quiet" infection. We call it quiet because you don't feel sick or uncomfortable.

Table 7-5 (continued)

What To Do	Comfort Measures	Avoiding Infections:
If you have some of these symptoms, please call your nurse-midwife. She will ask you to stop by the office or clinic to give a urine specimen. The urine specimen will be sent to a laboratory for testing. You will be contacted or asked to call the office in the next few days. If an infection is present, you will be given a prescription for medication. Please tell your nurse-midwife if you have any allergies to medications. A complete treatment may take 2 weeks but you should feel better in a few days. If you do not begin to feel better, call your nurse-midwife. You may be asked to take a different medication. Take all of the medication prescribed. After the medication treatment is finished you will probably be asked to give another urine specimen. This is done to check on whether or not the infection is cured.	After you have called your nurse-midwife and received her instructions, there are a number of things you may do to be more comfortable until your infection is cured: Drink at least 10 glasses of fluids each day. One glass of cranberry juice every 4 hours may help. Take several hot tub baths each day. Don't drink coffee, tea, colas, and alcohol or eat spicy foods. Place a hot water bottle or heating pad on your lower back or abdomen. Refrain from sexual intercourse, since this may aggravate the discomfort.	The following is a list of steps you may take to avoid future urinary tract infections: Go to the bathroom and urinate as soon as you feel the need. Drink lots of water and fruit juice each day. Avoid sexual intercourse that puts too much pressure on the bladder such as positioning yourself so that the penis enters from the rear. Require that your sexual partner's hands and penis are clean. Avoid having a lowered resistance to infection by getting enough sleep and eating well.

273

which muscles should be relaxed and contracted when she attempts to begin urination and then suddenly stopping urination. This start and stop action when repeated throughout the entire stream of urine will give her a sense of which muscles are to be worked. Ten repetitions each day of the stop and start action are suggested. Some women have increased the number of repetitions to as many as three hundred each day.

Menstrual disorders

Quite frequently, when providing gynecologic health care, nurse-midwives encounter women with complaints about the menstrual cycle, dysmenorrhea, or premenstrual syndrome. Information sharing, as a part of health education, has become one of the most important and sought after nurse-midwifery services. This section will focus on a suggested approach to preparing patients to recognize potential problems, when to seek consultation, and comfort measures to be utilized when indicated.

Menstrual cycle. Each woman should be taught to recognize the normal characteristics of her menstrual cycle. A simple explanation of the menstrual cycle, focusing on basic anatomy and physiology when indicated, may prove helpful in abolishing myths, misconceptions, and incorrect information. Explaining how to plot the monthly cycles on menstrual calendar cards is helpful in detecting normal characteristics as well as deviations in cycle length and amount of bleeding. Noting cycle length, duration, amount and character of blood flow, and related symptoms each month teaches a woman self-health monitoring. In this way deviations in the menstrual cycle may be more easily and systematically evaluated.

Any deviation from her normal menstrual pattern—increased menstrual blood loss, increased duration of menses, or a shorter interval between bleeding episodes—should be considered abnormal and the woman should be directed to seek consultation. Similarly, the cessation of menses or deviations to a longer cycle pattern, symptoms of anovulatory cycles, or a marked decrease in menstrual flow must be evaluated. It is hoped that teaching a woman to recognize the normal characteristics of her menstrual pattern, and alerting her to seek evaluation when deviations occur may prevent severe health problems.

Reassurance may be given by explaining that certain factors such as sleep patterns, nutritional status, presence of illness, emotional upsets, medications, intrauterine devices, fluctuations in body weight, excessive exercise, and seasonal variations may cause changes in a woman's menstrual pattern. Nonetheless, it is important for the patient to seek consultation with her nurse-midwife in the event of changes in the menstrual pattern.

Dysmenorrhea and premenstrual syndrome. Approximately 50 percent of women complain of menstrual pain during their lifetime.[66] Understandably, many seek medical consultation for this problem. There are two types of dysmenorrhea, primary and secondary. Primary dysmenorrhea is the development of painful menstruation within a few years of the menarche. It occurs in the absence of any underlying organic pathology. Secondary dysmenorrhea begins later in life and occurs as a result of pelvic pathology such as polyps, fiboids, pelvic inflammatory disease, endometriosis, and benign tumors. This discussion will focuse on primary dysmenorrhea.

Utilize the pelvic examination to teach the consenting woman about the location of her pelvic organs. Guide her hands over the abdomen as you help her identify the uterus and the general location of the adnexae. By using a mirror during the speculum exam, the woman is instructed in the location and appearance of the cervix, vagina, and external genitalia. After this instruction she will probably be better able to describe where discomfort occurs during dysmenorrhea or during any potentially abnormal pain.

Women must know of the normality of their complaint and the causes of dysmenorrhea. Explain that only recently studies have linked certain substances, prostaglandins, in the blood of ovulating women with symptoms of dysmenorrhea.[61,62] Inform the patient that when all supportive comfort measures fail, pharmacologic therapy may be considered when treating cases of unusual distress due to dysmenorrhea. This does not usually require the use of oral contraceptives, strong analgesics, or tranquilizers; antiprostaglandins may be used instead. Findings from several studies have shown that not only have antiprostaglandins aided in decreasing pain and disability, but they have also relieved the associated symptoms of nausea, vomiting, diarrhea, syncope, and flushing.[35,39] Inform your patient that aspirin is a mild antiprostaglandin and may prove to be helpful in some cases. Encourage her to make an appointment to discuss her particular complaint so that you may evaluate whether it is truly primary dysmenorrhea or another problem requiring evaluation and treatment.

Comfort measures must be suggested. In a study conducted by Ben-Menachem, relaxation therapy was utilized to treat ten high-school–aged girls suffering from dysmenorrhea. It was found that the treatment group experienced a significant decrease in complaints of symptoms of cramps, nausea, difficulty in concentrating, feelings of being unambitious, and irritability.[5]

The use of massage, heat, warm liquids, increased sleep, orgasm, yoga, meditation, and diet alterations may be suggested. The dietary approach includes a decrease in foods high in sodium, and an increase in natural diuretics. A natural diuretic effect is found in vitamin B. This improves the hepatic removal of estrogen, and helps by abolishing fatigue and tension. An increase in protein also may help. Teas made with the following herbs—either alone or in combination—are suggested to decrease cramps: golden seal root, red raspberry, black cokosh, queen of the meadow, marshmallow root, blessed thistle, lobelia, capsicum, and ginger.[40]

Symptoms in addition to pain may be noted, and these are now diagnosed as the premenstrual syndrome. All women who have experienced any of these symptoms are happy to know that the symptoms finally are recognized as a syndrome. Explain to your patient that, just as the name signifies, the premenstrual syndrome begins before the onset of menstruation. Reassure her that the supportive measures previously mentioned will also be helpful. Inform her that any of the following physical symptoms are reported to have been experienced during the premenstrual syndrome: lower abdominal pain, lower back discomfort, headaches, weight gain, bloating, insomnia, fatigue, breast tenderness and swelling, mild pelvic discomfort, diarrhea, anorexia, nausea, and thigh pain. This is not an all-inclusive list. In addition to the physical symptoms, she may also experience an apprehensive feeling of mental and emotional tension leading to anxiety, depression, and irritability.

The premenstrual syndrome usually presents about 3–7 days before onset of the period yet may occur as early as 10–14 days before menstruation. It usually peaks 24–48 hours before the menses and subsides in the same length of time after menses begin. Explain that this syndrome may occur from menarche to menopause. It usually begins mildly in adolescence and becomes full blown after 35 years of age.[30] The nurse-midwife may wish to discuss the suspected etiology of this syndrome with those women who are interested. It is thought to result from excessive sodium and fluid retention secondary to an altered estrogen–progesterone balance.

Breasts

All women must be taught how to conduct breast self-examination (BSE), and which findings require professional assessment. The woman must be motivated to perform any self-evaluation technique. The nurse-midwife's challenge is to motivate a woman to perform BSE on a regular basis, utilize the correct technique, and seek professional assessment when indicated.

The climate of the teaching interaction should be positive and non-judgmental. As Varney suggests, BSE may be quickly and thoroughly taught during an office visit while the nurse-midwife conducts the patients' breast examination.[99] This approach is perhaps most frequently used by nurse-midwives precisely because of the ease with which it works into the visit and the affordability of a systematic approach to teaching. Findings from a study of 180 lower socioeconomic women attending a southeastern urban clinic demonstrated that a teaching program employing the one-to-one instruction method of BSE with return demonstration yielded a significantly greater increase in BSE knowledge and exam accuracy. A marked improvement was noted in the subjects' ability to correctly answer questions on proper positioning of the examining hand and feeling the axillary areas for lumps. Additionally, the women improved in regularly checking the nipples for discharge and knowing the most appropriate time for BSE.[56]

The nurse-midwife approaching the discussion of BSE must find out more about the individual woman's experience with breast disease. Questioning about relevant family health history, breast disease among friends and any previous personal experience of breast disease may be helpful in detecting cancerphobia, the abnormal fear of cancer. Cancerphobia may inhibit her from performing regular BSEs or acting on abnormal findings. Since society treats the breast with such great sexual symbolism, the thought of breast removal due to cancer may present an overwhelming picture of mutilation. Among the incidental findings of the study previously mentioned, the researchers found that 31 percent of the 180 subjects revealed when questioned that they would choose the loss of a limb over the loss of a breast.[56]

While teaching BSE and attempting to motivate the patient to self-monitor her health status, the nurse-midwife may also discuss topics such as the woman's previous experiences with BSE, scientific facts regarding breast disease, when and how the exam should be done, demonstrating what to look and feel for during the exam, and what to do if abnormal or irregular findings are discovered. The nurse-midwife may ask the patient to demonstrate BSE and to verbalize important instructions.

Inquiring about whether or not the patient already performs the exam, and if so, requesting a demonstration of her technique, will provide the nurse-midwife with valuable information. It is always best to begin with the technique the woman uses and improve upon it when indicated. The areas that appear to be most frequently lacking in a woman's self-exam are inspection, proper hand technique, nipple evaluation, under arm palpation, and selection of the most appropriate time in the cycle to conduct the exam.

The BSE teaching session should include an explanation of the need for regularly conducted BSE. The nurse-midwife may wish to stress that the earlier cancer is detected and treatment instituted, the better the prognosis. In the early stages cancer is confined to the breast in about one-half of all cases. The curability of breast cancer therefore is likely when the lesion is small and the disease is still in an early stage.

It should also be stressed that not all breast lumps are cancerous, and that evaluation of a lump and rapid diagnosis is more readily available today than ever before. Cystic breast disease is the most common cause of palpable breast nodules and the etiology is unknown. The annual rate of breast cancer among women with cystic breast disease is 2.8/1000 person years. Characteristics of cystic breast disease may include the following:[29]

1. Nodules appear firm, mobile, and well defined on palpation.
2. Nodules may or may not be tender.
3. Nodules commonly appear premenstrually, with cyclic changes in growth caused by estrogen stimulation.
4. Nodules are usually multiple in number and bilateral in location.
5. Nodules infrequently present before 25 years of age, and peak in occurrence from 35–50 years of age.
6. Nodules occur most frequently on the left breast, located in the upper outer quadrant followed in frequency by the upper inner quadrant.

The timing of the exam, with respect to the menstrual cycle, is important. Most accurate results will be obtained shortly after the menstrual period since most women experience normal breast tenderness and lumpy quality on palpation premenstrually. This is thought to be caused by an imbalanced cyclical secretion of estrogen and progesterone.[29] According to Ajao the large breast is best evaluated at about the eighth day of the beginning of the menstrual cycle, because at this time the breast attains its smallest size during the cycle.[1] It is suggested that women who are not menstruating should examine their breasts at the first of each month in order to establish a routine. Changes are more easily detected by conducting BSE at the same time each month.

The woman should also be alerted about frequently encountered normal breast variations. During the patient's breast examination, in order to prevent any future alarm or anxiety, it is important to point out normal breast variations which may include:

1. one breast slightly larger than the other
2. accessory breast tissue
3. inverted nipples
4. rib protrusions
5. bilateral crescent shaped pads at the caudal end of the breast
6. fine nodularity evenly noted throughout the breast tissue
7. cyclic tenderness noted premenstrually

In teaching the technique of BSE the nurse-midwife and the woman may find it most helpful to keep the instructions complete but simple. Three parts of the BSE should be reinforced—inspection, palpation, and timing of the exam. After demonstrating the technique, suggest that the patient demonstrate BSE and use this opportunity to correct any errors and reinforce important points. Some women find it helpful to take home a written explanation to reinforce their learning. This is also a means of spreading information in the community since daughters, sisters, mothers, and grandmothers may choose to read your patient's pamphlet. The American Cancer Society provides useful pamphlets free of charge.

Early Detection of Pregnancy

The earliest possible detection of pregnancy is critical for various reasons. It is important for the pregnant woman to avoid certain medications, drugs, smoking, or diagnostic tests such as x-ray to safeguard the health of the unborn child. Early detection of an unwanted pregnancy may also offer the option of a safer, more accessible, and less costly termination if elected by an appropriately counseled woman. Early discontinued use of the IUD or oral contraceptives are necessary. The IUD has been linked in early pregnancy with the complications of spontaneous abortion and infection. Oral contraceptives have been known to cause congenital anomalies. Proper nutritional practices and the timely initiation of prenatal care are additionally important and reinforce the need for individuals to know when pregnancy is suspected and how to seek help.

Written information provided in the clinic or office and discussions with patients about the presumptive signs of pregnancy and the importance of seeking early consultation are valuable services. The earliest presumptive signs of pregnancy a woman may notice and should be instructed to observe for include the following:

1. cessation of menses
2. marked change in character of the menses
3. nausea and vomiting
4. frequency of urination
5. breast tingling, tenderness, or enlargement
6. nipple enlargement and increased pigmentation
7. increased fatigue
8. basal body temperature remains elevated
9. a positive home pregnancy test

Pelvic and Lower Abdominal Pain

It is probably safe to say that women usually seek medical consultation when acute pelvic or lower abdominal pain occurs. We know that problems may exist even with mild pain. Abnormal pelvic and lower abdominal pain can be detected more easily when women have been taught—during office visits or women's health classes—the basics of their anatomy, recognition of their normal menstrual pattern, and basic reproductive physiology. Patients should be prepared to notice where they are in their cycle when pain occurs, to evaluate potential precipitating physical or emotional causative factors, and to detect side effects of certain contraceptive methods.

The nurse-midwife who establishes a comfortable and therapeutic rapport with her patients makes the initial contact for the woman much easier. The woman feels welcome to call. She knows that the nurse-midwife will respond to her questions and concerns with interest and concern. A woman who is not well prepared to recognize her body's signals will find that the open and supportive attitude of her nurse-midwife makes a difficult experience more tolerable.

In the presence of pelvic or lower abdominal pain, the woman should be directed to come to the clinic or office for evaluation. Delaying evaluation and assistance may be dangerous. Once the nurse-midwife reviews common questions of historical importance the problem may be easily detected. If a diagnosis is not readily made, a process of elimination is used. When screening, the nurse-midwife collects a complete history, performs the necessary physical assessment, orders appropriate lab studies and consults with the physician. The physician may make the final diagnosis.

Explain to the patient that when pain symptoms occur it is important to review all possible causes which may include menstrual disorders, tumors of the reproductive system, urinary tract infections, sexually transmitted diseases, pelvic infection, a complication of the contraceptive method used, complications of early pregnancy, and other medical complications. Inform her that a blood count may be requested to note the presence and extent of any infectious disease.

Additional diagnostic tests may be necessary. A urine culture and sensitivity assist in ruling out an infection of the urinary tract and guide in the selection of antibiotic therapy. A gonorrhea culture detects the presence of this infection so that treatment can begin and the partner can be contacted. Microscopic evaluation of vaginal secretions may be needed to screen for certain vaginal infections which cause mild symptoms. For all women of reproductive age, a pregnancy test is critical in ruling out life-threatening circumstances of early pregnancy complications. Pelvic and abdominal ultrasound evaluation are helpful in screening for tumors, appendicitis, intact gestation, lost intrauterine device, or ectopic pregnancy. Finally, a Pap smear, if not recently obtained, may be indicated to screen for abnormal cytologic findings. If an accurate diagnosis is made based on the initial history and physical exam, this battery of tests will not be necessary. Yet, a combination of the above-mentioned tests may provide helpful information and safe evaluation.

The most acute problems require physician management and hospitalization. When infections are diagnosed a return office visit for repeat testing is required to ensure a cure. Returning after the next cycle to discuss the success or failure of supportive comfort measures and the possible need for pharmacologic therapy is indicated when menstrual disorders occur. When complications arise from the use of a particular contraceptive method, a discontinuation of that method may be necessary. Discontinuation of a method requires counseling in the selection of an acceptable, new method.

Sexually Transmitted Diseases

Today there is a wider range of sexually transmitted diseases (STD) than ever before recognized. These diseases are transmitted by an infected person during sexual contact. The following discussion will deal with several of the most well known infections—Gonorrhea, syphilis, and herpes simplex virus type 2.

Self-monitoring of health status is particularly important for the early detection of sexually transmitted disease for early cure, to avoid more severe health complications, and also to arrest the continued spread of STDs.

The most sexually active age group, 15–30 years old, is the population at greatest risk. Since the majority of women the nurse-midwife cares for fall within this age range, the focus on preparing women for early disease detection, treatment, and prevention is of particular importance. Furthermore, the vast and increasing number of infected people, estimated at over 10 million per year, signal that the STD problem is out of control.

Gonorrhea.   Gonorrhea, a gram-negative intracellular diplococci bacteria, known as *Neisseria gonorrhea*, has an incubation period of 2−6 days. It is difficult to control because in the early stages of the disease 50−80 percent of the infected women are symptom free. Once the disease progresses untreated, the woman experiences acute distress.

With changing attitudes toward sexual expression, new syndromes have begun and resulted in gonococcal organisms isolated from the body in other than genitourinary sites. Teaching a woman the traditional symptoms, if present at all, may therefore be insufficient. Table 7-6 lists the diverse symptoms of gonorrhea which each woman should be taught to recognize and to contact her nurse-midwife if any occur.

Table 7-6
Gonorrhea Symptoms that Patients Should Recognize

Early Symptoms

Urethritis and cervicitis
   Discomfort on urination, bladder irritability
   Profuse, creamy, thick, irritating urethral and vaginal discharge
   Vulvar pruritis

Proctitis
   Rectal itching, pain
   Mucoid or bloody rectal discharge
   Rectal pressure
   Diarrhea

Pharyngitis (transmitted by fellatio rather than kissing)
   Inflammed throat with or without purulent exudate
   Painful cervical lymphadenopathy

Conjuctivitis (resulting from direct contamination by a primary genital site)
   Purulent discharge from one or both eyes
   Inflammation, itching, burning of one or both eyes

Symptom descriptions of the more rare complications of untreated gonorrheal infections—arthritis-dermatitis syndrome, monoarticular septic arthritis, meningitis, and endocarditis—will not be discussed in this chapter. For the reader interested in pursuing this information, several references cited give descriptions of the disease processes, diagnostic procedures and treatment modalities recommended.[3,14,25,93]

The woman should be cautioned not to resume sexual intercourse until the disease has been cured. Varney suggests a series of three follow-up cultures, beginning 1−2 weeks after treatment, in order to evaluate whether or not the treatment has been effective.[82] Furthermore, it is important for the patient to know that she should not resume sexual activity with her previous partner until his treatment and cure have been completed.

Syphilis.   In 1978 an estimated 400,000 people in the United States were believed to have undetected and untreated syphilis.[96] Syphilis is caused by an organism known as *Treponema pallidum*. Evidence of the infection may not become apparent until 3–4 weeks after direct genital or oral–genital contact. The patients should be notified not only of the presenting symptoms of primary and secondary syphilis (see Table 7-7) but also of the importance of treatment for herself and her partner. She may also be informed that consultation with the nurse-midwife as well as the physician may be required since nurse-midwifery protocol varies in each setting.

Early detection and successful treatment is critical to avoid progressive disease causing systemic infection; damage to the brain, heart, and other vital organs; and possibly death. If undetected and untreated, syphilis infections will spread to others.

Table 7-7
Primary and Second-Stage Syphilis Symptoms that Patients Should Recognize

Primary stage	Secondary stage
Pimple or wart-like sore which becomes larger and surrounded by a zone of induration	Rashes and sores on other parts of the body
	Sore throat
Chancre—usually located on the labia majora, cervix, or external genitalia and causes no pain or itching	Hair falling out in patches
	Fevers
	Headaches
Chancre disappears in a few weeks	Condylomata
Leukorrheal discharge	Malaise
Abnormal bleeding in cases of cervical involvement	
Bilateral lymphadenopathy	

Herpes simplex virus.   Herpes simplex virus type 2 is incurable and is second only to gonorrhea as the most common STD.[27] There are occasions, however, when this disease may be spread not only by sexual intercourse. An estimated 300,000 new cases of genital herpes are reported each year, according to government health officials,[85] and adolescents and young single adults are most affected.

Herpetic lesions appearing below the waist were previously diagnosed as type 2 herpes simplex, and those above the waist were diagnosed as type 1. Type 1 herpes simplex is the cause of "fever blisters" and "cold sores". With changing mores in sexual expression, however, the herpetic lesions may present in various bodily locations.

When preparing patients to call in for consultation, the nurse-midwife must give the facts about herpes simplex virus type 2, the most important of which are shown in Table 7-8.

Health care providers should make specific safety tips available for all women to avoid the contraction and spread of STDs (Table 7-9).

Sexual Disorders

Two of the most frequently encountered complaints made by women regarding sexual function are dyspareunia and the inability to achieve or-

Table 7-8
Symptoms and Characteristics of Herpes Simplex Virus Type 2

Information for Patient

The symptoms appear within 3-7 days and sometimes in less than 24 hours after initial exposure.
Lesion
    Fluid-filled sores that look like blisters or severe ulcers, lasting from 1−4 weeks
Sensation
    Pain, burning, itching
Location
    Vagina, cervix, labia, vulva, buttocks, upper-inner thigh, anus, or mouth
Other symptoms
    Fever, enlarged lymph glands near the lesion, painful urination, flu-like symptoms, vaginal pain, pain on intercourse, increased vaginal discharge, headaches, or abnormal bleeding
Contagious
    While sores are open and wet, can be passed to other people or other areas of her body
Recurrence
    Outbreak at times of physical or emotional stress; prolonged intercourse; during menstruation
Number of outbreaks
    Limitless
Cure
    None
Symptomatic treatment
    Surface anesthetics, oral analgesics, sulfa creams to prevent infection of the sores, lubricated tampon placed between lips of affected labia
Tests
    Cytology smear and culture of sores, serologic tests for type I and II antibodies, screening for related diseases of hemophilus, trichomonas, gonorrhea, and syphilis
Future complications
    Linked with cancer of the cervix; pregnancy at risk for spontaneous abortion, and risk of cesarean birth to avoid fetal morbidity and mortality if infection is active

Table 7-9
Measures to Avoid Contraction and Spread of STDs

Information for Patient

Avoid casual sex unless condoms are used for protection from STDs.

Avoid having sex with someone who is suspicious of being infected.

Urinate and wash with soap and water after intercourse.

Ask the nurse-midwife about the correct use of condoms.

If an STD is diagnosed notify all sexual partners so that they may seek treatment and take measures to avoid spreading the disease.

Maintain good physical condition—get enough sleep, exercise, and eat a well-balanced diet.

Require sex partners to be clean.

Observe male partner's lips, mouth, and genitals for sores, reddened areas, warts, or discharge from an unerect penis.

Ask the nurse-midwife about certain vaginal creams, foams, and suppositories which may give some protection against STDs.

gasm. The nurse-midwife encountering patients with these complaints must be able to identify possible causes, provide appropriate treatment, offer suggestions for supportive measures, and initiate appropriate referrals when indicated.

The American Medical Association suggests that there are three types of dyspareunia: pain on entry, pain during coitus, and pain after coitus.[9] Pain on entry may be caused by any number of conditions. It may be due to vaginismus, which is a strong, involuntary tightening of the vaginal wall causing a spasm at the outer one-third of the vagina. This condition makes penetration very uncomfortable. Vaginismus may occur as a result of strong conflicts, fears, or negative conditioning about sexual intercourse. For women who experience vaginismus, suggesting a well-qualifed therapist may be helpful. In addition to therapy and counseling the following suggestions may aid the woman and her partner in attempting to alleviate discomfort:

1. Practice relaxation techniques.
2. Avoid penetration until maximal vaginal lubrication is achieved.
3. Use additional lubricants if necessary (vaginal creams, jellies, or saliva).
4. Use the superior position during intercourse to control depth and speed of penetration.

A vaginal or pelvic infection will also cause discomfort during intercourse. Vaginal infections such as monilia or trichomonas are particularly irritating to the introitus and vaginal wall. The friction of the penis against the vaginal wall or introitus becomes abrasive and causes an increase in the symptoms of burning and itching. Motion of the cervix during intercourse initiates deep pelvic pain in the presence of a pelvic infection.

It is possible for barrier methods along with foams, jellies, or creams to cause an allergic reaction creating local inflammation and irritation. Again, itching, burning, or pain especially during intercourse may signal the presence of a problem of this type.

Dyspareunia may also occur when adequate vaginal lubrication is missing. Certain circumstances may precipitate the lack or insufficient amount of vaginal lubrication, such as emotional stress, hormonal deficiency as seen in menopausal women or after birth in nursing mothers with diminished estrogen, painful episiotomy, and beginning penetration before sexual excitement is adequate. Relaxation, penetration after attaining adequate excitation, the use of additional lubrication, or altered positions are helpful supportive measures.

Dyspareunia during deep penetration may be caused by previous obstetric trauma to the ligaments, traumatic sexual intercourse, pelvic infection, endometriosis, cysts, or tumors. In the absence of disease, a simple change in position, open communication with the partner, and less vigorous sexual practices may alleviate the problem.

In the past, the inability to experience orgasm was described in medical texts as one aspect of frigidity. Since Master's and Johnson's research,[54a] much has been learned about the female response during sexual interaction. For instance, pain described as a vague ache in the lower abdomen and pelvic area occuring immediately following intercourse is now thought to be caused by vasocongestion. We have learned that effective supportive, comfort, and communication techniques are quite helpful in assisting couples with these problems. Your patient may find the suggestions in Table 7-10 helpful.

Table 7-10
Suggestions for the Patient Experiencing Dyspareunia or Inability to Achieve Orgasm

Self-Help Techniques

Explore and touch your body to aid in learning the location of sexual pleasure sites.
Practice bringing yourself to orgasm through masturbation.
Plan time for relaxed and undisturbed sexual interaction with your partner.
Concentrate totally on the sensations you are feeling.
Recall previous erotic or stimulating experiences.
Recall the sensation of previous orgasm if possible.
Do not repress sexual response.
Do not be afraid to ask your partner to stimulate you as best you know how.
Do not be rushed into penetration until you are adequately excited.
Communicate openly with your partner about the importance of being patient.
Provide your partner with the pleasurable sensations he seeks.
Be open to sexual experimentation as long as it is not painful or physically traumatic.
Remember the goal is mutual pleasuring and not necessarily orgasm.

Whenever dyspareunia or the inability to achieve orgasm occurs, women should be encouraged to seek consultation with their nurse-midwife. Causative problems may then be identified, treated, and supportive measures suggested. If in-depth problems are experienced, the nurse-midwife may wish to refer the woman to a certified sex therapist.

Complications of Contraceptive Methods

The nurse-midwife should prepare the patient to know, recognize, and seek help when complications of the selected contraceptive method occur. Because the nurse-midwife depends on the woman to take an active role in this aspect of her care, educational needs must be carefully considered. In addition to explanation and discussion during the office visit, a printed guide is helpful to reinforce the instruction. A guide may be helpful in several respects; it may point out that no method is perfect, some complications are more serious than others, back-up and alternative methods should be considered, and when professional help must be sought. The nurse-midwife's name and clinic, as well as her office or emergency telephone number, should also appear on the guide. An example of this type of guide is suggested in Table 7-11.

Available Resources for Meeting Individual Needs

Patients seek nurse-midwifery care for a variety of reasons. Discussing women's health related issues, including intimate problems of receiving support and health services from a professional provider who focuses on health maintenance, are only a few of the reasons. In attempting to meet these needs we find it difficult to be "all things to all people." At times appropriate referrals to professional organizations, peer support, and self-help groups geared toward a particular problem, need, or interest is truly indicated. Each office or clinic must have a listing of the most appropriate resources and referrals for women's health in the community or major cities nearby. These may provide patients with the opportunity to participate on a variety of levels—as a receiver of services, by working on committees that support community services, or by establishing self-help groups.

Some of the more well-known organizations to be included in such a list may be the nearest office of the American Cancer Society and their Reach to Recovery program for pre- and postoperative support services, the American Red Cross, the local offices of the county board of health. Planned Parenthood, or the National Organization for Women. The national offices of less well-known organizations dealing with specific areas of need may be contacted in order to secure the addresses and telephone numbers of local chapters. The list of organizations in Table 7-12 may be helpful.

Table 7-11

Guide to the Early Detection of Problems Associated with Certain Contraceptive Methods — For Patient Information

If you are using one of these contraceptive methods and you have any of the symptoms listed below your method, follow the instructions listed under "What To Do." Certain complications require that you switch to another method. Discuss with your partner and nurse-midwife which methods would be best for you in case a change is necessary.

Condoms, Foams, Jellies, Creams, or Suppositories	Diaphragm	IUD	Pill
Symptoms			
1. Itching, soreness, or redness on the lips or skin outside the vagina	1. Irritation in the vagina causing pain or burning	1. Very heavy vaginal bleeding lasting days longer than your normal period, and spotting between periods	1. Severe headaches
2. Recent discomfort during sex	2. Pain in the pelvis, cramps	2. Severe abdominal back or pelvic pain	2. Changes in your vision (blurring, flashing lights, spots, moments of blindness)
	3. Painful urination	3. Missed period	3. Chest pain or shortness of breath
	4. Pressure on your bladder	4. Discharge with very bad odor	4. Severe abdominal pain
	5. Pain during sex	5. Fever, chills, nausea, vomiting	5. Severe leg pain (calves or thighs)
	6. Vaginal discharge having a foul odor	6. Pain during sex	6. Temporary numbness or paralysis anywhere
		7. Unable to feel string	7. Severe depression
			8. One missed menstrual period

(continued)

Table 7-11 (continued)

	Condoms, Foams, Jellies, Creams, or Suppositories	Diaphragm	IUD	Pill
Possible problem (nos. given in parentheses correspond to symptom above)	(1) Allergy to either the rubber in the condom or to the jelly, foam, or suppository (2) Aggravation of the irritated tissue in the vagina or on the perineum; vaginal or pelvic infection	(1) Allergy to the rubber in the diaphragm or to the cream or jelly used (1,2,3,4,5) Diaphragm may not fit correctly; pelvic, bladder or vaginal infection (6) Vaginal infection; left diaphragm in too long — remove and clean it every 24– 48 hours	(1) IUD may be falling out, pelvic infection, tumors present (2) Pelvic infection, IUD in the abdomen instead of the uterus, tumors or cysts present, tubal pregnancy (3) Pregnancy (4,5) Pelvic, bladder or vaginal infection (6) Pelvic or vaginal infection; misplaced IUD (7) Short string or lost IUD in abdomen	(1) High blood pressure, migraine, stroke (2) High blood pressure, stroke (3) Blood clot in lungs or heart attack (4) Gallbladder disease, liver tumors, blood clot, inflammation of the pancreas (5) Blood clot in the lung (6) Stroke (7) Vitamin deficiency (B_6) (8) Pregnancy

What To Do			
Try switching brands of foam, jelly, cream, or suppository. Stop using these methods. Sit in a hot tub 2—3 times a day. Don't use vaginal sprays. Make an appointment to see the nurse-midwife. Don't douche for at least 2 days before your appointment. The nurse-midwife will examine you, help you select an acceptable form of contraception, and possibly take several specimens for laboratory tests (microscopic exam of vaginal discharge, gonorrhea culture).	Call your nurse-midwife for an appointment. Postpone having sex until after your appointment. Drink lots of liquids. You may need a new diaphragm of a different size or rim type. You will be examined for other possible problems like pelvic, vaginal, or bladder infections. Don't douche for 2 days before your appointment. During your examination, certain tests may be ordered: urine culture, gonorrhea culture, microscopic exam of vaginal secretions.	Call for an immediate appointment to see the nurse-midwife. Don't have sex if you are uncomfortable. If you think you have an infection, extra bleeding or can't feel the string, have your partner wear a condom. Don't douche before the appointment. In cases of heavy bleeding, possible infection, pregnancy, or pain you will probably be given an appointment for the same day you call. In cases of a lost string or discomfort during sex, you will probably be asked to come in within several days. During your examination certain tests may be ordered: Complete blood count, gonorrhea culture, pap smear, pregnancy test, ultrasound, microscopic exam of vaginal secretions, x-ray (if not pregnant and ultrasound not available). The IUD may be removed at this time. Consider which method you would like to use if the IUD is removed.	Call immediately; you will be given an appointment to be seen that same day. These symptoms are serious and life threatening. Do not continue to take your pills until an answer to your problem is found. Discuss with your partner and nurse-midwife other methods you would like to use if you must stop taking the pill.

Table 7-12
Informational Organizations for Patient Resources

Organization

Population Dynamics
  Zero Population Growth
  1314 Connecticut Avenue, N.W.
  Washington, D.C. 20036
  202-785-0100

Pro-Life/Birth Rights Groups
  Call local office of Catholic Charities or National Conference of Catholic Bishops
  Pro-Life Office
  202-659-6673

Infertility, Pre-Adoption, Child-Free Living
  "Resolve"
  P.O. Box 474
  Belmont, Massachusetts 02178
  617-484-2424
  Organization with local chapters providing counseling, medical and social referrals
    and peer group support services

Sexually Transmitted Diseases
  National Operation Venus Hotline
  800-523-1885
  National Hotline for Venereal Diseases
  800-227-8922
  Counseling and referral services

Women's Health Networking
  National Women's Mailing List
  1195 Valencia Street
  San Francisco, California 94110
  415-824-6800
  This organization provides membership or one time service for a very small fee.
    Computerized information is available on resources, providers of services, peer
    and self-help programs, women and culture, sports, legal assistance, women and
    violence, minority women, and health. Health information includes abortion,
    contraception, mental health, sterilization, drugs and alcohol, holistic health care,
    herbology, alternative care providers, pregnancy, and childbirth.

REFERENCES

1. Ajao OG: Benign breast lesions. J Natl Med Assoc 71:867−868, 1979
2. Allen F: Cultural attitudes toward contraception: A Tower of Babel, in Keith L, Kent D, Berger G, et al: The Safety of Fertility Control. New York, Springer, 1980, pp 35−41
3. Aurelian L: Genital herpes update. Fem Patient 11:19−25, 1979
4. Beasley WB: Coping with family planning in a rural area. Obstet Gynecol 41:155, 1973
5. Ben-Menachem M: Treatment of dysmenorrhea: A relaxation therapy program. Int J Gynaecol Obstet 17:340−342, 1980
6. Bibb BN: The effectiveness of non-physicians as providers of family planning services. JOGN Nurs 8:137−143, 1979
7. Burlow H: The condom and gonorrhea. Lancet 2:811−812, 1977
8. Britt SQ: Fertility awareness: Four methods of natural family planning. JOGN Nurs 6:9−17, 1977
9. Committee on Human Sexuality: Problems of Female Sexual Response in Human Sexuality. New York, American Medical Association, 1972
10. Curtis EM: Oral contraceptive feminization of a normal male infant. Obstet Gynecol 23:295, 1964
11. Cutright P: The teenage sexual revolution and the myth of an abstinent past. Fam Plann Perspect 4:24−31, 1972
12. DeLora J, Warren C: Sexuality and social process, in DeLora J, Warren C: Understanding Sexual Interaction. Boston, Houghton Mifflin, 1977, pp 105−129
13. DeLora J, Warren C: Incestuous and monogamous sexual interactions, in DeLora J, Warren C: Understanding Sexual Interaction. Boston, Houghton Mifflin, 1977, pp 243−267
14. Diagnosis and treatment of syphilis. ACOG Tech Bull 30:1−8, 1975
15. Dickey RP: Managing Contraceptive Pill Patients (ed 2). Minneapolis, Anderberg-Lund Printing, 1980
16. Doll R: The long-term effects of steroid contraceptives. J Biosoc Sci 2:376−389, 1970
17. Dosseter J: Drug interactions with oral contraceptives. Br Med J 11:467−467, 1975
18. Edmonson HA, Henderson B, Benton B: Liver cell adenomas associated with the use of oral contraceptives. N Engl J Med 294:471−472, 1979
19. Elder N: Natural family planning: The ovulation method. J Nurs Mid 23:25−30, 1978
20. Eurad J, Burton B, Erickson D: Amenorrhea following oral contraception. Am J Obstet Gynecol 124:88, 1976
21. Fasal E, Paffenbarger RS: Oral contraceptives as related to cancer and benign lesions of the breast. J Nat Cancer Inst 55:767−773, 1975
22. Felman Y: A plea for the condom, especially for teenagers. JAMA 241:2517−2518, 1979
23. Fleckstein L, Joubert J, Lawrence R, et al: Oral contraceptive patient information. JAMA 235:1331−1336, 1976

24. Freeman EW, Huggins GR, Mudd EH, et al: Adolescent contraceptive use: Comparisons of male and female attitudes and information. Am J Public Health 70:790−797, 1980
25. Garagusi VF: Gonorrhea in genital and non-genital sites. Fem Patient 3:14−17, 1978
26. Gibbs R: The IUD and PID: Is the contraceptive the culprit? Contemp OB-GYN 11:163−167, 1978
27. Gordon S, Scales P, Everly K: Sexually Transmitted Diseases, in The Sexual Adolescent, Communicating With Teenagers About Sex (ed 2). North Scituate, Duxbury Press, 1979, pp 109−122
28. Gorline LL: Teaching successful use of the diaphragm. Am J Nurs 10:1732−1735, 1979
29. Gray MJ: The reproductive years, in Romney SL, Gray MJ, Little AB, et al: Gynecology and Obstetrics. The Health Care of Women (ed 2). New York, McGraw-Hill, 1981, pp 412−434
30. Green TH: Functional menstrual disorders, in Green TH: Essentials of Clinical Practice (ed 3). Boston, Little, Brown and Company, 1977, pp 145−181
31. Green TH: Pelvic inflammatory disorders and venereal diseases, in Green TH: Essentials of Clinical Practice (ed 3). Boston, Little, Brown and Company, 1977, pp 247−283
32. Green TH: Disorders of pelvic support, in Green TH: Essentials of Clinical Practice (ed 3). Boston, Little, Brown and Company, 1977, pp 539−564
33. Green TH: Premarital examination, marital counseling, and conception control, in Green TH: Essentials of Clinical Practice (ed 3). Boston, Little, Brown and Company, 1977, pp 577−605
34. Guttmacher Institute: Planned Births, the Future of the Family, and the Quality of American Life. New York, Planned Parenthood, 1977, pp 12−24
35. Hanson FW: Naproxen sodium in dysmenorrhea—its influence in allowing continuation of work/school activity. Obstet Gynecol 52:583−587, 1978
36. Hatcher RA, Stewart GK, Stewart FS, et al: The condom, in Hatcher RA, Stewart GK, Stewart FS, et al: Contraceptive Technology 1980−1981. New York, Irvington Publishers, 1980, pp 86−90
37. Hatcher RA, Stewart GK, Stewart FS, et al: Abortion, in Hatcher RA, Stewart GK, Stewart FS, et al: Contraceptive Technology 1980−1981. New York, Irvington Publishers, 1980, pp 139−156
38. Hatcher RA, Stewart GK, Stewart FS, et al: Sterlization, in Hatcher RA, Stewart GK, Stewart FS, et al: Contraceptive Technology 1980−1981. New York, Irvington Publishers, 1980, pp 157−173
39. Henzl MR: The treatment of dysmenorrhea with neproxen sodium: A report on two independent double-blind trials. Am J Obstet Gynecol 127:818−823, 1977
40. Herb Reference Guide: BiWorld Publishers, 1979, pp 1−13
41. Hunt M: Sexual Behavior in the 1970's. Chicago, Playboy Press, 1974, pp 186−195
42. Inman WH, Vessey MP, Westerholm B, et al: Thromboembolic diseases and the steroidal content of oral contraceptives. Br Med J 2:203−209, 1970
43. Janz D, Schmidt D: Anti-epileptic drugs and failure of oral contraceptives. Lancet 1:1133, 1974

44. Jensen, MD, Bensen RC, Bobak IM: Genetics and genetic counseling, in Jensen MD, Bensen RC, Bobak IM: Maternity Care, The Nurse and the Family. Saint Louis, Mosby, 1977

45. Jick J, Dinan B, Rothman K: Oral contraception and nonfatal myocardial infarction. JAMA 239:1403–1406, 1978

46. Kapstrom AB: How long dare I put off having a baby? RN 9:61–64, 1980

47. Katchadourian HA, Lunde D: Sex and morality, in Katchadourian HA: Fundamentals of Human Sexuality (ed 2). New York, Holt, Rinehart and Winston, 1975, pp 527–553

48. Kerwin DR: Nutritional concerns for women, in Kerwin DR: Maternal Infant and Child Nutrition. North Carolina, Health Sciences Consortium, 1981, pp 1–38

49. Kistner RW: The pill and IUD: Not perfect but still the best we have. Mod Med 42:36–44, 1974

50. Lenton EA, Weston GA, Cooke ID: Problems in using basal body temperature recording in an infertility clinic. Br Med J 1:803–805, 1977

51. Lesak-Gorline L: Teaching successful use of the diaphragm. Am J Nurs 10:1732–1735

52. Liebow E: Tally's Corner. Boston, Little, Brown and Company, 1967, 14–32

53. Manisoff M, Tyrer LB: The nurse practitioner's role in family planning, in Keith LG (ed): The Safety of Fertility Control. New York, Springer, 1980, pp 27–34

54. Manisoff M: Impact of family planning nurse practitioners. JOGN Nurs 8:73–77, 1979

54A. Masters WH, Johnson VE: Female Orgasm, in: Human Sexual Response. Boston, Little, Brown and Co., 1966, pp 127–140

55. McCusker MP: The subfertile couple. JOGN Nurs 11:157–162, 1982

56. McLendon MS, Fulk C, Starnes D: Effectiveness of breast self-examination teaching to women of low socioeconomic class. JOGN Nurs 11:7–10, 1982

57. Moghissi KS: Accuracy of basal body temperature for ovulation detection. Fertility Sterility 27:1415–1421, 1976

58. Morton JH: Experience with a maternity and infant care project. Am J Obstet Gynecol 3:107, 1970

59. National Center for Health Statistics, Washington, D.C., United States Bureau Digest 2:20, 1978

60. Perez A: First ovulation after childbirth: The effect of breastfeeding. Am J Obstet Gynecol 114:1041, 1972

61. Pickles VR: A plain muscle stimulant in the menstrum. Nature 180:1198, 1957

62. Pickles VR: Prostaglandins in the human endometrium. Int J Fertil 12:335, 1967

63. Planned Parenthood Association—Chicago: Contraception. Chicago, Planned Parenthood Association, 1979

64. Population Institute: Focus: All in the family. Population Issues 3:3–6, 1977

65. Pritchard JA, MacDonald PC: Family planning, in Pritchard JA, MacDonald PC: Williams Obstetrics. New York, Appleton-Century-Crofts, 1980, pp 1015–1016

66. Roberts SJ: Dysmenorrhea. Nur Pract 5:9–10, 1980

67. Roe DA: Nutrition and the contraceptive pill, in Winick M: Nutritional Disorders of American Women. New York, Wiley, 1977, pp 46–52

68. Rosenheim E: Sexual attitudes and regulations in Judaism, in Money J, Musaph H (ed): Handbook of Sexology. New York, Excerpta Medica, 1977, pp 64–80

69. Ross C, Piotrow PT: Birth control without contraceptives. Popul Rep (I) 1:1974
70. Ryan GM, Sweeney PJ: Attitudes of adolescents toward pregnancy and contraception. Am J Obstet Gynecol 137:358–364, 1980
71. Sabagh G: Fertility planning status of Chicano couples in Los Angeles. Am J Public Health 70:56–61, 1980
72. Scanzoni J: Gender roles and process of fertility control. J Marriage Fam 38:687, 1976
73. Serious adverse effects of oral contraceptives and estrogens. Med Letter 18:21–23, 1976
74. Settledge DS, Baroff S, Cooper D: Sexual experience of young teenage girls seeking contraceptive assistance for the first time. Fam Plann Perspect 5:223, 1973
75. Shangold MM: Do women's sports lead to menstrual problems? Contemp OB-GYN 17:52–62, 1979
76. Siegler AM: Applying the new technology for tubal sterilization. Contemp OB-GYN 14:77–80, 1979
77. Singer A, Reid BL: Does the male transmit cervical cancer? Contemp OB-GYN 13:173–180, 1979
78. Skillman TG: Oral contraceptive use: Its risks and benefits. Hosp Formul 8:622–630, 1980
79. Smiciklas-Wright H, Ippolito R, Collins J: Nutrition counseling at planned parenthood centers. Public Health Rep 94:239–242, 1979
80. Spellacy WN: Carbohydrate metabolism in male infertility and female fertility-control patients. Fertil Steril 27:1132, 1976
81. Spellacy WN: Contraception for the high-risk woman. Contemp OB-GYN 14:119–125, 1979
82. Spence MR: Testimony presented to the sexually transmitted disease work group. U.S. Department of Health, Education and Welfare. Washington, D.C., January 10, 1978
83. Speroff L: Infertility in men: What the gynecologist needs to know. Contemp OB-GYN 14:188–200, 1979
84. Sporken P: Marriage and sexual ethics in the Catholic Church, in Money J, Musaph H (ed): Handbook of Sexology. New York, Excerpta Medica, 1977, pp 20–32
85. St. John RK, Jones OG: Nonreported sexually transmitted diseases. Paper presented at American Public Health Association annual meeting, November, 1977
86. Steinman ME, Farr JD: Nurse practitioner acceptance in private OB-GYN practice. JOGN Nurs 9:240–242, 1980
87. Stolley PD, Tonascia JA, Tockman MS, et al: Thrombosis with low-estrogen oral contraceptives. Am J Epidemiol 102:197–208, 1975
88. Stone MT: Female sterilization: The nurse's role. Issues H Care Women 1:45–60, 1979
89. Swan SH, Brown WL: Oral contraceptive use, sexual activity, and cervical carcinoma. Am J Obstet Gynecol 139:52–57, 1981
90. Toddywalla VS, Joshi L, Virkar K: Effect of contraceptive steroids on human lactation. Am J Obstet Gynecol 127:245, 1977

91. Tripp CA: The homosexual matrix. New York, McGraw Hill, 1975, pp 40–46
92. Uhlenberg P: Fertility patterns within the Mexican-American population. Soc Biol 20:30–39, 1973
93. United States Department of Health, Education and Welfare, Public Health Service: VD Fact Sheet 1976 (ed 33). Atlanta, Center for Disease Control, 1977
94. United States Department of Health, Education and Welfare, Medical Device and Drug Advisory Committee on Obstetrics and Gynecology: Second Report on Intrauterine Contraceptive Devices. Washington, D.C., December, 1978, pp 18–23
95. Van Gennep FO: Sexual ethics in Protestant churches, in Money J, Musaph H (ed): Handbook of Sexology. New York, Exerpta Medica, 1977, 94–98
96. Varney H: Screening for antepartal complications, in Varney H: Nurse-Midwifery. Boston, Blackwell Scientific, 1980, pp 133–150
97. Varney H: Natural methods of family planning, in Varney H: Nurse-Midwifery. Boston, Blackwell Scientific, 1980, pp 405–410
98. Varney H: IUD management, in Varney H: Nurse-Midwifery. Boston, Blackwell Scientific, 1980, pp 426–436
99. Varney H: Breast examination, in Varney H: Nurse-Midwifery. Boston, Blackwell Scientific Publications, 1980, pp 485–496
100. Vaughn B: Contraceptive failure among married women in the United States. Fam Plann Perspect 9:251–258, 1977
101. Vorherr H: Human lactation and breast feeding, in Larson BL (ed): Lactation: A Comprehensive Treatise. New York, Academic Press, 1978, pp 30–46
102. Wessler S, Gitel S, Wan L, et al: Estrogen containing oral contraceptive agents: A basis for their thrombogenicity. JAMA 236:2179–2182, 1976
103. Westoff C: The modernization of U.S. contraceptive practice. Fam Plann Perspect 4:9–12, 1972
104. Worthington B: Nutrition during pregnancy, lactation and oral contraception. Nurs Clin N Am 14:281, 1979
105. Zabin L, Kantner J, Zelnik M: The risk of adolescent pregnancy in the first months of intercourse. Fam Plann Perspect 11:215–222, 1979
106. Zacharias L, Wurtman R, Schatzoff M: Sexual maturation in contemporary American girls. Am J Obstet Gynecol 108:833–846, 1970
107. Zelnik M, Kantner J: Some preliminary observations on preadult fertility and family formation. Stud Fam Plann 3:59–65, 1972
108. Zelnik M, Kantner J: Contraceptive patterns and premarital pregnancy among women aged 15–19 in 1976. Fam Plann Perspect 10:135–142, 1978

Appendix 7-1

Contraceptive Method Suitability Based on Health Status Characteristics

Health Status Characteristics	Foam and Condoms	Diaphragm	Natural Family Planning	IUD	Oral Contraceptives
Acne	Suitable	Suitable	Suitable	Suitable	Use estrogen-dominant agents (norethynodrel or ethynodiol diacetate), which suppress subaceous gland activity. Avoid androgen-dominant pills (nogestrel, norethindrone acetate), which cause or aggravate acne.[15]

Allergies	Suggest natural-skin condoms, or change in foam brand if allergic reaction occurs. On rare occasions some women are allergic to semen and/or sperm; this method would prevent allergic reactions of urticaria.	Suitable unless allergic to rubber or jelly	Suitable	Not suitable if allergic to copper and considering Cu7 or CuT	Suitable

(continued)

297

Appendix 7-1 (continued)

Health Status Characteristics	Foam and Condoms	Diaphragm	Natural Family Planning	IUD	Oral Contraceptives
Anatomic Problems	Suitable	Not suitable in cases of inadequate pelvic muscle support; abnormally short or long length of anterior vaginal wall; damaged pelvic floor; no palpable notch behind the symphasis pubis; unusually small cervix; severe displacement of the uterus by cystocele, rectocele, anteflexion, retroversion or uterine prolapse[28]	Suitable	Not suitable in cases of congenital or surgically induced malformations distorting the uterine cavity or hampering safe and proper placement of the IUD	Suitable

Anemia (iron deficiency)	Suitable	Suitable	Suitable	Not suitable in cases of Hgb<10mg, Hct<30%, due to potential for increased menstrual blood loss	Suitable May cause decreased menstrual blood loss Counsel women on increased need for B_6, B_{12}, riboflavin, folic acid, zinc, and Vitamin C. [65]
Athlete, serious	Suitable	Suitable	Not suitable in cases of amenorrhea May experience increased amenorrhea, possibly due to combination of stress, training, competition, weight loss, or insufficient body fat, which cause a reverting back to pre-midpuberty gonadotropin secretion patterns. [75]	Suitable unless having problems with amenorrhea and infertility prior to insertion	Not suitable in cases of previous history of amenorrhea Problems in establishing ovulatory cycles on pill discontinuation may occur.

(continued)

Appendix 7-1 (continued)

Health Status Characteristics	Foam and Condoms	Diaphragm	Natural Family Planning	IUD	Oral Contraceptives
Cancer (Breasts, uterus)	Suitable	Suitable	Not suitable in cases of disease or therapy-induced alterations in cervical mucus, or basal body temperature findings	Not suitable in cases of cancer of the uterus	Not suitable: Increased hazard of developing thrombosis in cancer patients. Tumor growth may accelerate. Increased tendency for preexisting carcinoma of breast, vagina, liver, cervix or uterus to recur
Cardiovascular death, family history of (<50 years)	Suitable	Suitable	Suitable	Suitable	Not suitable: At greater risk of cardiovascular disease
Cerebrovascular/ coronary artery disease	Suitable	Suitable	Suitable	Not suitable in cases of valvular heart disease which may increase susceptibility to subacute bacterial endocarditis	Not suitable: At risk for stroke or heart attack.

| Chronic stress | Suitable | Suitable | Not suitable in cases of: Irregular working/life schedule and demands making basal body temperature technique difficult and inaccurate. Syndrome of anovulatory amenorrhea with normal estrogen levels similar to polycystic ovary syndrome[75]. Anxiety due to need for periodic sexual intercourse abstinence and planned sex and worry about method failure and risk of pregnancy | Suitable | Suitable |

(continued)

Appendix 7-1 (continued)

Health Status Characteristics	Foam and Condoms	Diaphragm	Natural Family Planning	IUD	Oral Contraceptives
Diabetes Mellitus (Subclinical, clinical not requiring insulin, and juvenile)	Suitable	Suitable	Not always suitable due to greater incidence of infertility and irregular cycles causing difficulty and inaccuracy with basal body temperature and calendar method techniques	Not always suitable: Impaired response to infection	Not suitable: Steriods alter carbohydrate metabolism by decreasing insulin activity.[80] Blood insulin and glucose levels may rise causing overt and irreversible insulin dependency.[81] At greater risk of thromboembolic disease

Condition					
Dysfunctional uterine bleeding	Suitable	Suitable	Not suitable: Makes correct evaluation of cervical mucus, calendar method and basal body temperature techniques impossible to interpret Requires avoidance of intercourse during bleeding, treated as possible "breakthrough" accompanying ovulation	Not suitable: Diagnosis must rule out uterine/cervical carcinoma, fibroids.	Not suitable: Diagnosis must rule out adnexal uterine, cervical or vaginal carcinoma.
Ectopic pregnancy (history)	Suitable	Suitable	Suitable	Not suitable: Significant risk of repeated ectopic Compromised fertility	Suitable

(continued)

Appendix 7-1 (continued)

Health Status Characteristics	Foam and Condoms	Diaphragm	Natural Family Planning	IUD	Oral Contraceptives
Epilepsy	Suitable	Suitable	Suitable	Suitable	Not suitable: Potential for increased cerebrovascular disease Several anticonvulsant medications (phynytoin, primidone, phenobarbital) cause significant decrease in oral contraceptive effectiveness.[43]
Gallbladder Disorder	Suitable	Suitable	Suitable	Suitable	Not suitable: Increased tendency to develop gall stones while on pill
Gastrointestinal disturbances	Suitable	Suitable	Not suitable: Will cause inaccurate temperature graph	Suitable	Not suitable: Vomiting and diarrhea may cause incomplete absorption of pill and thus not inhibit ovulation.

Hyperlipidemia (type II) and Hypercholesterol-emia	Suitable	Suitable	Suitable	Suitable	Not suitable: At coronary risk May increase chances of fatal/non-fatal myocardial infarction Pills containing estrogen and progesterone cause increased plasma lipids and lipoproteins[33]
Hypertension	Suitable	Suitable	Suitable		Not suitable: Mechanism causing rise in plasma renin and angiotensin levels is estrogen induced. Fluid retention causes increase in aldosterone level.[33]
Hypertension (continued)					Acceleration of antherogenesis causes greater risk of thromboembolic disease.

(continued)

Appendix 7-1 (continued)

Health Status Characteristics	Foam and Condoms	Diaphragm	Natural Family Planning	IUD	Oral Contraceptives
Infertility (history)	Suitable: In cases of females producing antibodies which agglutinate sperm, condoms are used for 3–6 months to present the release of sperm antigens into the vagina. This may lower the antibody titre and conception becomes possible. [36]	Suitable	Suitable: Extremely helpful in planning pregnancy and evaluating cycles for ovulation Irregular cycles may cause difficulty with calendar method.	Not Suitable	Not suitable: When use of estrogen—progestin contraception is discontinued, ovulation may not return.
Impaired liver function	Suitable	Suitable	Suitable	Suitable	Not suitable: Progestogen component of pill interferes with bile secretion in women with impaired liver function causing increased bromosulfophthalein retention leading to jaundice.

| Medication interaction | Suitable | Suitable | Not always suitable: May cause temperature variations Synthetic estrogen progesterone may cause abnormal cervical mucus patterns for up to 3–6 months postdiscontinuation. May cause drying effect on mucus secretions and hence difficult interpretation of cervical mucus | Suitable | Not always suitable: Medications known to decrease oral contraceptive efficiency are: anticonvulsants (phenytoin, primidone, phenobarbital)[43] antibiotics (ampicillin, chloramphenicol, sulphameth, oxypyradizine)[17] others (phenacetin analgesics containing meprobamate, chloriazepoxide)[17] |
| Menopausal/peri-menopausal | Suitable | Suitable | Not suitable: Cycles irregular Changes in vaginal/cervical secretions | Suitable | Not suitable: Women over 35 years old are at greatest risk of cardiovascular disease while on the pill. |

(continued)

Appendix 7-1 (continued)

Health Status Characteristics	Foam and Condoms	Diaphragm	Natural Family Planning	IUD	Oral Contraceptives
Menstrual disorders	Suitable	Suitable	Not suitable: Problems in predicting ovulation may occur when cycles are irregular, when >1 ovulation in a cycle, anovulatory, or when temperature chart is irregular. Cycles increasing in length may have more fertile than safe days. Evaluation of thyroid/prolactin levels indicated in cases of oligoamenorrhea.	Not suitable in cases of menorrhagia, or dysmenorrhea unless using the Progestasert	Suitable in cases of dysmenorrhea, endometriosis, or hypermenorrhea

Mental retardation	Not suitable: Method requires repeated motivation for consistent and careful use and dependence on partner.	Not suitable unless able to follow instructions for correct usage; requires motivation	Not suitable: Requires repeated motivation Requires understanding of method, techniques and interpretation	Not always suitable due to impaired ability to check for danger signals and seek appropriate assistance	Not suitable: Mental impairment may hamper ability to understand, recognize danger signs and seek appropriate help when needed. Requires motivation May be unable to utilize method correctly
Migraine headaches	Suitable	Suitable	Not suitable if migraines cause emotional tension and upset, lack of sleep, or irregular sleeping hours because these factors may affect basal body temperature and make prediction of ovulation difficult	Suitable	Not suitable due to sodium and water retaining effects of estrogen and potential for increased incidence of headaches

(continued)

Health Status Characteristics	Foam and Condoms	Diaphragm	Natural Family Planning	IUD	Oral Contraceptives
PAP smear abnormality (endometrial hyperplasia, cervical intraepithelial neoplasia or cancer) Class III or greater	Suitable	Suitable	Not always suitable due to alterations in cervical mucus changes, or possible basal body temperature irregularity causing ovulation prediction problems	Not suitable	Not suitable: Women with dysplasia of the cervix at the time of pill initiation are more likely to develop carcinoma *in situ* than other users.[15]
PID (history)	Suitable if recent gonorrhea infection, have partners use condoms until cure is confirmed	Suitable	Suitable	Not suitable: Increased risk of acute PID among IUD wearers Severe repeated attacks of PID lead to tube damage and sterility[53]	Suitable
Pregnancy (suspected or known)	Suitable	Suitable	Not suitable: Reliability of charts and temperature questionable	Not suitable: In cases of pregnancy may cause spontaneous abortion, infection, hemorrhage	Not suitable: In cases of unrecognized pregnancy the pill may have teratogenic effects on the fetus.[65]

Psychic depression	Suitable only if partner is reliable	Not suitable unless able to exhibit continued motivation for consistent, correct use	Not suitable: May experience temperature variations May be unable to follow rules of method Requires established daily routine May be unable to abstain from coitus and required times	Suitable unless severely impaired and unable to check for danger signs and seek appropriate assistance	Not suitable: Depressive neurosis may increase. May be related to vitamin B_6 deficiency Depression may be adversely affected by the protestin component of the pill which causes tiredness and other pregnancy symptoms.[15]
Psychological preparedness (especially in adolescence)	Not always suitable if unable to demand partner use a condom May not wish to protect self with use of foam. Requires repeated motivation	Not suitable: Requires repeated motivation Requires self-manipulation of genitals and practice	Not suitable: Requires willingness to part with sexual spontaneity Requires keeping careful records Requires willingness to follow rules of methods, correct techniques, and interpretation of data	Suitable if woman accepts potential side effects: cramping, increased menstrual flow, leukorrhea; follows practice of routine string checks; reliable in seeking help when danger signs occur; will use back-up method when indicated	Not suitable if unable to take pills correctly, call in for refill when needed, or seek help when danger signs occur

(continued)

Appendix 7-1 (continued)

Health Status Characteristics	Foam and Condoms	Diaphragm	Natural Family Planning	IUD	Oral Contraceptives
Sexually transmitted diseases and vaginitis	Suitable: Condoms provide effective protection against transmission of STDs. Foam decreases transmission of gonorrhea and trichomoniasis.	Not suitable: Provides no protection from STD or vaginitis	Not suitable: Provides no protection from STD Infection causes changes in vaginal secretions which makes ovulation difficult to predict.	Not suitable: While infection (gonorrhea) is active there is an increased change of developing pelvic inflammatory disease. Provides no protection from STD.	Not suitable when in contrast with an infected partner as it provides no protection from STD. Pills cause increased occurence of vulvovaginitis which may be resistent to treatment.[33]
Smoking	Suitable	Suitable	Suitable	Suitable	Not suitable: In women 40–44 years old there is an increased incidence of fatal and non-fatal myocardial infarction.[45]

Pre- and Postsurgery	Suitable	Suitable unless surgery causes anatomic malformations interfering with correct fit of diaphragm.	Not suitable in immediate postoperative phase due to possible alterations in temperature, menstrual cycle, and vaginal secretions	Suitable unless surgery is conducted.	Not suitable: Immobilization of an extremity postoperatively causes hazard of thromboembolic disease. Discontinue at least 4 weeks preoperatively to avoid circulatory problems.
Thrombophlebitis, pulmonary embolism, cerebral thrombosis	Suitable	Suitable	Suitable unless current problem is causing temperature fluctuations.	Suitable only if the woman is not taking anticoagulants.	Not suitable: 4-fold greater incidence of these problems when on the pill (3–6/ 100,000 each year) Pills cause alterations in clotting time, fibrinogen and other coagulation factors. Risk is greater on sequential pills — suggesting estrogen component related to etiologic role.[33]

(continued)

Appendix 7-1 (continued)

Health Status Characteristics	Foam and Condoms	Diaphragm	Natural Family Planning	IUD	Oral Contraceptives
Thyroid dysfunction	Suitable	Suitable	Not suitable: May have associated amenorrhea, irregular cycles making data difficult to interpret	Not suitable in cases of compromised fertility and wish for future childbearing	Suitable: No evidence of any fundamental effect on thyroid function. May cause alteration in protein-bound iodine and luetanol extractable iodine secondary to the increase of thyroxine binding proteins[33]
Uterine fibroid tumors	Suitable	Suitable	Suitable	Not suitable: May cause excessive bleeding	Suitable: Reduction in fibroid tumors is directly related to increasing progestin dose and activity and decreasing estrogen dose.

Varicose veins	Suitable	Suitable	Suitable	Suitable	Not suitable: May cause increased incidence of superficial thrombosis due to vein dilitation. Progesterone causes dilation of smooth muscle structures such as vein walls.
Weight—low body fat and poor nutritional status	Suitable	Suitable	Not Suitable: Subject to hypostrogenic amenorrhea resulting from inadequate gonadotropin stimulation (22% of body fat required to maintain/restore menstruation)[75]	Not suitable in cases of malnutrition, anemia, menstrual irregularity, infertility.	Suitable if vitamin and mineral deficiencies are supplemented.

315

Index

```
        a
        b
   3 c
   4 d
   5 e
   6 f
   7 g
   8 h
   9 i
 8 0 j
```